ADVANCES IN ELECTROCARDIOGRAMS – CLINICAL APPLICATIONS

Edited by **Richard M. Millis**

Advances in Electrocardiograms – Clinical Applications
Edited by Richard M. Millis

Published by InTech

Janeza Trdine 9, 51000 Rijeka, Croatia

Publishing Process Manager Petra Nenadic

Technical Editor Teodora Smiljanic

Cover Designer InTech Design Team

Additional hard copies can be obtained from orders@intechopen.com

Advances in Electrocardiograms – Clinical Applications, Edited by Richard M. Millis
p. cm.
ISBN 978-953-307-902-8

For EU product safety concerns:
IN TECH d.o.o., Prolaz Marije Krucifikse Kozulić 3, 51000 Rijeka, Croatia,
info@intechopen.com or visit our website at intechopen.com.

Meet the editor

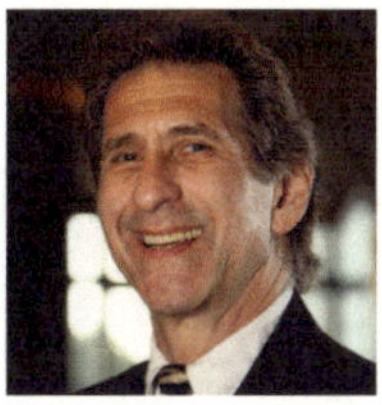

The author teaches physiology at The Howard University College of Medicine. He has authored/co-authored more than 70 scientific articles. His research on obesity,identified physiological correlates of heart rate variability. His report on nicotine played a crucial role in the development of the first smoke-free workplace in the US federal government. He developed the first database on antidotes to chemical and biological warfare agents, the first curriculum used to train physicians on chemical casualty care for the Persian Gulf War,and the first minority neuroscience fellowship program sponsored by the international Society for Neuroscience. He served as an evaluator for the National Institute of Mental Health's Advocacy for Individuals with Mental Illness program, and as a consultant at the National Institute of Drug Abuse on AIDS cofactors. He also helped with the development of the first doctor assistant training program in sub-Saharan Africa,Ethiopia, as well as biomedical curricula for the National University of Rwanda after the execution of many of it's professors during the Rwandan genocide.

Contents

Preface XI

Part 1 Cardiac Arrhythmias 1

Chapter 1 **The Prognostic Role of ECG in Arterial Hypertension 3**
Stavros Dimopoulos, Christos Manetos, Eleni Koroboki, John Terrovitis and Serafim Nanas

Chapter 2 **Electrocardiographic QT Interval Prolongation in Subjects With and Without Type 2 Diabetes – Risk Factors and Clinical Implications 13**
Jimenez-Corona Aida, Jimenez-Corona Maria Eugenia and Gonzalez-Villalpando Clicerio

Chapter 3 **The Prevalence and Prognostic Value of Rest Premature Ventricular Contractions 27**
Matthew D. Solomon and Victor Froelicher

Chapter 4 **Arrhythmias in Children and Young Adults 41**
Harinder R. Singh

Chapter 5 **Paced ECG Morphology – Reveals More than What It Conceals 77**
Ajay Bahl

Chapter 6 **Electrocardiograms in Acute Pericarditis 83**
Anita Radhakrishnan and Jerome E. Granato

Chapter 7 **The Remodeling of Connexins Localized at Pulmonary Vein – Left Atria in Triggering and Maintenance of Atrial Fibrillation 95**
Guo-qiang Zhong, Ri-xin Xiong, Hong-xing Song, Yun Ling, Jing-chang Zhang and Zhe Wei

Part 2 Myocardial Infarction 111

Chapter 8 **ECG in Acute Myocardial Infarction in the Reperfusion Era 113**
Massimo Napodano and Catia Paganelli

Chapter 9 **Mechanisms of Postinfarction Electrophysiological Abnormality: Sympathetic Neural Remodeling, Electrical Remodeling and Gap Junction Remodeling 133**
Guoqiang Zhong, Jinyi Li, Honghong Ke, Yan He, Weiyan Xu and Yanmei Zhao

Chapter 10 **Novel Porcine Models of Myocardial Ischemia/Infarction – Technical Progress, Modified Electrocardiograms Validating, and Future Application 175**
Jianxun Liu and Xinzhi Li

Part 3 Autonomic Dysregulation 191

Chapter 11 **The Emergence and Development of Physiological Regulatory Systems of Newborn Infants in a Neonatal Intensive Care Unit 193**
Motoki Bonno, Esmot Ara Begum and Hatsumi Yamamoto

Chapter 12 **Automated Detection and Classification of Sleep Apnea Types Using Electrocardiogram (ECG) and Electroencephalogram (EEG) Features 211**
Onur Kocak, Tuncay Bayrak, Aykut Erdamar, Levent Ozparlak, Ziya Telatar and Osman Erogul

Chapter 13 **Low Heart Rate Variability in Healthy Young Adult Males 231**
Richard M. Millis, Stanley P. Carlyle, Mark D. Hatcher and Vernon Bond

Chapter 14 **The Role of Exercise Test After Percutaneous Coronary Intervention 245**
Iveta Mintale, Milana Zabunova, Dace Lurina, Inga Narbute, Sanda Jegere, Ilja Zakke, Vilnis Taluts Dzerve and Andrejs Erglis

Part 4 Cardiotoxicology 269

Chapter 15 **Toxic and Drug-Induced Changes of the Electrocardiogram 271**
Catalina Lionte, Cristina Bologa and Laurentiu Sorodoc

Chapter 16 **Electrocardiogram (ECG) Abnormality Among Residents in Arseniasis-Endemic and Non-Endemic Areas of Southwestern Taiwan – A Study of Gene-Gene and Gene-Environment Interactions 297**
Ya-Tang Liao, Wan-Fen Li, Chien-Jen Chen, Wei J. Chen, Hsiao-Yen Chen and Shu-Li Wang

Chapter 17 **Abnormal Electrocardiogram in Patients with Acute Aluminum Phosphide Poisoning 319**
Amine Ali Zeggwagh and Maha Louriz

Preface

A number of heart diseases in humans are rooted in the structure-function relationships of the lower animal hearts. These relations are observable during human embryonic organogenesis. The hearts of invertebrates and lower vertebrates are similar to the embryonic tubular hearts of higher vertebrates. These primitive ancestral hearts possess cardiac myocytes that are electrically coupled by gap junctions such as those in mammalian and human hearts. The highest pacemaker activity occurs at the receiving end of the primitive ancestral heart, thereby, resulting in waves of peristaltic contractions similar to those in gastrointestinal tracts. This tubular arrangement gives rise to atrial and ventricular chambers with well-developed and well-coupled cardiac myocytes with low pacemaker activity, producing the rapid conduction and contraction of mammalian and human hearts. The forming chambers are made up of rapidly proliferating myocytes with a surrounding area of slowly proliferating trabecular myocardium. This slowly proliferating trabecular myocardium does not differentiate into normal myocardium of the heart chambers because it remains poorly developed. The tightly coupled electrically by highly organized gap junctions and intercalated discs give rise to the ventricular conduction system. Thus, the human ventricular conduction system arises from the embryonic myocardium, and permits rapid conduction of cardiac excitation, and subsequent contraction of the pumping chambers of the heart.

In contrast, to vertebrates, many invertebrates lack an autonomic nervous system for organizing cardiac signaling and insuring responsiveness to a wide variety of complex physiological stimuli. In lower vertebrates, the vagus nerve arises from the brain as a cranial nerve and innervates the pacemaker cells of the heart. When stimulated, the vagus slows the rate at which the cardiac phases of depolarization and repolarization are produced. In higher vertebrates with well- developed heart chambers, specialized for receiving (atria) and pumping (ventricles), the atrial pacemaker cells are innervated by vagal parasympathetic, as well as by sympathetic nerve fibers. This arrangement appears to subserve sophisticated tuning of the heart rate, and pumping activity (contractility) to immediate changes in the physiological state of the animal, insuring adequate flow of nutrients to the various tissue compartments, especially to the complex brains and other vital organs of mammals. In mammals, vagal innervation of pacemaker cells in the sinoatrial node appears to arise from two main sources, the dorsal vagal nucleus in the dorsal brainstem and the nucleus ambiguous in the ventral brainstem. The vagal fibers from the dorsal vagal nucleus appear to be driven mainly by baroreceptor and other cardiovascular inputs. The signaling of these vagal fibers produces variability in the rate of sinoatrial node depolarization associated mainly with changes in blood pressure. The vagal fibers,which arise from the nucleus ambiguous, appear to be driven mainly by respiratory inputs and produces variability in the rate of the sinus node depolarization - known as heart rate variability or respiratory sinus arrhythmia.

The measurement and analysis of heart rate variability has been introduced trough *Advances in Electrocardiogram - Methods and Analysis*. In the present book, *Advances in Electrocardiograms - Clinical Applications*, the reader will be presented with clinical applications of heart rate variability, as well as a wide range of pathophysiological conditions associated with abnormal electrocardiograms. From electrolyte disturbances to toxic exposures; from hypertension and myocardial infarction to cardiomyopathies; from sleep apneas to heart failures. Being mindful that the roots of many electrocardiographic abnormalities develop during embryonic organogenesis of the heart, will lead to improved recognition, diagnosis and treatment of cardiac diseases.

Richard M. Millis, PhD
Editor
Dept. of Physiology & Biophysics
The Howard University College of Medicine
USA

Part 1

Cardiac Arrhythmias

1

The Prognostic Role of ECG in Arterial Hypertension

Stavros Dimopoulos[1], Christos Manetos[1], Eleni Koroboki[2], John Terrovitis[3] and Serafim Nanas[1]
[1]1st Critical Care Medicine Department, "Evangelismos" Hospital,
[2]Hypertensive Center, Clinical Therapeutics, "Alexandra" Hospital,
[3]3rd Cardiology Department, "Laiko" Hospital,
University of Athens, Athens,
Greece

1. Introduction

Hypertension is very common and affects around 50 million Americans of which about 30% are not yet diagnosed. Hypertension is an under-diagnosed syndrome causing damage to the various target organs with no symptoms or only mild symptoms, also called a "silent killer" for this reason. Early diagnosis of arterial hypertension remains an important element in evaluating cardiovascular risk factors in general population. It is well established that isolated arterial hypertension increases the risk of left ventricular hypertrophy (LVH) and sudden death and prognostic indexes are necessary for risk stratification of these patients. The electrocardiogram (ECG) is a simple, non-invasive, low-cost method that can detect LVH, ventricular arrhythmias and ventricular repolarization abnormalities and confers useful prognostic information for patients with arterial hypertension

2. Prognostic data

It is well known that left ventricular hypertrophy (LVH) is associated with an increased incidence of ventricular arrhythmia and sudden cardiac death. Systemic arterial hypertension is one of the most important causes of pathological LVH and there is evidence indicating that hypertensive patients with LVH are at increased risk of sudden cardiac death (Haider 1998, Korren 1991). These patients are characterized by a high incidence of ventricular arrhythmias (Gallinier 1997, Messerli 1999, Dimopoulos 2009) and this observation has led to the logical hypothesis that these arrhythmias may be the cause of sudden cardiac death in these patients. However, the exact mechanism by which LVH, ventricular arrhythmias and sudden cardiac death are linked to each other has not been fully clarified yet. Premature ventricular beats, multiform beats, couplets and non-sustained ventricular tachycardia are commonly found in ECGs of hypertensive patients, are associated with LVH, and have a negative prognostic value (Gallinier 1997, Messerli 1999). Furthermore, ventricular repolarization abnormalities in the 12-lead surface ECG such as QT-interval prolongation, increased QT dispersion (Dimopoulos 2008,2009), T wave axis

(Salles 2008) and T wave alternans (Hennersdorf 2001) have all been associated with ventricular arrhythmias and sudden cardiac death in arterial hypertension; however further research is required to establish their prognostic significance.

2.1 LVH

In arterial hypertension, LVH is a physiologic and expected response to pressure or volume overload and it is a well known marker of increased cardiovascular morbidity. Previous studies have extensively shown that antihypertensive agents can partially reverse LVH and their efficacy is well documented (Haider 1998, Kannel 1969,1970, Sokolow & Lyon 1949, Deverreux & Reichek 1982, Okin 2004,2009). Development of the typical strain pattern in response to LVH may reflect true subendocardial ischemia in the absence of coronary artery disease, since the increases in coronary artery blood flow (through coronary artery dilatation and capillary recruitment) are inadequate to compensate the demand posed by increased LV mass and wall thickness, in the setting of LVH. The increased mass of the left ventricle (representing both myocardial interstitial fibrosis and/or myocyte hypertrophy) can cause abnormalities of the QRS complex and QT-interval. Although the ECG has a low sensitivity (less than 50%) for detecting LVH, when LVH is identified by ECG, the specificity is higher than 90%. From these observations several criteria have been proposed so far, however none is considered to have optimal accuracy (Sokolow & Lyon 1949, Hancock 2009). A variety of ECG abnormalities have been described, as shown in Tables 1,2,3:

R or S in any limb lead ≥20mm
R waves in aVL > 11mm
R in lead I + S in III > 25mm
S waves in V1 or V2 ≥ 30mm
R waves in V5 or V6 ≥ 30mm
S waves in V1 + R waves in V5 or V6 > 35mm
R waves in aVL+ S waves in V3 > 28mm (men) and 20 mm (women)
Total QRS voltage from all 12 leads ≥175mm
Onset of intrinsicoid deflection >0.05 seconds in V5 or V6
Increased duration of the QRS complex ≥0.09 seconds
Left axis deviation ≥-30°

Table 1. Abnormalities in the QRS complex

Terminal negativity of the P wave in V1 1mm X 1mm

Table 2. Left atrial abnormality

ST depression and T inversion in leads with tall R waves (left ventricular strain)

Table 3. Abnormalities in the ST segment and T wave

The following are the most frequently used criteria for the diagnosis of LVH, including the Sokolow-Lyon Index, Romhilt and Estes score, Cornell voltage criteria, Cornell product, total QRS voltage (Table 4,5,6,7,8):

S waves in V1 + R waves in V5 or V6 > 35mm
R waves in aVL > 11mm

Table 4. Sokolow-Lyon Index

Score of ≥ 5 points predicts LVH, score of 4 points = probable LVH
3 points each
1) P wave from left atrial abnormality 2) any increase in voltage of the QRS complex (R or S in any limb lead ≥20mm or S waves in V1 or V2 ≥ 30mm or R waves in V5 or V6 ≥ 30mm) 3) ST-T abnormalities any shift in the ST segment but without digitalis
2 points (left axis deviation ≥-30°)
1 point each (duration of the QRS complex ≥0.09 seconds or intrinsicoid deflection ≥0.05 seconds in V5 or V6 or ST-T abnormalities with digitalis)

Table 5. Romhilt and Estes score

R waves in aVL+ S waves in V3 > 28mm (men) and 20 mm (women)

Table 6. Cornell voltage criteria

Cornell voltage criteria x QRS duration in ms ≥ 2440 (in women 6 mm is added to Cornell voltage)

Table 7. Cornell product

Total QRS voltage from all 12 leads ≥175mm

Table 8. Total QRS voltage

Various epidemiological studies have previously demonstrated the importance of LVH for predicting cardiovascular events and sudden cardiac death. In the Framingham Heart Study the 3.4% of 5581 participants with ECG LVH and ST depression and T-wave flattening or inversion had a 3-fold increased risk for developing coronary heart disease after adjusting for age, gender, and blood pressure, (Kannel 1969, 1970). Similar results were found in the Copenhagen City Heart Study with enrollment of 11,634 participants with no evidence of ischemic heart disease at initial evaluation. In this study it was shown that ST depression and/or T-wave inversion (as defined by the Minnesota code) remained strongly predictive for cardiac events in multivariate analyses (Larsen 2002). The left ventricular (LV) strain-pattern of ST segment depression and T-wave inversion on the left precordial leads of the standard resting ECG is now considered a valid marker of the presence of anatomic LV hypertrophy (LVH) (Salles 2006). The presence of typical ECG strain pattern is also independently associated with increased LV wall thickness and mass and independently associated with other adverse factors: increased 24-hour systolic blood pressure, prolonged maximum QTc-interval duration, higher serum creatinine and fasting glycemia, physical inactivity, as well as with the presence of two types of important target organ damage (CHD and peripheral arterial disease). In the Losartan Intervention For Endpoint reduction in hypertension (LIFE) study, it was demonstrated that therapy with losartan was more effective than atenolol in preventing CV morbidity and mortality with nearly identical reductions in systolic and diastolic pressure in both treatment arms. The presence of typical strain on the ECG in hypertensive patients with ECG LVH also identified patients at higher risk of CV morbidity and mortality in the setting of antihypertensive therapy associated with large decreases in systolic and diastolic pressure. The increased CV risk associated with ECG strain was independent of the improved prognosis with losartan therapy in the LIFE trial and persisted after adjusting for the greater baseline severity and prevalence of ECG LVH and the higher prevalence of other CV disorders in patients with strain pattern. The development of new ECG strain between baseline and year 1 during the LIFE study identified patients at increased risk of cardiovascular morbidity and mortality and all-cause mortality in the setting of antihypertensive therapy associated with substantial decreases in both systolic and diastolic pressure. The increased risk associated with new ECG strain was independent of the improved prognosis with losartan therapy and with regression of ECG LVH in LIFE (Okin 2004,2009). These findings suggest that more aggressive therapy may be warranted in hypertensive patients who develop new ECG strain to reduce the risk of cardiovascular morbidity, cardiovascular and all-cause mortality, and sudden death. The relationship of cardiovascular risk to ECG strain pattern on a single ECG has been demonstrated in population-based studies and in patients with hypertension.

2.2 Ventricular arrhythmias, Lown score

Previous studies have shown an increased incidence of number and severity of ventricular arrhythmias in patients with hypertensive LVH (Galinier 1997, Messerli 1999, Dimopoulos 2008, Hennersdorf 2001). The average number of premature ventricular beats (PVB), and their severity according to a modified Lown's score (a: absence of PVB; b: PVB $< 30/h$; c: PVB $\geq 30/h$; d: multiform; e: couplets; f: nonsustained ventricular tachycardia; g: R on T = RR / QT ≤ 0.75) during a 24-hours ECG Holter are independent predictors of echocardiographically determined LVMI in normotensive and hypertensive elderly patients, as demonstrated in a previous study (Dimopoulos 2008). In that study, patients with arterial hypertension had a higher Lown's score compared with normotensive subjects, and this increase was found to be higher in those hypertensives with LVH. The elderly population group had a greater number of PVB in contrast to younger subjects. Elderly patients were also characterized by a higher Lown's score and a greater LVMI. Another study has previously shown that patients with LVH present frequent and complex ventricular premature beats and that the presence of non-sustained ventricular tachycardia has negative prognostic value in this population (Galinier 1997). However, the role of ventricular arrhythmias in arterial hypertension is still under investigation, with no clear evidence for high prognostic significance.

2.3 Silent ischemia

Transient changes of ST-segment (ST depression) is a phenomenon commonly observed in patients with arterial hypertension; although reported prevalence varied widely (from 15 to 80%-Stramba 1998, Asmar 1996), it seems that the true value is around 20% (Uen 2006). These findings on ECG are interpreted as silent ischemia, due to the absence of angina pectoris or other angina equivalent symptoms and are attributed to transient mismatch of myocardial blood flow to the myocardial demands. It seems that more than 90% of these episodes, identified in the Holter electrocardiogram (ECG) of hypertensive patients, are silent. When transient ST depressions are detected, the risk of cardiovascular events increases (Uen 2006, Sigurdson 1996, Szlachcic 1992). It is also well known that there is a circadian rhythm of transient ST depressions with a distinct peak in the early hours of the morning, similar to the peak period of myocardial infarction or sudden cardiac death (Asmar 1996). The ST depression is significantly more frequent in patients with known coronary heart disease, positive Sokolow index, as well as in patients who complain of dyspnea, have a smoking history or are on diuretics. The ST-segment depression is also observed more frequently in men than in women. The prevalence of ST-segment depression in patients with coronary heart disease is influenced by the severity of coronary heart disease (Uen 2006, Sigurdson 1996, Szlachcic 1992). This phenomenon is characterized by a significant rise of blood pressure, heart rate and double product before the appearance of ST depression. These parameters reach their peak during the ST depression. After ST depression resolution, they return to lower values. Apart from the systolic blood pressure, however, the other two parameters will remain significantly elevated compared with the mean 24-hour values. Other clinical predictors for the occurrence of cardiac ischemia during daily life are risk factors for silent ST-depression, indicating the presence of ischemic heart disease. A study showed that 24-hours ambulatory blood pressure monitoring (ABPM) has high predictive value, in contrast to office-based blood pressure measurements, for silent ST-segment depression. Interestingly, the office-based measurements, apart from the pulse pressure, are not predictive of the occurrence of ST-segment depression either in treated or in untreated hypertensive and normotensive hypertensive individuals. To what extent the 24-hours mean values of the ST segment depression analysis reflect the severity of ischemic heart disease or have prognostic significance regarding the development of an ischemic event remains so far unknown, although a study has previously reported that silent ischemia may be predictive of adverse outcome in arterial hypertension (Schillaci 2004).

2.4 QT-interval and QT-dispersion

Increased left ventricular mass, as mentioned before has a high prevalence in patients with arterial hypertension, particularly in the elderly and has been associated with increased cardiovascular risk, including sudden death, (Haider 1998, Koren 1991, Dimopoulos 2009, Kannel 1969,1970, Bednar 2001, Okin 2000). The increased electrical instability due to non-uniform left ventricular mass distribution has been suggested as a possible mechanism linking LVH and cardiovascular death. QT interval prolongation has been implicated in the origin of ventricular arrhythmias, possibly because of less uniform recovery of ventricular excitability in the setting of regional differences in cardiac sympathetic nervous system activity. In addition, the increased inhomogeneity of ventricular repolarization, induced by LVH, can be indirectly detected by QT dispersion, a relatively simple measurement of 12-lead electrocardiogram (ECG) variability, and this index has been recently shown to be related to poor prognosis in large population studies (Okin 2000, Salles 2005, Elming 1998, Bruyne 1998, Sheehana 2004). Interestingly, heterogeneous ventricular repolarization was initially recognized in standard ECGs as early as 1934; however only recently QTc interval dispersion was identified as a marker of arrhythmia risk and sudden cardiac death in patients after myocardial infarction or with heart failure (Barr 1994, Glancy 1995, Anastasiou-Nana 2000). Furthermore, other studies subsequently demonstrated the presence of increased QT-dispersion in patients with systemic arterial hypertension, associated with ventricular arrhythmias and LVH (Dimopoulos 2008, Clarkson 1995, Mayet 1996). QTc dispersion (QT-dispersion corrected for HR) was found to be an independent predictor of echocardiographically determined LVMI in normotensive and hypertensive elderly patients (Dimopoulos 2008). Patients with arterial hypertension had an increased

QTc dispersion compared with normotensive subjects, and this increase was found to be higher in those hypertensive patients with LVH. In a prospective study, patients with QTcD ≥45 ms had a higher rate of major cardiovascular events, higher LVMI, increased values of systolic and diastolic blood pressure, higher number of PVB and higher Lown's score than patients with QTcD <45 ms (Dimopoulos 2009) . After adjustment for multiple known predictors of adverse outcome, QT interval corrected for heart rate remained associated with both all-cause and cardiovascular mortality. Increased QTc interval dispersion was also a significant predictor of cardiovascular mortality in LIFE trial (Saaden & Jones 2001). This additive risk prediction suggests that increased QTc and QTc interval dispersion on the surface ECG reflect different aspects of abnormal ventricular repolarization. However only few studies have investigated the prognostic role of QT-dispersion and QT-interval in arterial hypertension (Galinier 1997, Dimopoulos 2009, Oikarinen 2004, Saaden & Jones 2001). Antihypertensive therapy with angiotensin-converting enzyme inhibitors, calcium antagonists and beta-blockers has been shown beneficial in terms of QT-dispersion normalization and/or LVH decrease (Tomiyama 1998, Karpanou 1998, Galetta 2005,Lim 1999). Beta blockers are associated with a reduction in both QT and QTc interval dispersion, raising the possibility that a reduction in dispersion of ventricular repolarization may be an important antiarrhythmic mechanism of beta blockade.

The direct linking mechanism between QT-dispersion, ventricular arrhythmias, LVH and adverse outcome has not been fully clarified yet. Increased QTc dispersion has been associated with increased regional heterogeneity of ventricular repolarization and it has been considered as a possible noninvasive surrogate marker of susceptibility to malignant ventricular arrhythmias and cardiovascular mortality in large population studies and, in cardiac patients (Okin 2000, Elming 1998, Bruyne 1998, Sheehana 2004, Barr 1994, Glancy 1995, Anastasiou 2000). The degree of myocardial interstitial fibrosis induced by either systemic arterial hypertension and/or by ageing, as well as the inhomogeneous myocyte hypertrophy caused mainly by arterial hypertension, might play an important role in increasing action potential duration and amplitude in different myocardial regions (Dimopoulos 2008,2009). These myocardial electrical abnormalities may affect ventricular repolarization and might be the main cause of increased QTc dispersion in hypertensives. In order to maximize reproducibility of QT-dispersion measurements, it is important to follow certain methodological rules that are reported below.

All 12-leads ECGs are obtained at a speed of 25 mm/sec. The ECG registration should be a simultaneous 12-lead ECG. QT intervals are measured manually on all possible leads. QT interval is defined as the interval from the onset of the QRS complex to the end of the T wave, which is defined as its return to the T-P baseline. If U wave is present, the QT interval is measured to the nadir of the curve between the T and U waves. QT intervals are then corrected with the Bazett's formula to compensate for its known dependence on heart rate: $QTc = QT / \sqrt{RR}$. Measurements on QT and RR intervals should be carried out in 3 consecutive cardiac cycles in all leads, and average values are then obtained. QTc dispersion is determined as the difference between the maximal and minimal QTc interval in different leads. No subject should have fewer than 9 measurable ECG leads. Various studies have also demonstrated the predictive value of the QT interval and QTc interval dispersion measured automatically by computerized ECG for noninvasive risk stratification in a population-based sample.

It should be mentioned that there are some methodological difficulties related to QT dispersion measurements, including the circadian variation of the QT interval. The QTc interval dispersion has obvious predictive value, but inter- and intraobserver varialbility limits the wider clinical use. In perspective, it is important to decrease measurement errors by improving measurement technique, define precisely normal values and demonstrate predictive value in studies with large number of patients with arterial hypertension.

2.5 T wave axis

Two electrocardiographic markers of ventricular repolarization abnormalities have been recently proposed: spatial T-wave axis deviation and T (peak)-T (end)-interval duration. In a cross-sectional study (Salles 2008), 810 treatment-resistant hypertensive patients were evaluated. Maximum T(peak)-T(end)-interval duration (Tpe(max)) was considered prolonged if it was beyond the upper quartile value (120 ms), and the spatial T-wave axis on the frontal plane was considered abnormally deviated if >105 degrees or < 15 degrees. Tpe(max)-interval prolongation, as well as QTc-interval prolongation, was found to be associated with body mass index, 24-h systolic blood pressure (SBP), indexed LVM, serum potassium, and heart rate. Abnormal T-axis deviation was associated with male gender, presence of coronary heart disease, serum creatinine, 24-h SBP, LVM, and serum potassium. All three repolarization parameters (T-wave axis deviation, T (peak)-T (end)-interval and QTc-interval) were shown to be associated with increased LVM, after adjustment for possible confounders. However, when included together into the same model, only abnormal T-axis and QTc-interval prolongation remained independently associated with LVM. All three parameters were also increased in patients with concentric hypertrophy. It seems that only abnormal T-wave axis deviation appears to have distinct and additive prognostic value compared with the more classic marker, the QTc interval. More investigational studies are needed to evaluate the prognostic value of T-wave axis abnormalities in arterial hypertension, prior to clinical application of this index.

2.6 T wave alternans (TWA)

An association between the occurrence of TWA and inducibility of tachyarrhythmias has been reported in a previous electrophysiological study (Rosenbaum 1994). Another significant study (Hennersdorf 2001) has evaluated the significance of TWA in 51 patients with arterial hypertension. The patient population was divided into a group of 11 consecutive patients who had survived arrhythmic events or cardiogenic syncope and a group of 40 consecutive patients without documented ventricular arrhythmias. Patients exercised with a gradual increase of workload to maintain a heart rate of at least 105/min. Workload was increased in a stepwise fashion to avoid a sudden increase of the heart rate, which could provoke a false positive test result. After recording 254 consecutive heartbeats, ECG signals were digitally processed by a spectral analysis method and analyzed. The beat domain power spectrum of the T wave (J point 160 ms through end of the T wave) was calculated every 16 beats from sequential overlapping 128-beat sequences. The magnitude of the TWA was measured at a frequency of 0.5 cycles per beat. The results of this study showed that the prevalence of TWA was higher in patients with LVH. There was also a significant correlation between patients with a positive TWA and a survived arrhythmic event. None of the patients without documented ventricular arrhythmias had a positive alternans tracing. The underlying mechanism of a positive TWA is not clear yet; it seems that there is an alteration in action potential morphology or dispersion of repolarization. The changes in morphology of the action potentials might lead to spatial inhomogeneity in refractoriness and may result in increased vulnerability to ventricular fibrillation. During repeated episodes of ischemia, action potential alternans was detectable in 95% of the cases with ventricular fibrillation. The dispersion of repolarization is closely related to the temporo-spatial pattern of depolarization-repolarization, which can alternate on a beat-to-beat basis. The temporo-spatial dispersion of cellular refractoriness seems to predispose the myocardium to wave front fractionation and subsequent reentry. It is noteworthy that the TWA can be influenced by various conditions such as ischemia, hypothermia, heart rate, and sympathetic tone. Drugs such as procainamide and amiodarone reduce magnitude of alternans and sotalol can lead to the conversion of TWA from negative to positive. In the case of cardiomyopathies, the development of small areas of scars and ischemia is considered to be of pathological relevance for the development of alterations in action potentials or dispersion of repolarization. Whether T wave alternans can be used as a clinical marker of susceptibility for sudden cardiac death and cardiovascular events is under research.

3. Conclusions

The electrocardiographic findings in patients with arterial hypertension are valuable tools for risk stratification of these patients, by predicting cardiovascular events and sudden cardiac death. The ECG strain pattern, an old parameter of well established value, should always be searched as it provides additional prognostic information beyond the one derived from echocardiographic LVH and LVM. Also among hypertensive patients with left ventricular hypertrophy, the presence of non-sustained ventricular tachycardia on ECG Holter monitoring identifies patients with a high risk of mortality, who need more aggressive care. Silent ischemia on ECG Holter should be taken into account as ST depression episodes have a high prevalence (about 20%) in hypertensive patients. ST depression and T-wave inversion may reflect true subendocardial ischemia in the absence of coronary artery disease. The prolonged QT interval and increased QT interval dispersion have been associated with LVH and ventricular arrhythmias and seem to contain significant predictive value, but inter- and intraobserver varialbility limit their wider clinical applicability. The analysis of T wave axis and T wave alternans might also be helpful for risk stratification in patients with arterial hypertension. However, the clinical usefulness of these indices in arterial hypertension and their possible role in monitoring medical treatment is under investigation and further research is needed prior to its clinical application.

4. References

Anastasiou-Nana et al., 2000, Relation of dispersion of QRS and QT in patients with advanced congestive heart failure to cardiac and sudden death mortality. *Am J Cardiol*, Vol.85, (2000), pp. 1212-1217

Asmar et al., 1996, Prevalence and circadian variation of ST-segment depression and its concomitant blood pressure changes in asymptomatic systemic hypertension. *Am J Cardiol*, Vol. 77, (1996), pp.384–390

Barr et al., 1994, QT dispersion and sudden unexpected death in chronic heart failure. *Lancet*, Vol. 343, (1994), pp. 327-329

Bednar et al., 2001, The QT interval, *Prog Cardiovasc Dis.*, Vol. 43, (2001), pp.1- 45

Bruyne et al., 1998, QTc Dispersion Predicts Cardiac Mortality in the Elderly. The Rotterdam Study, *Circulation*, Vol 97, (1998), pp. 467-472

Clarkson et al., 1995, QT dispersion in essential hypertension. *QJM*, Vol. 88, (1995), pp. 327–332

Devereux & Reichek, 1982, Repolarization abnormalities of left ventricular hypertrophy. Clinical, echocardiographic and hemodynamic correlates. *Journal of Electrocardiology*, Vol.15, No.1, (1982), pp.47-53

Dimopoulos et al., 2009, Prognostic Evaluation of QT-Dispersion in Elderly Hypertensive and Normotensive Patients. *PACE*, Vol.32, (2009), pp. 1381–1387

Dimopoulos et al., 2008, QT Dispersion and Left Ventricular Hypertrophy in Elderly Hypertensive and Normotensive Patients. *Angiology*, Vol.59, No.5 (October-November 2008), pp.605-612

Elming et al., 1998, The prognostic value of the QT interval and QT dispersion in all-cause mortality and morbidity in a population of Danish citizens. *Eur Heart J*, Vol. 19, (1998), pp. 1391–1400

Galetta et al., 2005, Effect of nebivolol on QT dispersion in hypertensive patients with left ventricular hypertrophy. *Biomed Pharmacother*, Vol. 59, No. 1-2, (January-February 2005), pp. 15-19

Galinier et al., 1997, Prognostic value of ventricular arrhythmias in systemic Hypertension. *Journal of Hypertension*, Vol.15, No.12, (December 1997), pp. 1779-1783

Glancy et al., 1995, QT dispersion and mortality after myocardial infarction. *Lancet*, Vol. 345, (1995), pp. 945-948

Haider et al., 1998, Increased left ventricular mass and hypertrophy are associated with increased risk for sudden death. *Journal of the American College of Cardiology* Vol.32, No.5, (November 1, 1998), pp. 1454-1459

Hancock et al., 2009 AHA/ACCF/HRS Recommendations for the Standardization and Interpretation of the Electrocardiogram. Part V: Electrocardiogram Changes Associated With Cardiac Chamber Hypertrophy A Scientific Statement From the American Heart Association Electrocardiography and Arrhythmias Committee, Council on Clinical Cardiology; the American College of Cardiology Foundation; and the Heart Rhythm Society. *Circulation, Journal of the American Heart Association*, Vol.119, (February 19, 2009), pp.251-261

Hennersdorf et al., 2001, T Wave Alternans and Ventricular Arrhythmias in Arterial Hypertension, *Hypertension*, Vol.37 (2001), pp.199-203

Kannel et al., 1969, Left ventricular hypertrophy by electrocardiogram: prevalence, incidence, and mortality in the Framingham Study, *Annals of Internal Medicine*, Vol.71, No.1, (July 1, 1969), pp. 89–105

Kannel et al.,1970, Electrocardiographic left ventricular hypertrophy and risk of coronary heart disease: the Framingham Study. *Annals of Internal Medicine*, Vol.72, No.6, (June 1, 1970), pp. 813–822

Karpanou et al., 1998, Regression of left ventricular hypertrophy results in improvement of QT dispersion in patients with hypertension. *Am Heart* J, Vol. 136, No. 5, (November 1998), pp. 765-768

Koren et al., 1991, Relation of left ventricular mass and geometry to morbidity and mortality in uncomplicated essential hypertension. *Annals of Internal Medicine*, Vol.114, No. 5, (March 1, 1991), pp. 345-352

Larsen et al., 2002, Prevalence and prognosis of electrocardiographic left ventricular hypertrophy, ST segment depression and negative T-wave: The Copenhagen City Heart Study. *Eur Heart J*, Vol.23, (2002), pp. 315-324

Lim et al., 1999, Reduces QT Dispersion in Hypertensive Individuals. *Hypertension*, Vol. 33, (1999), pp. 713-718

Mayet et al., 1996, Left ventricular hypertrophy and QT dispersion in hypertension. *Hypertension*, Vol. 28, (1996), pp. 791–796

Messerli, FH.(1999), Hypertension and sudden cardiac death. *American Journal of Hypertension*, December 1999 Vol.12, No. 5, pp.181-188

Oikarinen et al., 2004, QRS duration and QT interval predict mortality in hypertensive patients with left ventricular hypertrophy: the Losartan Intervention for Endpoint Reduction in Hypertension Study. *Hypertension,* Vol. 43, No. 5, (May 2004), pp. 1029-1034

Okin et al., 2000, Assessment of QT Interval and QT Dispersion for Prediction of All-Cause and Cardiovascular Mortality in American Indians. The Strong Heart Study. *Circulation,* Vol. 101, (2000), pp.61-66

Okin et al., 2004, Electrocardiographic Strain Pattern and Prediction of Cardiovascular Morbidity and Mortality in Hypertensive Patients. *Hypertension,* Vol.44, No.1, (July 2004) pp. 48-54

Okin et al., 2009, Prognostic Value of Changes in the Electrocardiographic Strain Pattern During Antihypertensive Treatment: The Losartan Intervention for End-Point Reduction in Hypertension Study (LIFE), *Circulation*, Vol. 119 (2009) pp.1883-1891

Rosenbaum et al., 1994, Electrical alternans and vulnerability to ventricular arrhythmias. *N Engl J Med*, Vol. 330, (1994) pp. 235–241

Saadeh & Jones, 2001, Predictors of sudden cardiac death in never previously treated patients with essential hypertension: long-term follow-up. *Journal of Human Hypertension*, Vol. 15, (2001), pp. 677–680

Salles et al., 2005, Combined QT interval and voltage criteria improve left ventricular hypertrophy detection in resistant hypertension, *Hypertension,* Vol. 46, (2005), pp. 1207–1212

Salles et al., 2006, Importance of the Electrocardiographic Strain Pattern in Patients With Resistant Hypertension *Hypertension* Vol. 48, (2006) pp. 437-442

Salles et al., 2008, Muxfeldt ES Recent ventricular repolarization markers in resistant hypertension: Are they different from the traditional QT interval? *American Journal of Hypertension*, Vol.21, No.1 (January 2008) pp. 47-53

Schillaci et al., 2004, Prognostic significance of isolated, non-specific left ventricular repolarization abnormalities in hypertensive. *J Hypertens*, Vol.22 (2004), pp. 407–414

Sheehana et al., 2004, QT dispersion, QT maximum and risk of cardiac death in the Caerphilly Heart Study. *Eur J Cardiovasc Prevention Rehab* Vol. 11, (2004), pp.63–68

Sigurdson et al., 1996, Silent ST-T changes in an epidemiologic cohort study - a marker of hypertension or coronary heart disease, or both: The Reykjavik Study. *J Am Coll Cardiol*, Vol.27, (1996), pp.1140–1147

Sokolow & Lyon, 1949, The ventricular complex in left ventricular hypertrophy as obtained by unipolar precordial and limb leads. *Am Heart J.* Vol. 68, (1949), pp.161–186

Stramba et al., 1998, Prevalence of episodes of ST-segment depression among mild to moderate hypertensive patients in northern Italy: The Cardioscreen Study. *J Hypertens*, Vol.16, (1998), pp.681–688

Szlachcic et al., 1992, What is the role of silent coronary artery disease and left ventricular hypertrophy in the genesis of ventricular arrhythmias in men with essential hypertension? *J Am Coll Cardio,* Vol.19, (1992), pp.803–808

Tomiyama et al., 1998, Left ventricular geometric patterns and QT dispersion in borderline and mild hypertension: their evolution and regression. *Am J Hypertens,* Vol. 11, No. 3, (March 1998), pp. 286-292

Uen et al., 2006, Myocardial ischemia during everyday life in patients with arterial hypertension: prevalence, risk factors, triggering mechanism and circadian variability. *Blood Press Monit,* Vol.11, No.4 (August 2006) pp.173-182

2

Electrocardiographic QT Interval Prolongation in Subjects With and Without Type 2 Diabetes – Risk Factors and Clinical Implications

Jimenez-Corona Aida, Jimenez-Corona Maria Eugenia and Gonzalez-Villalpando Clicerio
National Institute of Public Health, Cuernavaca, Morelos, Laboratories of Biologicals and Reagents of Mexico, BIRMEX, Mexico City, Mexico

1. Introduction

Several studies have focused on the identification of patients at risk of sudden cardiac death, which is mostly due to depolarization and repolarization impairment. The measurement of QT interval indicates the total duration of ventricular myocardial depolarization and repolarization. Localized repolarization data can be obtained easily from the standard 12-lead electrocardiogram (ECG), a non-invasive method extensively used as a tool for cardiovascular risk assessment. [1,2] Non-uniform myocardial repolarization time may result from inhomogeneity, variation of action potential duration between the individual leads of the 12-lead ECG, or localized delay in activation due to slow conduction or altered conduction pathways. To ensure the recording of the earliest depolarization at the latest repolarization of the ventricular myocardium, the maximum QT interval should be measured from the beginning of the earliest QRS complex to the end of the latest T wave from all leads of a simultaneous 12-lead ECG. Nevertheless, the QT interval may reflect increased inhomogeneity of myocardial repolarization, resulting from delayed repolarization in some areas of the myocardium, and it can be caused by a uniform increase in action potential duration. A measure that can help differentiate between these two conditions is the QT dispersion. Using both the QT prolongation and the QT dispersion the individual lead variation and the interlead variation provide a measure of repolarization heterogeneity. [3]

The QT interval prolongation has been proposed as a marker of cardiovascular risk in the clinical setting and it has also been particularly associated with arrhythmias, sudden death and poor survival in apparently healthy subjects. [4,5] As for diabetic subjects, although some cross-sectional studies suggest that glycemic control, ischemic heart disease, and blood pressure, among other risk factors, are associated with the QT interval prolongation, its pathogenesis remains unclear. [6,8] Also, and increased mortality in newly diagnosed type 2 diabetes patients has been associated with QT interval prolongation. [9,10]

The aim of this study was to estimate the prevalence of QTc interval prolongation in diabetic and non-diabetic subjects, as well as to evaluate cross-sectionally and prospectively the associated risk factors of QTc interval prolongation and its clinical implications in subjects with and without type 2 diabetes who had not suffered from previous myocardial infarction corroborated on the ECG.

2. Methods

The Mexico City Diabetes Study is a prospective, population-based investigation designed to describe the prevalence and incidence of diabetes and cardiovascular risk factors in low-income urban population from Mexico City. The detailed methodology has been reported elsewhere. [11] Briefly, the sample size included 2282 men and non-pregnant women aged 35 to 64 years who completed a baseline interview and physical examination in 1989-1990. Two follow-up visits were carried out in 1994-1996 (n=1773) and in 1998-2000 (n=1764). All evaluations included medical history, physical examination, ECG, and several laboratory tests. Current smoking was defined as at least one cigarette per day in the last year. Physical examination included an anthropometric evaluation with participants wearing lightweight clothing and no shoes. Height was measured using a stadiometer with subjects standing on the floor with the back against a wall; weight was measured using a clinical scale. Body mass index (BMI) was calculated as weight/height^2 in kg/m^2. Waist circumference (WC) was measured considering the umbilicus as the landmark. Systolic (SBP) and diastolic blood pressure (DBP) were measured 3 times in the right arm of seated subjects (after resting for at least 5 min) using a random zero sphygmomanometer (Hawksley, London). We used the average of the last 2 readings as the BP of the participants. Hypertension was defined as SBP≥140 mmHg, DBP≥90 mmHg, or treatment with antihypertensive drugs. In every visit, participants completed a 75-g oral glucose tolerance test. Diabetes was defined according to the World Health Organization criteria with a fasting glucose ≥7mmol/l (126 mg/dl), 2-hour glucose ≥11.1 mmol/l (200 mg/dl), or treatment with oral antidiabetic drugs. [12] Fasting and 2-hour plasma glucose and insulin as well as fasting serum lipids and all other biomarkers were measured using previously reported methods [13] at the research laboratory of the Division of Clinical Epidemiology at the Medicine Department of the University of Texas Health Science Center at San Antonio, USA. Insulin resistance was estimated by the homeostasis model (HOMA-IR) as follows: [fasting insulin (units/ml) X fasting glucose (mmol/l)/22.5].

A resting standard 12-lead ECG was taken with the subject in a supine position at each examination. A standard interpretation of ECGs at a reading center (Wake Forest University, EPICARE Center) was made using the Minnesota Code. [14] Heart rate (HR), QRS duration, R amplitude in AVL lead (R-AVL), S amplitude in V3 lead (SV3), left ventricular hypertrophy (LVH), QT interval, and myocardial infarction, among other variables, were coded. Left ventricular hypertrophy (LVH) was defined as (R-AVL) + (SV3) ≥2600μv in men and ≥2200μv in women. Myocardial infaction was defined according to the following codes: Q-QS pattern with 1.1-1.2.7, Q-QS and T wave pattern 1.2.8-1.3, and wave T pattern with 5.1-5.3. QT interval was measured from the electrocardiogram tracing in lead II and defined as the first deflection of the QRS complex and the end as the point of maximal change in the slope as the T wave merges with the baseline. QT corrected (QTc) was calculated according to Bazzett's formula as QT/square root of (R–R interval). The same measurement instruments were used throughout the study.

The Institutional Review Boards of both The University of Texas Health Science Center and the Centro de Estudios en Diabetes approved the study protocol. Each participant gave informed consent. For this analysis, we included 1661 subjects, 218 with and 1443 without type 2 diabetes, without myocardial infarction at baseline corroborrated by ECG, who were followed-up for a median of time of 4.26 and 3.32 years, respectively.

2.1 Statistical analysis

Comparisons of clinical and laboratory features were made according to diabetes status at baseline. Proportions and means (standard deviation [s.d.]) were compared by Pearson Chi^2 and by T student, respectively, while medians (interquartile range [IQR]) were compared by Wilcoxon test. QTc interval was analyzed as continuous and dichotomous variable. Because of the normal distribution of the QTc interval, all analyses were carried out using the original units. QTc interval prolongation, using the Bazzett´s formula, was defined as an interval ≥430 msec in men and 450 msec in women. Partial Pearson correlation between QTc interval and some risk factors were estimated in diabetic and non-diabetic subjects, separately. To estimate the association between some cardiovascular risk factors and QTc interval prolongation in diabetic and non-diabetic subjects, both together and separately, multiple linear regression for cross-sectional analysis and generalized estimating equations regression models (GEE), with family normal identity link, for longitudinal analysis were carried out. Models were performed with the forward method considering the biological and statistical relevance. Results are given as regression β coefficients and 95% confidence interval (95%CI). P value equal or less than 0.05 was considered significant. All analyses were done with Stata/SE 9.0 (Stata statistical software: Release 9. College Station. Texas: Stata Corporation, 2005).

3. Results

Characteristics of the sample

A total of 1661 subjects (1443 non-diabetic and 218 diabetic subjects), aged 47.4±8.2 years at baseline were included. Table 1 shows comparisons of some QT interval risk factors between subjects with and without type 2 diabetes. Individuals with diabetes were older and had greater abdominal fat and upper-body fat accumulation, as well as higher BP levels, total cholesterol and fasting and 2-hour glucose levels compared with individuals without diabetes. The percentage of hypertension was higher for subjects with diabetes (27.1%) compared with non-diabetic subjects (13.0%); likewise, the proportion of individuals under antihypertensive medication was slightly greater in the diabetic group. Although the percentage of subjects who were under antihyperlipidemic medication was higher in subjects with diabetes compared with non-diabetic subjects, these differences were not significant. As for diabetic subjects, 136 (62.4%) were prevalent cases whereas 82 (37.6%) were incident cases, with a ratio 1:1.6. Mean of age at diagnosis of diabetes was 46.6 years (s.d. 8.0 years) and median of diabetes duration was 1.8 (IQR 25-75% 0-7.3).

Some characteristic on the ECG were compared between diabetic and non-diabetic subjects at baseline and during follow-up and are shown in table 2. The mean of heart rate, QRS duration, and R amplitude in AVL lead were significant higher in diabetic compared with non-diabetic subjects. Mean of QTc by the Bazzet´s formula was significantly higher ($p<0.001$) in diabetic (414.0 msec) than in non-diabetic (404.3 msec) individuals. The prevalence of longer QTc interval (≥430 msec in men and ≥450 msec in women) was greater in diabetic (10.1%) compared with non-diabetic subjects (4.0%). Prevalence was remarkably higher in both diabetic and non-diabetic men (16.3% vs. 4.5%, $p<0.001$) compared with

	Non-diabetic subjects	Diabetic subjects	p value
	n=1443	n=218	
Age (years)	46.6 (8.0)	52.5 (7.7)	<0.001
Age at diabetes diagnosis (years)	-	47.8 (8.3)	-
Women (no., %)	848 (58.8)	138 (63.3)	0.204
Current smoking (no., %)	487 (33.8)	65 (30.0)	0.269
BMI (kg/m^2)	28.0 (4.3)	29.1 (4.8)	0.001
Waist circumference (cm)			
Men	93.6 (9.1)	98.8 (11.7)	<0.001
Women	97.8 (13.4)	101.6 (11.5)	0.002
Hypertension (no., %)	188 (13.0)	61 (28.0)	<0.001
SBP (mmHg)	115.6 (16.1)	122.9 (18.6)	<0.001
DBP (mmHg)	72.5 (10.3)	75.4 (9.6)	<0.001
Total cholesterol (mmol/L)*	4.9 (4.2-5.6)	5.2 (4.5-5.9)	<0.001
HDL-C, (mmol/L)*			
Men	0.7 (0.6-0.9)	0.8 (0.7-0.9)	0.319
Women	0.9 (0.7-1.0)	0.9 (0.7-1.0)	0.334
Triglycerides (mmol/L)*	1.9 (1.4-2.8)	2.5 (1.8-3.6)	<0.001
Fasting glucose (mmol/L)*	4.7 (4.2-5.1)	8.9 (6.6-13.5)	<0.001
2-hour glucose (mmol/L)*	5.7 (4.6-6.8)	14.1 (11.6-18.8)	<0.001
Antihypertensive medication (no., %)†	67 (35.6)	27 (44.3)	0.227
Antihyperlipidemic medication (no., %)	4 (0.3)	1 (0.5)	0.638
Diabetes cases			
Prevalent	-	136 (62.4)	-
Incident	-	82 (37.6)	-
Hypoglycemic medication (no., %)	-	143 (65.9)	-
Diabetes duration (years)*	-	1.8 (0-7.3)	-
Duration of follow-up (years)*	3.32 (3.15-3.74)	4.26 (4.00-4.44)	0.0001

*Median (IQR 25-75).
†Only subjects with hypertension.
Missing values in non-diabetic subjects: WC, 26; HDL-C, 2; 2-hour glucose, 1; antihyperlipidemic medication, 37.
Missing values in diabetic subjects: current smoking, 1; WC, 3; triglycerides, 2; 2-hour glucose, 122; antihyperlipidemic medication, 9.

Table 1. Characteristic of the study population by diabetes status

women (6.5% vs. 3.7%, $p>0.05$). Similar differences were observed on the QTc interval as continuous and dichotomous variable during the follow-up. In addition, after stratifying by hypertension, prevalence of longer QTc interval was significantly higher in both diabetic (13.3%) and non-diabetic subjects (5.2%) with hypertension compared with diabetic (8.9%) and non-diabetic subjects (3.8%) without hypertension. When stratification was made by BMI<25 and BMI≥25, prevalence remained significantly higher in diabetic compared with non-diabetic subjects with normal weight (14% vs. 1.8%, respectively) and with overweigh/obesity (9.1% vs. 4.7%, respectively).

	Non-diabetic subjects	Diabetic subjects	p value
	n=1443 mean (s.d.)	n=218 mean (s.d.)	
At baseline			
Heart rate (bpm)	65.2 (9.2)	70.9 (12.0)	<0.001
QRS duration (msec)	90.9 (10.4)	88.9 (10.7)	0.007
R amplitude in AVL lead	294.4 (239.8)	346.8 (270.5)	0.003
S amplitude in V3 lead	879.9 (523.3)	917.2 (545.1)	0.330
LVH, no (%)	33 (2.3)	6 (2.8)	0.672
QT interval (msec)	390.0 (25.4)	384.3 (28.5)	0.002
QTc interval by the Bazzett´s formula (msec)	404.3 (22.5)	414.5 (23.8)	<0.001
QTc interval by the Bazzett´s formula ≥430 in men and ≥450 in women (no., %)	58 (4.0)	22 (10.1)	<0.001
At the end of follow-up			
Heart rate (bpm)	62.8 (9.5)	66.6 (9.4)	<0.0001
QRS duration (msec)	89.9 (10.9)	88.0 (15.2)	0.027
R amplitude in AVL lead	338.5 (224.5)	369.0 (233.4)	0.063
S amplitude in V3 lead	815 (434.7)	880.3 (503.5)	0.045
LVH, no (%)	20 (1.4)	6 (2.8)	0.130
QTc interval by the Bazzett´s formula (msec)	406.7 (22.3)	416.1 (21.6)	<0.001
QTc interval by the Bazzett´s formula ≥430 in men and ≥450 in women (no., %)	77 (5.3)	20 (9.2)	0.024

Missing values in non-diabetic subjects: S amplitude in V3 lead 1.
Bazzett´s formula: QT/square root of (R–R interval).

Table 2. QTc interval segment and other electrocardiographic parameters in subjects with and without type 2 diabetes

Figure 1 shows the relation between QTc interval and BMI in subjects with and without type 2 diabetes according to age. The values of QTc interval were slightly greater in subjects with greater BMI in both diabetic and non-diabetic individuals, regardless of age group. A similar trend was observed when BMI was substituted for WC. (Data not shown)

As for fasting glucose in diabetic subjects, a slight increment in the QTc interval was observed in subjects with higher levels of fasting glucose, particularly in subjects with levels between 12 mmol/l and 20 mmol/l. (Figure 2) For non-diabetic subjects, a modest increment in the QTc interval was observed when 2-hour glucose (≥6 mmol/l) and HOMA-IR (≥10 units) increased (Figure 3).

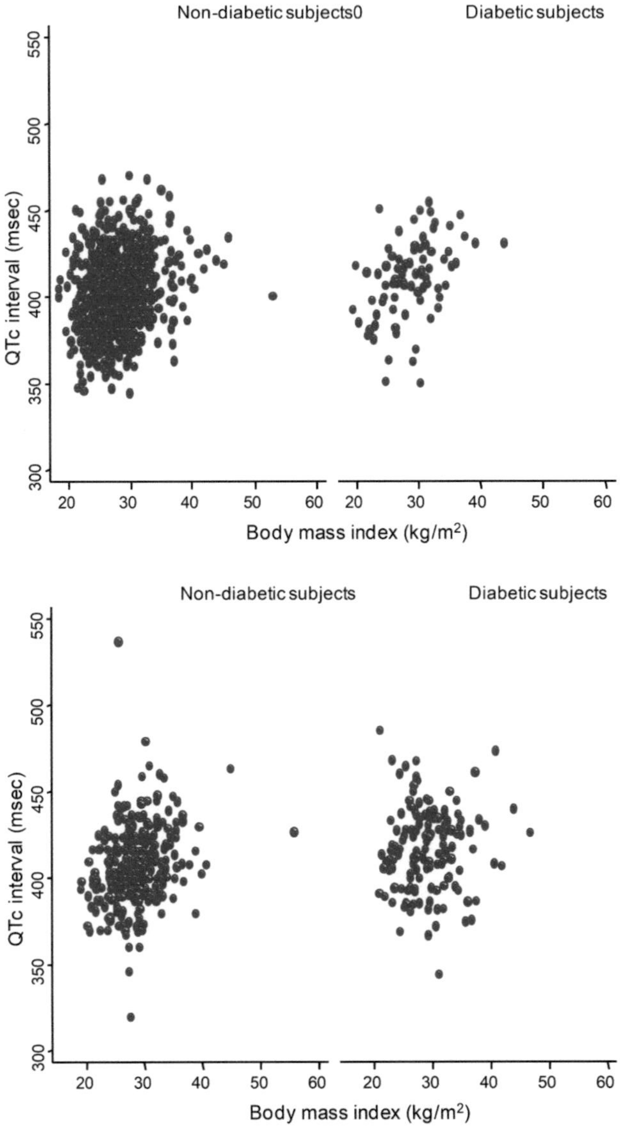

Fig. 1. Comparison between QTc interval level and BMI at baseline in subjects with and without type 2 diabetes stratifying by age <50 (upper panel) years and ≥50 years (bottom panel).

In diabetic subjects, partial Pearson correlations with QTc interval were statistically significant for age (rho=0.15, p=0.024), BMI (rho=0.19, p=0.006), and WC (rho=0.20, p=0.003). No significant correlation with diabetes duration was observed. In non-diabetic subjects, correlations with QTc interval were significant for age (rho=0.16, p<0.0001), SPB (rho=0.10, p=0.0002), DBP (rho=0.07, p=0.008), BMI (rho=0.23, p<0.0001), and WC (rho=0.21, p<0.0001). During follow-up, the correlation of QTc interval with BMI and WC remained significant (p<0.001) in both diabetic (BMI, rho=0.24 and WC, rho=0.25) and non-diabetic individuals (BMI, rho =0.23 and WC, rho=0.26).

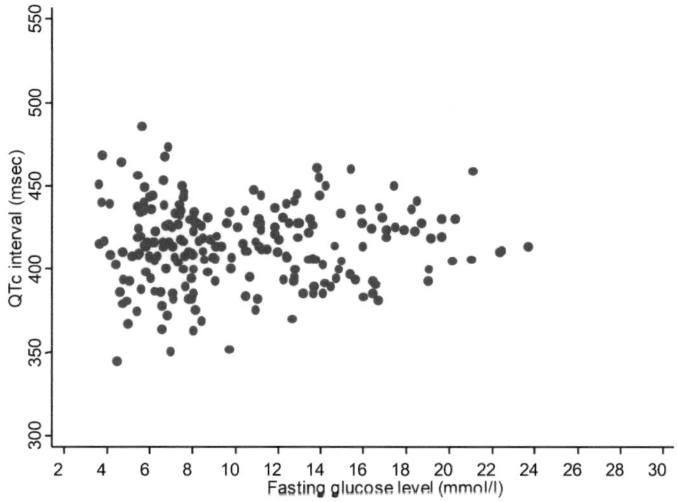

Fig. 2. Comparison between QTc interval level and fasting glucose level at baseline in subjects with type 2 diabetes.

Cross-sectional analysis

In the whole sample, QTc interval prolongation was significantly associated with age, sex, BMI, and diabetes. For each unit of change on age (year), the QTc interval increased 0.36 msec (95%CI 0.23; 0.49). For each unit of increment on BMI, the QTc interval increased 0.75 msec (95%CI 0.51; 1.00). Women had a greater QTc interval mean than men (difference of 13.36 msec (95%CI 11.36; 15.76). Regarding diabetes, the difference on the QTc interval between diabetic and non-diabetic subjects was 6.33 msec (95%CI 3.24; 9.43). Models stratified by diabetes status were also performed. In diabetic subjects, risk factors significantly associated with QTc interval were sex and BMI, whereas age had a borderline significance. For each unit of increment on BMI, the QTc interval increased 0.72 msec (95%CI 0.07; 1.37). Women had a greater QTc interval than men (difference of 15.93 msec, 95%CI 9.50; 22.35). In non-diabetic subjects, risk factors significantly associated with QTc interval were age (beta=0.35, 95%CI 0.21; 0.50), sex (beta=13.69, 95%CI 11.27; 16.10), BMI (beta=0.62, 95%CI 0.33; 0.91), hypertension (beta=4.18, 95%CI 0.14; 8.22), and HOMA-IR (beta=0.43, 95%CI 0.08; 0.78) (Table 3).

Longitudinal analysis

When the whole sample was considered, the progression of QTc interval prolongation was significantly associated with age, sex, BMI, hypertension, and diabetes. The QTc interval prolongation increased with age (beta= 0.33, 95%CI 0.24; 0.42) and BMI (beta= 0.73, 95%CI 0.56; 0.90). Women had a greater QTc interval prolongation than men (difference of 11.84 msec, 95%CI 10.09; 13.59), as did diabetic compared with non-diabetic subjects (difference of 6.58 msec, 95%CI 4.02; 9.13). In a model restricted to diabetic subjects, the QTc interval was predicted by sex (beta= 11.18, 95%CI 6.27; 16.10), BMI (beta= 0.84, 95%CI 0.38; 1.30), and fasting glucose (beta= 0.42, 95%CI 0.11; 0.74). In non-diabetic subjects, predictors of QTc

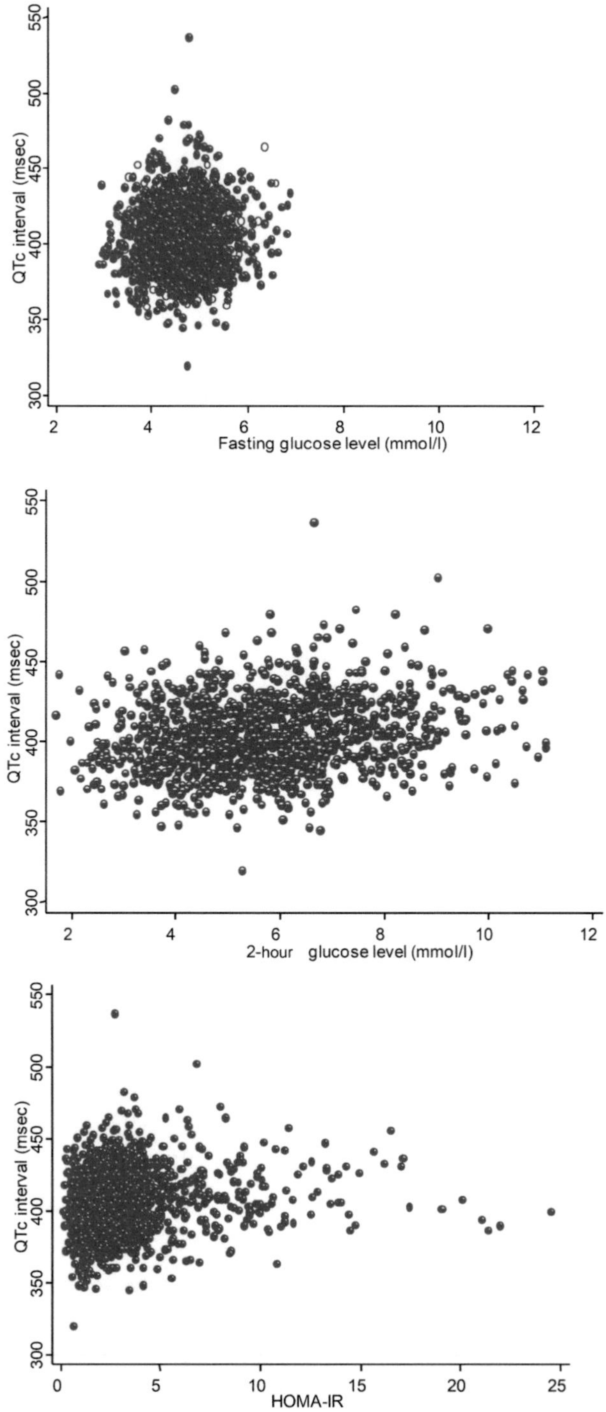

Fig. 3. Comparison between QTc interval level and fasting glucose, 2-hour glucose and HOMA-IR levels at baseline in subjects without type 2 diabetes.

	Non-diabetic subjects N=1368		Diabetic subjects N=218		Whole sample N=1661	
	Beta (95%CI)	p	Beta (95%CI)	p	Beta (95%CI)	p
Age (years)	0.35 (0.21;0.50)	<0.001	0.37 (-0.04;0.79)	0.077	0.36 (0.23;0.49)	<0.0001
Women	13.69 (11.27;16.10)	<0.001	15.93 (9.50;22.35)	<0.001	13.56 (11.36;15.76)	<0.0001
BMI (kg/m^2)	0.62 (0.33;0.91)	<0.001	0.72 (0.07;1.37)	0.030	0.75 (0.51;1.00)	<0.0001
Hypertension	4.18 (0.14;8.22)	0.043	0.93 (-6.02;7.88)	0.792	3.11 (-0.47;6.69)	0.088
HDL-C (mmol/L)	-2.50 (-7.68;2.68)	0.344	-5.56 (-18.67;7.54)	0.404	-2.69 (-7.33;1.94)	0.255
Fasting glucose (mmol/L)	-	-	0.44 (-0.25;1.13)	0.209		
HOMA-IR	0.43 (0.08;0.78)	0.016	-	-	-	-
Diabetes	-	-	-	-	6.33 (3.24-9.43)	<0.0001
Diabetes duration (years)	-	-	0.28 (-0.29;0.85)	0.331	-	-
Antihypertensive medication	-2.26 (-8.68;4.17)	0.491	-	-	-1.21 (-6.64;4.23)	0.664
Hypoglycemic medication	-	-	-4.45 (-11.91;3.00)	0.240	-	-

Table 3. Risk factors associated with the QT interval prolongation in subjects with and without type 2 diabetes. Cross-sectional analysis

interval prolongation were age (beta=0.34, 95%CI 0.25; 0.44), sex (beta=12.23, 95%CI 10.29; 14.18), BMI (beta=0.64, 95%CI 0.44; 0.83), hypertension (beta=3.72, 95%CI 1.57; 5.87), HOMA-IR (beta=0.45, 95%CI 0.16; 0.75) (Table 4). Antihypertensive therapy had a negative effect in QTc prolongation. In a multivariate model with diabetes duration equal or greater than 1 year, the increment of QT interval prolongation remained similar for fasting glucose (beta=0.38, 95%CI 0.06; 0.70, p=0.021), whereas a significant increment with diabetes duration was observed (beta=0.42, 95%CI 0.04; 0.80, p=0.032). (Data not shown)

4. Discussion

The methods used in the Mexico City Diabetes Study meet the accepted international criteria in terms of study protocol, diagnostic algorithms, and particularly electrocardiographic interpretations. [11] The ECGs were interpreted without disclosure of clinical or laboratory data, in a reference center recognized as a gold standard for this procedure. A rigorous quality control procedure was followed along the study. In this population, there is a high prevalence of cardiovascular risk factors, namely overweight,

	Non-diabetic subjects N=1368		Diabetic subjects N=216		Whole sample N=1661	
	Beta (95%CI)	p	Beta (95%CI)	p	Beta (95%CI)	p
Age (years)	0.34 (0.25; 0.44)	<0.0001	0.22 (-0.8; 0.53)	0.151	0.33 (0.24; 0.42)	<0.0001
Women	12.23 (10.29; 14.18)	<0.0001	11.18 (6.27; 16.10)	<0.0001	11.84 (10.09; 13.59)	<0.0001
BMI (kg/m²)	0.64 (0.44; 0.83)	0.0001	0.84 (0.38; 1.30)	<0.0001	0.73 (0.56; 0.90)	<0.0001
Hypertension	3.72 (1.57; 5.87)	0.001	1.67 (-1.80; 5.14)	0.345	2.63 (0.74; 4.52)	0.006
Fasting glucose (mmol/L)	-	-	0.42 (0.11; 0.74)	0.009	-	-
HOMA-IR	0.45 (0.16; 0.75)	0.002	-	-	-	-
Diabetes	-	-	-	-	6.58 (4.02; 9.13)	<0.0001
Diabetes duration (years)	-	-	0.24 (-0.12; 0.61)	0.191	-	-
Antihypertensive medication	-3.57 (-6.50; -0.64)	0.017	-	-	-1.27 (-3.78; 1.24)	
Hypoglycemic medication	-	-	-3.00 (-8.41; 2.41)	0.277	-	-

Models were run by using generalized estimating equations with family normal and identity link.

Table 4. Risk factors associated with the QT interval prolongation in subjects with and without type 2 diabetes. Longitudinal analysis

obesity, diabetes, hypertension, and dyslipidemia. [15-17] This circumstance offers a unique opportunity to study the effect of the above-mentioned factors on the QTc interval as a proxy for the repercussions of the electrophysiologic phenomena on the heart cycle. Our findings clearly show the deleterious effects of the identified cardiovascular risk factors on the QTc interval, particularly those related to insulin resistance.

In the present study, prevalence of QTc interval prolongation was higher in diabetic that in non-diabetic subjects without previous myocardial infarction detected by ECG, independently of age and sex. As expected, subjects with diabetes had 6 times the risk of developing QTc interval prolongation compared with non-diabetic subjects. In multivariate models, QTc interval prolongation was consistently predicted by sex, BMI, and fasting glucose in diabetic subjects. In non-diabetic subjects, age, sex, BMI, hypertension, HOMA-IR, and antihypertensive medication predicted QTc interval prolongation. In both groups, results were largely unchanged when WC was used in place of BMI, or when 2-hour glucose was included instead of fasting and HOMA-IR in diabetic and non-diabetic subjects, respectively.

Several studies have demonstrated that the prevalence of prolonged QTc interval is higher in subjects with type 2 diabetes (26%) than in subjects without. [18-21] Also, the QTc interval prolongation has been associated with a high risk of ischemic heart disease, ventricular fibrillation, and sudden death (range 2 to 5) in several studies, even in subjects with short duration of diabetes. [10] In our study, we observed a significantly higher proportion of prolonged QTc interval in diabetic compared with non-diabetic subjects (10.1% vs. 4.0%). After adjustment for other risk factors, the mean difference on the QTc interval between diabetic and non-diabetic subjects was 6.33 msec. It has been suggested that this difference relates to the sympathetic activity present in diabetes, which reduces both the ability to regulate heart rate and the heart rate variability. [19,20]

As for diabetes duration, it has been reported as a risk factor for chronic complications, including QTc interval prolongation, the latter being related to neuropathy in subjects with diabetes. [19] In our study, neither at baseline nor at follow-up duration of diabetes was significantly associated with QTc interval, which could be explained, in part, by the high proportion of new cases at baseline (37.6%). When the analysis was restricted to subjects with diabetes duration equal or greater than 1 year, QTc interval prolongation was predicted by duration, independently of other risk factors, despite the short median duration of the disease in subjects with previous diagnosis of diabetes (median 5.4 years, IQR 2.1-10.6).

We found a significant prospective association between fasting plasma glucose and prolonged QTc interval in diabetic subjects, even after adjustment for other risk factors. Some studies have reported an association between fasting glucose and QTc interval, particularly in individuals in the normal high level or with impaired fasting glucose, after adjustment for diabetes duration, among other risk factors. [21-22] However, other studies have not found any significant association. [23] As for non-diabetic subjects, we noted an independent association between HOMA-IR and QT-interval prolongation. These results showed an important degree of insulin resistance, maybe related to overweight and obesity in this population, and both predicted QTc interval prolongation. No association was observed with fasting plasma glucose in this group. By contrast, previous studies have reported an association between plasma glucose and QT interval in healthy subjects [24], even after hyperglycemic clamp insulin release, which suggests that the effect of glucose on the QTc interval is not mediated by insulin.

The association of higher BMI with the prolongation of the QTc interval observed in the non-diabetic group is not clearly seen in the diabetic group, probably because of the effect of weight loss as a result of poor metabolic control. It is particularly interesting the finding that HOMA-IR index has a significant association with the prolongation of the QTc duration in both the cross-sectional and the prospective analyses. The pathophysiologic implications direct our attention to the cellular effects of insulin resistance in the electrophysiology that mediates the depolarization and repolarization of the myocardium. Somewhat surprisingly, we could not show a demonstrable effect of therapy for diabetes or hypertension in the QTc duration.

Some of the limitations with the QT interval evaluation relate to the lack of accuracy and reproducibility of the measurements, since there is no standard method for analysis and lead selection. The definition for the end of the QT interval is unclear as well, and may represent a changing T wave morphology that could provide a measure of altered disparity of repolarization. [25,26] Nevertheless, its application as a non-invasive and cost-effective screening tool is invaluable for cardiovascular risk stratification of population. On the other hand, because of the lack of QT interval dispersion measurement in this study, we were not able to determine the type of variation on repolarization.

5. Conclusion

In this study, in addition to specific cardiovascular risk factors associated with the QTc interval prolongation in diabetic and non-diabetic subjects, general excess of body weight measured by BMI was a significant risk factor for both groups. Our findings clearly show the deleterious effects of the identified cardiovascular risk factors on the QTc interval, particularly those related to insulin resistance. In diabetic subjects, the lack of metabolic control (measured by fasting glucose level) predicted strongly the QTc prolongation, whereas in non-diabetic subjects the presence of insulin resistance (HOMA-IR) predicted it. Given the cardiovascular clinical implications of QTc interval in subjects with and without diabetes, further interventional researches are needed to confirm whether the metabolic control in diabetic subjects and the decrease of insulin resistance in non-diabetic subjects together with weight reduction can prevent QTc interval prolongation.

6. Acknowledgments

The authors would like to thank the residents of the neighborhoods that participated in the study. The Research Grant RO1HL 24799 of the National Heart Lung and Blood Institute, Bethesda, MD, USA, supported this work. Funding from The Consejo Nacional de Ciencia y Tecnologia, CONACYT, Grants 2092/M9303, F677-M9407, 3502-M9607 helped in some parts of the study. The Fundacion Mexicana para la Salud provided administrative support.

7. References

[1] Gardner MJ, Montague TJ, Armstrong CS, Horacek BM, Smith ER. Vulnerability to ventricular arrhythmias: Assessment by mapping of body surface potential. Circulation. 1986; 73:684-692.

[2] Abildskov JA, Green LS. The recognition of arrhythmia vulnerability by body surface electrocardiographic mapping Circulation. 1987; 75(4 Pt2):III79-85.

[3] Mirvis DM. Spatial variation of QT intervals in normal persons and patients with acute myocardial infarction. J Am Coll Cardiol. 1985; 5:625-631.

[4] Schouten EG, Dekker JM, Meppelimk P, Kok FJ, Vanderbroucke JP, Pool J. QT interval prolongation predicts cardiovascular mortality in an apparently healthy population. Circulation. 1991; 84:1516-1523.

[5] Shin HS, Lee WY, Kim SW, Jung CH, Rhee EJ, Kim BJ, Sung KC, Kim BS, Kang JH, Lee MH, Park JR. Sex difference in the relationship between insulin resistance and corrected QT interval in non-diabetic subjects. Circ J. 2005;69:409-413.

[6] Kumar R, Fisher M, Macfarlane PW. Review: Diabetes and the QT interval: time for debate. British Journal of Diabetes & Vascular Disease. 2004; 4:146-150.

[7] Okin PM, Devereux RV, Lee ET, Galloway JM, Howard BV. Electrocardiographic repolarization complexity and abnormality predict all-cause and cardiovascular mortality in diabetes. The Strong Heart Study. Diabetes. 2004; 53:434-440.

[8] Salles GF, Cardoso CRL, Deccache W. Multivariate associates of QT interval parameters in diabetic patients with arterial hypertension: importance of left ventricular mass and geometric patterns. Journal of Human Hypertension. 2003; 17:561–567.

[9] Ziegler D, Zentai CP, Perz S, Rathmann W, Haastert B, Döring A, Meisinger C; KORA Study Group. Prediction of mortality using measures of cardiac autonomic

dysfunction in the diabetic and nondiabetic population: the MONICA/KORA Augsburg Cohort Study. Diabetes Care. 2008; 31:556-561.

[10] Naas AAO, Davidson NC, Thompson C, Cummings F, Ogston SA, Jung RT, Newton RW, Struthers AD. QT and QTc dispersion are accurate predictors of cardiac death in newly diagnosed non-insulin -dependent diabetes: cohort study. BMJ. 1998; 316:745-746.

[11] Stern MP, Gonzalez C, Mitchell BD, Villalpando E, Haffner SM, Hazuda HP. Genetic and environmental determinants of type II diabetes in Mexico City and San Antonio. Diabetes. 1992; 41:484-492.

[12] World Health Organization: Definition, Diagnosis and Classification of Diabetes Mellitus and its Complications: Report of a WHO Consultation. Part 1: Diagnosis and Classification of Diabetes Mellitus. Geneva, World Health Organization, 1999.

[13] Haffner SM, Kennedy E, Gonzalez C, Stern MP, Miettinen H. A Prospective analysis of the HOMA model: The Mexico City Diabetes Study. Diabetes Care. 1996; 19:1138-1141.

[14] Prineas R, Crow R, Blackburn H. The Minnesota Code Manual of Electrocardiographic Findings. Littleton, MA, John Wrigth-PSG, Inc., 1982

[15] Gonzalez-Villalpando C, Stern MP, Villalpando E, Hazuda H, Haffner S, Lisci E. Prevalence of diabetes and glucose intolerance in an urban population at a low-economic level. Rev Invest Clin. 1992; 44:321-328.

[16] Haffner S, Gonzalez-Villalpando C, Hazuda HP, et al. Prevalence of hypertension in Mexico City and San Antonio, Texas. Circulation 1994; 90:1542-1549.

[17] Gonzalez-Villalpando C, Stern MP, Arredondo-Perez B, Martinez-Diaz S, Haffner S. Undiagnosed hypercholesterolemia: A serious health challenge. The Mexico City Diabetes Study. Arch Med Res 1996; 27:19-23.

[18] Veglio M, Bruno G, Borra M, Macchia G, Bargero G, D'Errico N, Pagano GF, Cavallo-Perin P. Prevalence of increased QT interval duration and dispersion in type 2 diabetic patients and its relationship with coronary heart disease: a population-based cohort. J Intern Med. 2002; 25:317-324.

[19] Weik, Dorian P, Newman D, Langer A. Association between QT dispersion and autonomic dysfunction in patients with diabetes mellitus. JACC. 1995; 26:859-863.

[20] Psallas M, Tentolouris N, Cokkinos A, Papadogiannis D, Cokkinos DV, Katsilambros N. QT dispersion: comparison between diabetic and non-diabetic individuals and correlation with cardiac autonomic neuropathy. Hellenic J Cardiol. 2006; 47:255-262.

[21] Brown DW, Giles WH, Greenlund KJ, Valdez R, Croft JB. Impaired fasting glucose, diabetes mellitus, and cardiovascular disease risk factors are associated with prolonged QTc duration. Results from the Third National Health and Nutrition Examination Survey. J Cardiovasc Risk. 2001; 8:227-233.

[22] Cardoso CR, Salles GF, Deccache W. Prognostic value of QT interval parameters in type 2 diabetes mellitus: results of a long-term follow-up prospective study. J Diabetes Complications. 2003; 17:169-178.

[23] Cardoso C, Salles G, Bloch K, Deccache W, Siqueira-Filho AG. Clinical determinants of increased QT dispersion in patients with diabetes mellitus. Int J Cardiol. 2001; 79(2-3):253-262.

[24] Marfella R, Nappo F, DeAngelis L, Siniscalchi M, Rossi F, Giugliano D. The effect of acute hyperglycaemia on QTc duration in healthy man. Diabetologia. 2000; 43:571-575.

[25] Statters DJ, Malik M, Ward DE, Camm AJ. QT Dispersion: Problems of Methodology and Clinical Significance. J Cardiovasc Electrophysiol. 1994; 5:672-85.

[26] Kautzner J, Yi G, Camm AJ, Malik M. Short- and long-term reproducibility of QT, QTc, and QT dispersion measurement in healthy subjects. Pacing Clin Electrophysiol. 1994; 17(5 Pt 1):928-937.

3

The Prevalence and Prognostic Value of Rest Premature Ventricular Contractions

Matthew D. Solomon and Victor Froelicher
Stanford University,
USA

1. Introduction

This chapter discusses research conducted to evaluate the prognostic significance of premature ventricular contractions (PVCs) on a routine electrocardiogram (ECG), and to evaluate their relationship to heart rate, heart failure and sport participation. Identifying parameters to help risk stratify patients and provide prognostic implications can help identify individuals who may benefit from early diagnosis and intervention. Our discussion utilizes research from a large database of computerized 12-lead ECGs, including 45,402 members of the US Veterans Administration, of which 352 were known to have heart failure. In addition, 750 athletes were analyzed. Echocardiograms and treadmill tests were performed on all those with heart failure and echocardiograms were part of the annual physical exam of the college athletes.

Briefly, there were 1731 patients with PVCs (3.8%) in the total veteran population. Twenty-nine of the 352 with heart failure exhibited a PVC (8%) and 5 of the 750 athletes exhibited a PVC (0.7%). Compared to patients without PVCs, those with PVCs had significantly higher all-cause (39% vs. 22%, $p<0.001$) and cardiovascular mortality (20% vs. 8%, $p<0.001$). PVCs remain a significant predictor even after adjustment for age and other ECG abnormalities. The presence of multiple PVCs or complex morphologies did not add significant additional prognostic information. Those patients with PVCs had a significantly higher heart rate than those without PVCs (mean±SD: 78.6±15 vs. 73.5±16 bpm, $p<0.001$). When patients were divided into groups by heart rate (<60, 60-79, 80-99 and >100 bpm) and by the presence or absence of PVCs, mortality increased progressively with heart rate and doubled with the presence of PVCs. Using regression analysis, heart rate was demonstrated to be an independent and significant predictor of PVCs.

We identified 352 patients (64 ± 11 years; 7 females) with a history of clinical HF undergoing treadmill testing for clinical reasons at the VAPAHCS (1987-2007). Patients with rest PVCs were defined as having ≥1 PVC on the ECG prior to testing (n=29; 8%).During a median follow-up period of 6.2 years, there were 178 deaths of which 76 (42.6%) were due to CV causes. At baseline, compared to patients without rest PVCs, those with rest PVCs had a lower ejection fraction (EF) (30% vs. 45%) and the prevalence of EF≤35% was higher (75% vs. 41%). They were more likely to have smoked (76% vs. 55%).The all-cause and CV mortality rates were significantly higher in the rest PVCs group (72% vs. 49%, $p=0.01$ and 45% vs. 20%, $p=0.002$; respectively). After adjusting for age, beta-blocker use, rest ECG findings, resting heart rate (HR), EF, maximal systolic blood pressure, peak HR and exercise capacity, rest PVCs was associated with a 5.5 -fold increased risk of CV mortality (p=0.004). Considering the presence of PVCs during exercise and/or recovery did not affect our results. All five athletes with at least one PVC on a routine screening ECG as part of the annual physical exams had normal echocardiograms and no clinical manifestations of heart disease. Thus, we concluded that PVCs on a resting ECG are a significant and independent predictor of all-cause and cardiovascular mortality. Increased heart rate predicts mortality in patients with and without PVCs and the combination dramatically increases mortality. These findings together with the demonstrated independent association of heart rate with PVCs suggest that a hyper-adrenergic state is present in patients with PVCs and that it likely contributes to their adverse prognosis. In patients with heart failure the presence of PVCs on a resting ECG is associated with a significant increase in risk of CV death independent of age and exercise capacity. PVCs are rare in young athletes and do not appear to be associated with cardiac disease.

2. Background

Premature ventricular contractions (PVCs) are common electrocardiographic findings in patients with and without structural heart disease. Prior evidence suggests that the presence of PVCs has prognostic value but it is unclear what underlying process they represent. A surprising observation in some studies has been an apparent association between higher mean resting heart rates and the presence of PVCs. Activation of the sympathetic nervous system is an important factor in the genesis of ventricular arrhythmias (Anderson, 2003; Podrid, Fuchs & Candinas, 1990). Enhanced automaticity, triggered activity, and reentry are all mechanisms generating rhythm abnormalities; all three mechanisms are markedly potentiated by the action of catecholamines. We sought to make use of our large database of electrocardiogram (ECG) data to confirm the prognostic significance of PVCs and analyze the interaction between heart rate and PVCs. We hypothesized that both elevated heart rate and the presence of PVCs are markers of sympathetic nervous system (SNS) activity and would, therefore, be correlated with each other and predictive of mortality. This would support the other lines of evidence suggesting that the sympathetic nervous system is active in the genesis of PVCs.

3. Research methods

3.1 Study population

All initial ECGs of consecutive veterans (outpatient and inpatient) who obtained ECGs for any reason at the Palo Alto VA Medical Center from April 1987 until December 1999 were considered in the study. From these 46,959 ECGs, those with atrial fibrillation and paced rhythms were excluded, leaving 45,402 for analysis.

3.2 Electrocardiography

Computerized 12-lead resting 10-second ECG recordings were digitally recorded on the Marquette MAC system. Only the initial ECG was considered for patients with multiple ECGs in the database. Most of the ECG analysis was performed using the GE/Marquette ECG analysis program (www.gemedicalsystems.com). PVCs were defined as at least one QRS complex that was premature, ectopic shaped and had a QRS duration of greater than 120 ms. All ECGs classified as having PVCs were manually over-read by two cardiologists.

Of the ECGs originally classified as having PVCs present, 14% were found to be misclassified as having PVCs when none were present. The most common reason for these errors was misclassification of artifact or of aberrantly-conducted supraventricular beats. All the misclassified patients were reclassified into the 'PVC absent' group, leaving 1731 patients for analysis in the 'PVC present' group.

The 'PVC present' ECGs were then reviewed to categorize the patterns and morphologic characteristics of confirmed PVCs. These characteristics included presence of multiple PVCs on a single 10-sec ECG, presence of couplets or salvos (≥3 consecutive PVCs), presence of bigeminal or trigeminal rhythm, and presence of multiform PVC morphologies. For the purposes of this study, complex PVCs were defined as repetitive PVCs (≥2 consecutive) and multiform morphologies. Non-sustained ventricular tachycardia was rarely documented on these short recordings and the few short runs of 3 or more consecutive beats were not analyzed separately.

Heart rate was determined by the program by counting all QRS complex templates in 10 seconds and multiplying by six. When PVCs were present, the R-R interval between the normal, dominant sinus QRS complexes (NN) was manually measured except when the pattern of PVCs made it impossible (i.e., bigeminy). This NN interval was used to calculate the intrinsic sinus rate.

An 'abnormal' ECG was defined as the presence of one or more of the following: pathologic Q waves, left or right bundle branch block, intraventricular conduction delay, Wolff-Parkinson-White syndrome, right or left ventricular hypertrophy (Romhilt-Estes), left atrial enlargement, or abnormal ST segments. All remaining ECGs were classified as 'normal'.

3.3 Follow-up

The Social Security Death Index and California Health Department Service were used to ascertain vital status as of 12/31/00. Cause of death was available from the latter and deaths determined by the Social Security Death Index were classified by review of the Veteran's Affairs clinical data base. All-cause death and cardiovascular death were used as endpoints. Mean follow-up was 5.5 years. Data regarding cardiac interventions or events was not available.

3.4 Statistical methods

Number Crunching System SoftwareÔ (Kaysville, UT) was used for all statistical analyses after transferring the data from a Microsoft ACCESS© (Redmond, WA) database. Unpaired two-tailed t tests were used for univariate comparison of variables. Cox proportional hazard analysis was performed to evaluate those with and without PVCs and those with multiple and complex PVCs. Multivariate Cox hazard function analysis was performed to demonstrate if the various PVC characteristics were independently and significantly associated with time until death after considering age and other ECG abnormalities. Analysis was repeated using data from only those patients with normal ECGs. Kaplan Meier survival analysis was again performed after patients were divided into groups by heart rate (<60, 60-79, 80-99 and >100 bpm) and by the presence or absence of PVCs. Multivariate regression analysis was performed with heart rate as the dependent variable and with the following independent variables: age, gender, abnormal/normal ECG classification, in- or outpatient status and PVCs present or not. Logistic regression was performed with PVCs as the dependent variable and with the following independent variables: age, gender, abnormal/normal ECG classification, PVCs present or absent and in- or outpatient status.

4. Results

After exclusion of patients with atrial fibrillation and paced rhythms, there were 43,671 patients without PVCs and 1731 patients with PVCs (3.8%). Demographic and ECG characteristics of the groups are shown in Table I. The group with PVCs was older than those without PVCs (mean age ± SD: 65 ± 12 vs. 56 ± 15, P<0.001). As this was a VA study, the patients are 90% male but there was a slightly higher percentage of men among those with PVCs (90% vs. 94%, p=0.01). There were no significant differences between height, weight or BMI. Patients with PVCs had a significantly higher prevalence of Q waves, LVH, LAE, bundle branch blocks and ECGs classified as abnormal. Of the ECG characteristics evaluated, only RVH was similar between the groups.

Variable	Total N=45,402	No PVCs N=43,671	PVCs N=1,731	P-value
Demographics				
Age	56±15	56±15	65±12	<0.001
Males	90.0%	90%	94%	0.01
Height	69±4	69±4	69±4	0.3
Weight	182 ± 40	182 ± 40	184 ± 41	0.1
BMI	27±6	27±6	27±6	0.4
Outpatients	73%	73%	70%	0.004
ECG Findings				
Heart rate	73.7 ± 16	73.5 ± 16	78.6 ± 15	<0.001
Q Wave	13%	11%	23%	<0.001
LVH	5%	5%	8 %	<0.001
RVH	0.3%	0.3%	0.3%	0.6
RBBB	4%	3%	7%	<0.001
LBBB	1%	1%	3%	<0.001
LAE	4%	3.8%	10.7%	<0.001
Abnormal ECG	24%	23%	43%	<0.001

Age, height (inches), weight (pounds), BMI and heart rate are presented as the mean ± SEM.
BMI = body mass index; ECG = electrocardiogram; LAE = left atrial enlargement; LBBB = left bundle branch block; LVH = left ventricular hypertrophy; PVC = premature ventricular contraction; RBBB = right bundle branch block; RVH = right ventricular hypertrophy

Table I. Demographics and ECG findings in patients with and without PVCs.

Those patients with PVCs had a significantly higher heart rate than those without PVCs (mean ± SD: 78.6 ± 15 vs. 73.5 ± 16 bpm, P<0.001). This heart rate difference persisted when patients were sub-grouped by gender, race, outpatient vs. inpatient status and those with otherwise normal ECGs (i.e., least likely to have structural heart disease). Those patients with PVCs always had a significantly higher mean heart rate. Further analysis of heart rate differences showed that women had a significantly lower mean HR than men (71.1 ± 13.7 vs 74.0 ± 16.2, p<0.001), outpatients had a lower mean heart rate than inpatients (72.5 ± 15.0 vs 76.9 ± 17.7, p<0.001), and those with an otherwise normal ECG had a lower heart rate than those with an abnormal ECG (73.2 ± 15.6 vs 75.2 ± 16.8, p<0.001).

Variable	Single PVCs N=911	Multiple PVCs N=815	P- Value	Non-complex PVCs N=1527	Complex PVCs N=199	P- Value
Demographics						
Age	65±12	66±11	0.05	65±12	68±10	<0.001
Height	69±3	69±3	0.26	69±3	70±3	0.30
Weight	186±39	186±39	>0.9	186±39	184±37	0.52
BMI	27±6	27±6	0.4	27±6	27±6	0.36
Outpatients	68%	68%	0.89	68%	67%	0.68
ECG Findings						
Heart rate	77±16	81±15	<0.001	79±16	84±14	<0.001
Q Wave	25%	23%	0.32	23%	31%	0.007
LVH	8 %	9%	0.59	8%	11%	0.18
RVH	0.3%	0.5%	0.60	0.3%	1.5%	0.009
RBBB	7%	7%	0.81	7%	7%	0.85
LBBB	3%	3%	0.77	3%	3%	0.81
LAE	10%	11%	0.81	10.5%	10.6%	>0.9
Abnormal ECG	48%	47%	0.72	47%	54%	0.04

Age, height (inches), weight (pounds), BMI and heart rate are presented as the mean ± SEM.
BMI = body mass index; ECG = electrocardiogram; LAE = left atrial enlargement; LBBB = left bundle branch block; LVH = left ventricular hypertrophy; PVC = premature ventricular contraction; RBBB = right bundle branch block; RVH = right ventricular hypertrophy.

Table II. Demographics and ECG findings in patients with single versus multiple and non-complex versus complex PVCs.

Multiple PVCs (≥2 PVC per ECG) were present in 47% patients with PVCs. Of these 10% were couplets or salvos, 21% had multiform morphologies, and 15% had ventricular bigeminal or trigeminal patterns. The demographics and prevalence of ECG abnormalities for these patients are shown in Table II. Patients with multiple PVCs were older than those with only single PVCs present on the ECG. Those with complex forms were older than those with non-complex morphologies. There were no statistically significant differences in the prevalence of Q waves, LVH, right or left bundle branch block between those patients with or without multiple PVCs. Patients with complex PVCs had statistically significantly more Q waves on their ECGs than those without complex PVCs (p=0.007).

The average annual all-cause mortality in the total population was 3.9% with mortality in those with PVCs (6.7%) significantly higher than for those without PVCs (3.8%) (Table III). The average annual CV mortality in the total population was 1.5% (39% of the deaths) with CV mortality in those with PVCs (3.5%) significantly higher than for those without PVCs (1.4%). Those with complex PVCs had an annual CV mortality rate of 5.1%. The hazard ratios for patients with all types of PVCs were significantly increased when compared to patients having no PVCs on an ECG. The age-adjusted hazard ratios in patients with any PVCs versus those with no PVCs was 1.39 (95% CI 1.29 - 1.50) for all cause mortality and 1.81 (95% CI 1.62 - 2.01) for cardiovascular mortality. There was no statistically significant difference in mortality between patients who had multiple (≥2) PVCs per ECG and those with only single PVCs. The age-adjusted hazard ratio for complex PVCs (versus no PVCs) for all-cause and cardiovascular mortality in all patients was 1.6 (95% CI 1.3-1.9) and 2.1 (95% CI 1.6-2.8), respectively. Patients with complex PVCs appeared to have increased all-cause and CV mortality as compared to those with non-complex PVCs but the difference in survival did not achieve statistical significance. Similar findings resulted when the analysis was limited to patients with normal resting ECGs. After considering age, BMI, and ECG findings in a Cox hazard model, the presence of any resting PVCs were found to be independent predictors of mortality with a hazard ratio of 2.0 (95% CI 1.1-2.8)

	Total N=45,402	**No PVCs N=43,671**	**PVCs N=1,731**	**P-value**
All-cause mortality	23%	22%	39%	<0.001
Annual all-cause mortality	3.9%	3.8%	6.7%	<0.001
CV mortality	8.3%	7.9%	19.6%	<0.001
Annual CV mortality	1.5%	1.4%	3.5%	<0.001

CV = cardiovascular; PVC = premature ventricular contraction.

Table III. Mortality in patients with and without PVCs.

When patients were divided into groups by heart rate (<60, 60-79, 80-99 and >100 bpm) and by the presence or absence of PVCs, mortality increased progressively with heart rate and doubled with the presence of PVCs (Table IV, Figure 1). Cardiovascular mortality ranged from a low of 6.3% in those with heart rates less than 60 bpm and no PVCs to a high of 26.1% in those with a heart rate > 100 bpm and PVCs. Within each heart rate group, there was a significant increase in mortality when PVCs were present (p<0.001). The differences in event free survival between groups is also clearly demonstrated with Kaplan-Meier cumulative survival curve (Figure 2). The PVC and heart rate stratifications performed similarly when patients were divided into those with normal and abnormal ECGs. Cox regression analysis (controlled for age, gender, outpatient vs. inpatient status and normal vs. abnormal ECG) demonstrates that PVCs (RR 1.61, 95% CI 1.44-1.80, $p<0.001$) and heart rate (RR 1.02 for each 1 bpm increase, 95% CI 1.01-1.02, $p<0.001$) are independent predictors of cardiovascular mortality.

	Heart Rate <60	Heart Rate 60-79	Heart Rate 80-99	Heart Rate >99
		Without PVCs		
# of patients	8,077	22,090	10,677	2,827
CV mortality	6.3%	7.3%	9.4%	11.3%
Annual CV mortality	1.1%	1.3%	1.7%	2.0%
		With PVCs		
# of patients	150	832	596	153
CV mortality	12.0%	17.1%	23.3%	26.1%
Annual CV mortality	2.2%	3.1%	4.2%	4.7%

CV = cardiovascular; PVC = premature ventricular contraction

Table IV. Cardiovascular mortality by heart rate group.

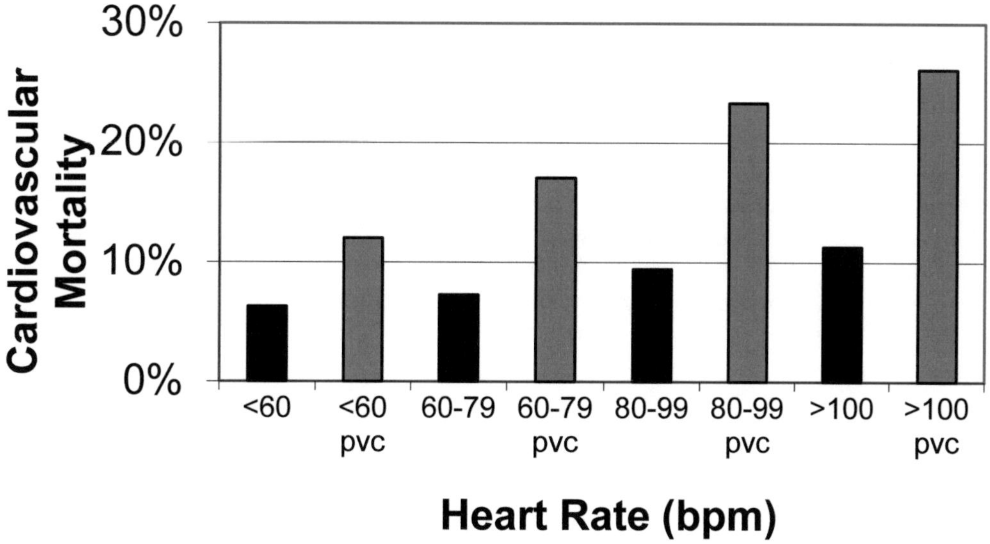

Fig. 1. Differences in cardiovascular mortality between patients without PVCs (black) and those with PVCs (gray) are shown. Within each heart rate group, there is a significant increase in mortality when PVCs are present ($p<0.001$). Mortality also increases as heart rate increases in both patients with and without PVCs ($p<0.001$). PVC = premature ventricular contraction

Logisitic regression controlled for age, gender and normal vs. abnormal ECG was performed to confirm that heart rate was a significant and independent predictor of the presence of PVCs (OR 1.40 for each 20 bpm, 95% CI 1.33 to 1.48, $p<0.001$).
Although patients with PVCs were older than those without PVCs (univariate analysis above), age alone cannot explain the different heart rates because regression analysis showed that resting heart rate did not change significantly with age (slope of less than 1 bpm per decade). When multiple regression analysis was performed to evaluate predictors of heart rate, age did not demonstrate a statistically significant contribution.

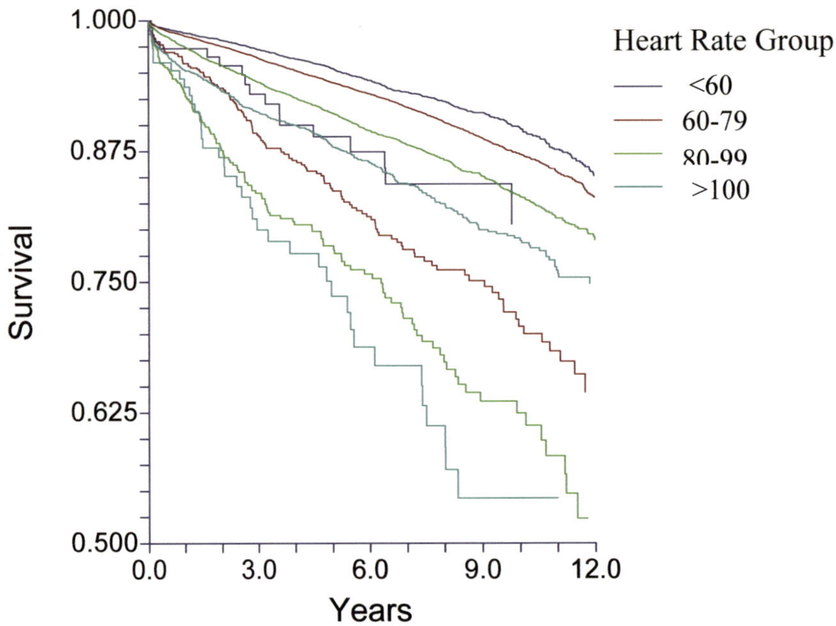

Fig. 2. Kaplan-Meier cumulative survival curves demonstrate decreasing survival with increasing heart rate among patients without PVCs and more significant declines in survival in those with PVCs. The curves followed a consistent order with increasing mortality with increasing rate and with the matching color coded line with PVCs exhibiting an increased mortality. PVC = premature ventricular contraction

5. Discussion

5.1 PVCs

The "PVC hypothesis" that PVC suppression would prevent sudden death was popularized by Lown and others in the 1960's and 1970's and was accepted as dogma well into the late 1980's. It was based on seemingly sound logic that that sudden death in myocardial infarction survivors is due to ventricular fibrillation (Nikolic & Bishop 1982; Pratt, Francis & Luck, 1983) and that PVCs precede and therefore identify those patients who are susceptible to these episodes (Lown, 1971). It was assumed that the suppression of PVCs with antiarrhythmic drugs would be beneficial but the disappointing results of the CAST trials (CAST Investigators, 1989, 1992) negated the causal role theory of PVCs. In fact, the negating of the "PVC hypothesis" by the CAST results is a classic example of why hypothetical mechanisms cannot replace the evidence based approach. Partly due to these results, PVCs are generally ignored on a routine ECG. But, PVCs may still have an important role in risk stratification even if treatment with antiarrhythmic medications is not appropriate.

A higher prevalence of PVCs has been seen in patients with coronary artery disease (Bikkina, Larson, & Levy, 1992), hypertension (Vogt et al., 1990), accompanying ECG abnormalities (Fisher & Tyroler, 1973), and nearly every form of structural heart disease. PVCs also increase with age (Flegg, 1988; Kostis et al., 1982). In the acute phase of myocardial infarction, PVCs are seen in 80-90% of patients and have been related to residual ischemia (Mukharji et al., 1984), degree of coronary narrowing (Minisi et al., 1988), degree of left ventricular involvement (Bigger et al., 1984; Tracy et al., 1987), and age of infarction (Kostis et al., 1987).

In patients without established cardiovascular disease, there have been conflicting findings with some authors concluding that PVCs are benign in this population (Fleg & Kennedy, 1992; Rodstein, Wolloch, & Gubner, 1971) and others reporting increased mortality (Abdalla et al., 1987; Bikkina, Larson, & Levy, 1992; Rabkin, Mathewson & Tate, 1981) although the methods used to determine true absence of coronary artery disease varied greatly between studies. Our results are consistent with the Framingham Heart Study of 6,033 men and women who underwent one hour ambulatory electrocardiography (Bikkina, Larson, & Levy, 1992). After adjusting for age and traditional risk factors for coronary artery disease, there was a significant and independent association between asymptomatic ectopy in men without clinically apparent coronary heart disease and the risk for all-cause mortality (RR 2.3) as well as death from coronary heart disease (RR 2.1). Such an association was not seen in women or in men with known coronary artery disease.

The idea that looking at the frequency and morphology of PVCs might provide additional predictive power has been investigated. Ismaile et al. reported findings from a prospective study of 15,637 apparently healthy white men who underwent screening for the Multiple Risk Factor Intervention Trial (MRFIT) (Abdalla et al., 1987). They used 2 minute resting rhythm strips and concluded that the presence of frequent or complex PVCs is associated with a significant and independent risk for sudden cardiac death (RR 4.2; RR 3.0 for the presence of any PVCs). Our study confirms the risk predicted by any PVC but only shows a non-significant trend towards worse outcome with complex or multiple PVCs. This may be because we looked at all-cause and cardiovascular mortality but did not limit our outcome to sudden death.

5.2 Heart rate

Gillman et al. evaluated 4,530 untreated hypertensives using 36-year follow-up data from the Framingham Study (Gillman et al., 1993). Regression analysis, after adjustment for age and systolic blood pressure, showed that there was a two-fold increase in cardiovascular mortality for each heart rate increment of 40 beats/min. In a French study of 19,386 subjects undergoing routine health examinations, resting tachycardia was demonstrated to be a predictor of non-cardiovascular mortality in both genders, and of cardiovascular mortality in men, independent of age and blood pressure (Benetos et al., 1999). Heart rate on the initial ECG after acute myocardial infarction has also been shown to be an independent predictor of prognosis (Hathaway et al., 1998). Our results add to the evidence that heart rate is an important prognostic variable.

Several large studies confirm our finding of heart rate not being related to age (Gillum, 1988; Morcet et al., 1999; Simpson et al., 2002; Spodick et al., 1992). There are conflicting reports in the literature as to the association of gender and heart rate. Some studies suggest that heart rate is higher in women (Gillum, 1988; Morcet et al., 1999) while others confirm our finding of heart rate being lower in women (Simpson et al., 2002).

5.3 PVCs and heart rate

Few studies have evaluated the relationship of resting PVCs with increased heart rate on an ECG. The Atherosclerosis Risk In Communities (ARIC) study reported the prevalence of PVCs in 15,792 individuals aged 45-65 years on a longer than normal ECG recording of 2-minutes (Simpson et al., 2002). PVCs were present in 6% of these middle-aged adults and faster sinus rates were directly related to PVC prevalence.

The relationship of PVCs to heart rate has been described in a series of studies using Holter monitoring. The relationship between the frequency of PVCs and underlying heart rate was reported in patients with frequent PVCs; the most frequent relationship was an increase in PVCs with increasing heart rate (Acanfora et al., 1993; Winkle, 1982) It has also been shown that there are three reproducible trends characterizing the dynamic behavior of PVCs: a tachycardia-enhanced pattern (28%), a bradycardia-enhanced pattern (24%), and an indifferent pattern in the remainder of patients (48%) (Pitzalis et al. 1997). Another study suggested that beta-blockers were most effective in reducing PVC frequency in the tachycardia and indifferent groups (Pitzalis et al., 1996). Propafenone has also been shown to be most effective in tachycardia-enhanced patients (Saikawa et al., 2001).

5.4 Sympathetic nervous system

Several lines of evidence suggest that activation of the sympathetic nervous system (SNS) plays a primary role in the generation of PVCs, ventricular arrhythmias and sudden cardiac death (Grassi et al., 2003; Podrid, Fuchs & Candinas, 1990). Circulating catecholamines and increased heart rate are known to interact with all three major mechanisms involved in the generation of arrhythmias: enhanced automaticity, triggered automaticity, and reentry (Stein et al., 1998). Substantial experimental data from animal studies shows that activation of the SNS is a strong stimulus for the development of ventricular tachyarrhythmias. It is well established that medications with beta-blocking properties help to decrease the frequency of PVCs (Krittayaphong et al, 2002) and prevent sudden death (JAMA, 1982; Pederson, 1985). Decreased sympathetic tone and improvement of cardiac autonomic regulation appear to play a major role in the ability of beta-blockers to reduce PVCs (Acanfora et al., 2000).

Studies of genetic disorders, animal models, and spontaneous human arrhythmias have helped to create a better understanding of this relationship.1 Infusion of nerve growth factor into animal models, designed to mimic long-term elevations of sympathetic activity and signaling, resulted in apoptosis, hypertrophy, and fibrosis. In human studies, changes in heart rate have been shown to occur prior to the onset of PVCs and ventricular arrhythmias (Anderson et al., 1999; Nemec, Hammill & Shen, 1999; Pitzalis et al, 1997; Sapoznikov, Luria & Gotsman, 1999). The propensity for PVCs and ventricular arrhythmias is highest when there are superimposed effects of short-, intermediate, and long-term changes. Parasympathetic inhibition of SNS activity may be part of a normal regulatory process that is lost in patients with severe heart failure and other disorders.

Some investigators have proposed the nerve sprouting hypothesis of ventricular arrhythmia to explain arrhythmic events seen in patients with a history of myocardial infarction (Chen et al, 2001). The theory is that myocardial damage results in nerve injury which is followed by sympathetic nerve sprouting and regionally increased sympathetic tone. The increased SNS activity in the local area of remodeled myocardium results in PVCs, ventricular tachycardia/fibrillation and sudden death. Support for this hypothesis was provided by an evaluation of cardiac nerves in explanted native hearts of human transplant recipients (Cao et al., 2000). Infusion of nerve growth factor into the left stellate ganglion of dogs was also shown to result in increased development of ventricular arrhythmias (Cao et al., 2000). The recurring theme of research in this area is that the response to injury results in heterogeneous sympathetic innervation which is highly arrhythmogenic (Verrier & Antzelevitch, 2004).

5.5 Study limitations

The population in our study included a relatively diverse group of all consecutive inpatients and outpatients who had a 12-lead ECG for any reason; the only exclusion criteria were the presence of atrial fibrillation or a paced rhythm. This differs from many previous studies of either more narrowly defined high-risk populations of patients referred to electrophysiologists or more broadly defined low-risk community epidemiological cohorts. These differences may be an advantage as our study is clinically based and includes all patients at our facility referred for an ECG. Base-line clinical data, laboratory studies and diagnostic tests such as echocardiograms or cardiac catheterizations were not available. Information on medications, especially beta-blockers, would have been very useful. The ECGs were obtained over the span of more than a decade during which time there were changes in practice patterns and beta-blocker usage. However, there is no reason to think that beta-blocker usage would be less in those with PVCs (such that this would explain their higher heart rate). We also lack other markers of sympathetic activity to confirm our hypothesis. An important limitation of the study is that PVCs are identified on a single 10 second ECG recording. This 'snapshot' might not be expected to provide as much clinically meaningful information as longer term ambulatory ECG monitoring but, the extremely large number of patients available for analysis allows significant results to be obtained. The 4% prevalence of PVCs found in our study compares favorably with a rate of 2-7% in previous epidemiologic studies including those using 2-min rhythm strips. (Crow et al., 1975; Fisher & Tyroler, 1973; Kostis et al., 1987; Simpson et al., 200).
Overall, this is a retrospective analysis and, as such, should be considered hypothesis generating rather than conclusive evidence of a cause and effect relationship. The predictive models generated here should be validated using other electrocardiographic databases and in prospective evaluations.

6. Conclusions

Our study suggests that the simple 12-lead ECG provides valuable information and can complement more advanced strategies for arrhythmic risk stratification. The presence of any PVC on a single ECG is a powerful predictor of all-cause and cardiovascular mortality. The presence of multiple or complex PVCs was not a significantly better predictor although there was a trend towards worse prognosis in patients with complex forms. These observations are true even in those patients with otherwise normal baseline ECGs.

Regression analysis demonstrates that heart rate is a significant and independent predictor of the presence of PVCs. Our findings support the hypothesis that activation of the sympathetic nervous system is an important factor in the genesis of PVCs and ventricular arrhythmias. The presence of elevated heart rate is a significant prognostic factor and the combination of increased heart rate and PVCs dramatically increases mortality.

7. References

No authors listed. A randomized trial of propranolol in patients with acute myocardial infarction. I. Mortality results. JAMA. 1982;247:1707-14.

Abdalla IS, Prineas RJ, Neaton JD, et al. Relation between ventricular premature complexes and sudden cardiac death in apparently healthy men. Am J Cardiol 1987;60:1036-42.

Acanfora D, De Caprio L, Di Palma A, et al. Relationship between ventricular ectopic beat frequency and heart rate: study in patients with severe arrhythmias. Am Heart J 1993;125:1022-9.

Acanfora D, Pinna GD, Gheorghiade M, et al. Effect of beta-blockade on the premature ventricular beats/heart rate relation and heart rate variability in patients with coronary heart disease and severe ventricular arrhythmias. Am J Ther 2000;7:229-36.

Anderson KP. Sympathetic nervous system activity and ventricular tachyarrhythmias: recent advances. Ann Noninvasive Electrocardiol 2003;8:75-89.

Anderson KP, Shusterman V, Aysin B, et al. Distinctive RR dynamics preceding two modes of onset of spontaneous sustained ventricular tachycardia. (ESVEM) Investigators. Electrophysiologic Study Versus Electrocardiographic Monitoring. J Cardiovasc Electrophysiol 1999;10:897-904.

Benetos A, Rudnichi A, Thomas F, et al. Influence of heart rate on mortality in a French population: role of age, gender, and blood pressure. Hypertension 1999;33:44-52.

Bigger JT, Jr, Fleiss JL, Kleiger R, et al. The relationships among ventricular arrhythmias, left ventricular dysfunction, and mortality in the 2 years after myocardial infarction. Circulation 1984;69:250-8.

Bikkina M, Larson MG, Levy D. Prognostic implications of asymptomatic ventricular arrhythmias: the Framingham Heart Study. Ann Intern Med 1992;117:990-6.

Cao JM, Chen LS, KenKnight BH, et al. Nerve sprouting and sudden cardiac death. Circ Res 2000;86:816-21.

Cao JM, Fishbein MC, Han JB, et al. Relationship between regional cardiac hyperinnervation and ventricular arrhythmia. Circulation 2000;101:1960-9.

Chen PS, Chen LS, Cao JM, et al. Sympathetic nerve sprouting, electrical remodeling and the mechanisms of sudden cardiac death. Cardiovasc Res 2001;50:409-16.

Crow RS, Prineas RJ, Dias V, et al. Ventricular premature beats in a population sample. Frequency and associations with coronary risk characteristics. Circulation 1975;52:III211-5.

Effect of the antiarrhythmic agent moricizine on survival after myocardial infarction. The Cardiac Arrhythmia Suppression Trial II Investigators. N Engl J Med 1992;327:227-33.

Fisher FD, Tyroler HA. Relationship between ventricular premature contractions on routine electrocardiography and subsequent sudden death from coronary heart disease. Circulation 1973;47:712-9.

Fleg JL. Ventricular arrhythmias in the elderly: prevalence, mechanisms, and therapeutic implications. Geriatrics 1988;43:23-9.

Fleg JL, Kennedy HL. Long-term prognostic significance of ambulatory electrocardiographic findings in apparently healthy subjects greater than or equal to 60 years of age. Am J Cardiol 1992;70:748-51.

Gillman MW, Kannel WB, Belanger A, et al. Influence of heart rate on mortality among persons with hypertension: the Framingham Study. Am Heart J 1993;125:1148-54.

Gillum RF. The epidemiology of resting heart rate in a national sample of men and women: associations with hypertension, coronary heart disease, blood pressure, and other cardiovascular risk factors. Am Heart J 1988;116:163-74.

Grassi G, Seravalle G, Bertinieri G, et al. Behaviour of the adrenergic cardiovascular drive in atrial fibrillation and cardiac arrhythmias. Acta Physiol Scand 2003;177:399-404.

Hathaway WR, Peterson ED, Wagner GS, et al. Prognostic significance of the initial electrocardiogram in patients with acute myocardial infarction. GUSTO-I Investigators. Global Utilization of Streptokinase and t-PA for Occluded Coronary Arteries. JAMA 1998;279:387-91.

Kostis JB, Byington R, Friedman LM, et al. Prognostic significance of ventricular ectopic activity in survivors of acute myocardial infarction. J Am Coll Cardiol 1987;10:231-42.

Kostis JB, McCrone K, Moreyra AE, et al. The effect of age, blood pressure and gender on the incidence of premature ventricular contractions. Angiology 1982;33:464-73.

Krittayaphong R, Bhuripanyo K, Punlee K, et al. Effect of atenolol on symptomatic ventricular arrhythmia without structural heart disease: a randomized placebo-controlled study. Am Heart J 2002;144:e10.

Lown B, Wolf M. Approaches to sudden death from coronary heart disease. Circulation 1971;44:130-42.

Minisi AJ, Mukharji J, Rehr RB, et al. Association between extent of coronary artery disease and ventricular premature beat frequency after myocardial infarction. Am Heart J 1988;115:1198-1201.

Morcet JF, Safar M, Thomas F, et al. Associations between heart rate and other risk factors in a large French population. J Hypertens 1999;17:1671-6.

Mukharji J, Rude RE, Poole WK, et al. Risk factors for sudden death after acute myocardial infarction: two-year follow-up. Am J Cardiol 1984;54:31-6.

Nemec J, Hammill SC, Shen WK. Increase in heart rate precedes episodes of ventricular tachycardia and ventricular fibrillation in patients with implantable cardioverter defibrillators: analysis of spontaneous ventricular tachycardia database. Pacing Clin Electrophysiol 1999;22:1729-38.

Nikolic G, Bishop RL, Singh JB. Sudden death recorded during Holter monitoring. Circulation 1982;66:218-25.

Pedersen TR. Six-year follow-up of the Norwegian Multicenter Study on Timolol after Acute Myocardial Infarction. N Engl J Med 1985;313:1055-8.

Pitzalis MV, Mastropasqua F, Massari F, et al. Dependency of premature ventricular contractions on heart rate. Am Heart J 1997;133:153-61.

Pitzalis MV, Mastropasqua F, Massari F, et al. Holter-guided identification of premature ventricular contractions susceptible to suppression by beta-blockers. Am Heart J 1996;131:508-15.

Podrid PJ, Fuchs T, Candinas R. Role of the sympathetic nervous system in the genesis of ventricular arrhythmia. Circulation 1990;82:I103-13.

Preliminary report: effect of encainide and flecainide on mortality in a randomized trial of arrhythmia suppression after myocardial infarction. The Cardiac Arrhythmia Suppression Trial (CAST) Investigators. N Engl J Med 1989;321:406-12.

Pratt CM, Francis MJ, Luck JC, et al. Analysis of ambulatory electrocardiograms in 15 patients during spontaneous ventricular fibrillation with special reference to preceding arrhythmic events. J Am Coll Cardiol 1983;2:789-97.

Rabkin SW, Mathewson FA, Tate RB. Relationship of ventricular ectopy in men without apparent heart disease to occurrence of ischemic heart disease and sudden death. Am Heart J 1981;101:135-42.

Rodstein M, Wolloch L, Gubner RS. Mortality study of the significance of extrasystoles in an insured population. Circulation 1971;44:617-25.

Saikawa T, Niwa H, Ito M, et al. The effect of propafenone on premature ventricular contractions (PVC): an analysis based on heart rate dependency of PVCs. Jpn Heart J 2001;42:701-11.

Sapoznikov D, Luria MH, Gotsman MS. Changes in sinus RR interval patterns preceding ventricular ectopic beats: assessment with rate enhancement and dynamic heart rate trends. Int J Cardiol 1999;69:217-24.

Simpson RJ, Jr, Cascio WE, Schreiner PJ, et al. Prevalence of premature ventricular contractions in a population of African American and white men and women: the Atherosclerosis Risk in Communities (ARIC) study. Am Heart J 2002;143:535-40.

Spodick DH, Raju P, Bishop RL, et al. Operational definition of normal sinus heart rate. Am J Cardiol 1992;69:1245-6.

Tracy CM, Winkler J, Brittain E, et al. Determinants of ventricular arrhythmias in mildly symptomatic patients with coronary artery disease and influence of inducible left ventricular dysfunction on arrhythmia frequency. J Am Coll Cardiol 1987;9:483-8.

Stein KM, Karagounis LA, Markowitz SM, et al. Heart rate changes preceding ventricular ectopy in patients with ventricular tachycardia caused by reentry, triggered activity, and automaticity. Am Heart J 1998;136:425-34.

Vogt M, Motz W, Scheler S, et al. Disorders of coronary microcirculation and arrhythmias in systemic arterial hypertension. Am J Cardiol 1990;65:45G-50G.

Verrier RL, Antzelevitch C. Autonomic aspects of arrhythmogenesis: the enduring and the new. Curr Opin Cardiol 2004;19:2-11.

Winkle RA. The relationship between ventricular ectopic beat frequency and heart rate. Circulation 1982;66:439-46.

4

Arrhythmias in Children and Young Adults

Harinder R. Singh
Assistant Professor, Pediatrics, Pediatric Electrophysiologist and Associate, Cardiology, The Carman and Ann Adams Department of Pediatrics, Children's Hospital of Michigan, USA

1. Introduction

One of the challenges that physicians taking care of children face is the interpretation of an electrocardiogram (ECG). The findings on ECG should be seen in the light of a patient's clinical presentation. In this evidence-based chapter, we will explore the most common pediatric arrhythmias, including sinus arrhythmia, premature beats, brady-arrhythmias, escape rhythms and tachy-arrhythmias including different types of atrial, junctional and ventricular tachycardias. The objective of this chapter is to familiarize the reader with ECG interpretation of common pediatric arrhythmias in children and young adults.

2. Sinus arrhythmia

2.1 *Definition*: Sinus arrhythmia is the normal variation in the rate of the sino-atrial (SA) node that is mainly associated with the respiratory phases.
2.2 *Incidence*: It is common in children and the incidence decreases with age(Kaushal and Taylor 2002).
2.3 *Mechanism*: It occurs due to change in sinus node function related to changes in the autonomic tone. Inspiration and expiration are associated with increased and decreased heart rate due to decreased and increased parasympathetic tone, respectively(Coker et al. 1984). Sinus arrhythmia disappears with conditions associated with elevated sympathetic tone causing increased heart rate.
2.4 *Clinical presentation*: Auscultation reveals irregular heart rhythm which varies with respiration.
2.5 *ECG*: ECG reveals sinus rhythm with variation in P-P interval preceding the change in R-R intervals without any significant change in P-R interval (Figure 1).
2.6 *Management*: No work-up is needed because sinus arrhythmia is a normal variant with excellent prognosis.

3. Ectopic complexes (premature beats)

3.1 Premature atrial contractions

3.1.1 *Definition*: Premature atrial contraction (PAC), or atrial premature beat, is a premature discharge arising from an atrial focus other than the sino-atrial (SA) node.
3.1.2 *Incidence*: PACs were reported in 14% of full-term infants on 24-hour ECGs (Southall et al. 1980). Among 10-13 year old boys with healthy hearts, 13% had singlet PACs (Scott et al.

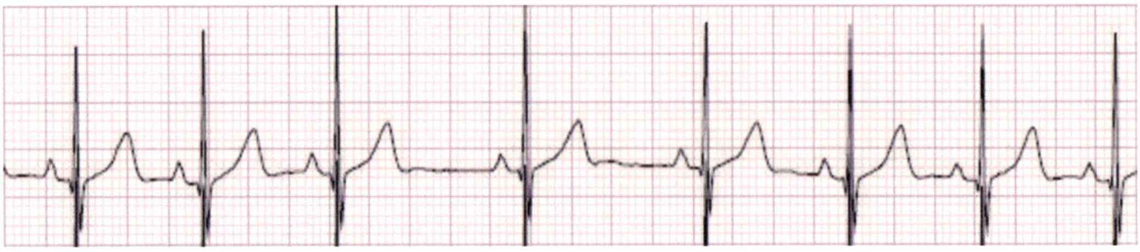

Fig. 1. Sinus arrhythmia

1980). On 24-hour ECG monitoring, 64% of young women (Sobotka et al. 1981) and 56% of male adolescents had PACs (Brodsky et al. 1977). Frequent causes of PACs include intake of caffeine, nicotine, alcohol, and other stimulants. PACs can be associated with atrial enlargement, electrolyte abnormalities, mechanical trauma, chronic pulmonary disease, and heart failure.

3.1.3 *Mechanism*: PACs can occur either due to a re-entry mechanism, (Wallace and Daggett 1964) automaticity outside of the SA node, or triggered activity (Wit and Cranefield 1977).

3.1.4 *Natural history*: PACs can give rise to atrial fibrillation and flutter, especially in older post-operative patients(Jideus et al. 2006). They may subside with removal or correction of the inciting stimuli. Control of congestive heart failure, ischemic heart disease, pulmonary disease, and electrolyte abnormalities may decrease the incidence of PACs.

3.1.5 *Clinical presentation*: Patients with PACs may be asymptomatic or perceive them as palpitations. They may be incidentally detected as irregular heart rhythm on auscultation.

3.1.6 *ECG*: A PAC presents as a P-wave that appears earlier than expected on an ECG. The P-wave morphology may appear different. The PR interval in a PAC is often different than the previous PR interval. PACs can have three possible outcomes: 1) block at the AV node due to AV nodal refractoriness (Figure 2a), 2) conduct normally through the AV node (Figure 2b), or 3) conduct with aberrancy due to His-bundle refractoriness (Figure 2c). There is no compensatory ventricular pause.

3.1.7 *Work-up*: A 12-lead ECG is usually adequate for evaluation; however, Holter monitoring may be performed.

3.1.8 *Management and Prognosis*: Control of exogenous factors will decrease the incidence of PACs. No physical restrictions need to be imposed on children without heart and/or lung disease, or electrolyte abnormalities. Beta blocker like bisoprolol decreased PACs by 50%, although 25% of these patients had adverse reactions associated with beta blockade (Sugimoto et al. 1986). Prognosis is excellent for patients with PACs with normal hearts and needs no treatment.

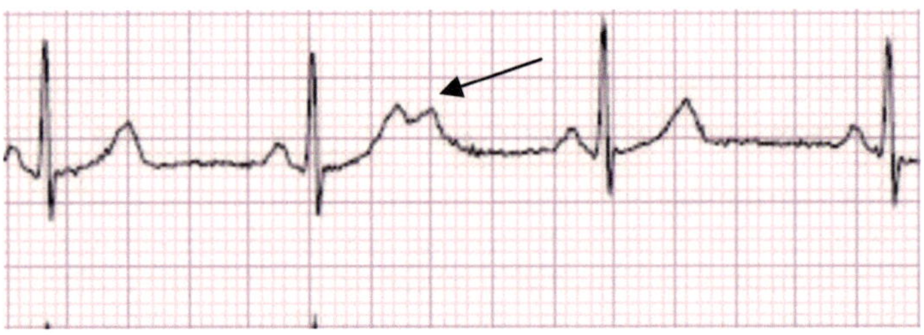

Fig. 2.a Premature atrial complex that is blocked

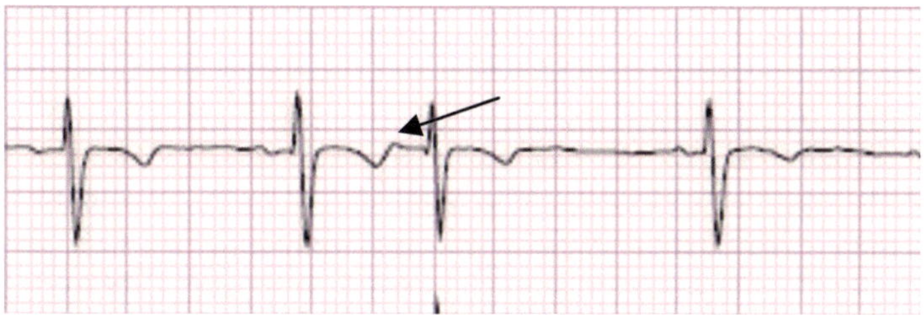

Fig. 2.b Premature atrial complex that is normally conducted

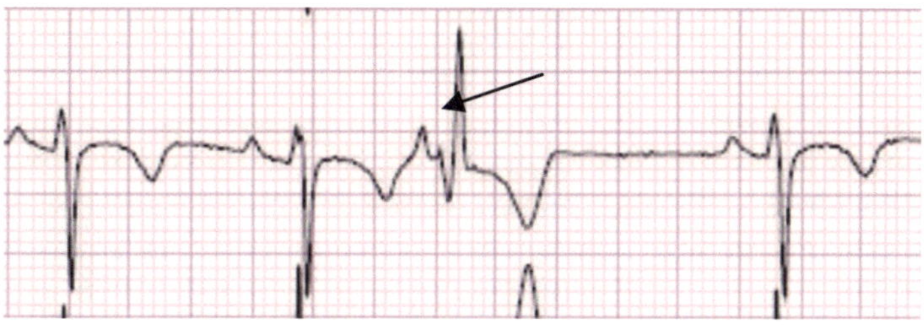

Fig. 2.c Premature atrial complex that is conducted with aberrancy

3.2 Premature ventricular contractions

3.2.1 *Definition*: A premature ventricular contraction (PVC) or ventricular premature beat (VPB) is an early ventricular beat that originates below the bifurcation of the bundle of His. It is characterized by a premature wide QRS complex that is morphologically different compared to the baseline QRS complexes (Sherron et al. 1985; Olgin and Zipes 2005b).

3.2.2 *Incidence*: PVCs follow a bi-modal distribution and are seen in 18% of neonates, 20% of toddlers, 16% of school children, 20-30% of adolescents and subsequent increases in late adulthood (Southall et al. 1980). On 24-hour ECG monitoring of subjects without heart disease, 54% of young women (Sobotka et al. 1981) and 50% of young males had PVCs (Brodsky et al. 1977). Surgically-corrected Tetralogy of Fallot patients have an incidence of 6-48% (Vaksmann et al. 1990),(Chandar et al. 1990).

3.2.3 *Mechanism*: Three mechanisms inducing PVCs include: automaticity, re-entry, and triggered activity. PVCs can result from mechanical, electrical, and chemical stimulation leading to ventricular depolarization. Abnormalities in metabolism, electrolytes, or iatrogenic causes can initiate PVCs in children. Both slow and fast heart rates are associated with PVCs (Sherron et al. 1985).

3.2.4 *Natural history*: PVCs increase with age and are more common in males (Silka and Garson 1999). In the absence of heart disease, PVCs are inconsequential under the age of 30 years but influence risk of sudden death in those over 30 years (Chiang et al. 1969). PVCs may be present in those with increased vagal tone such as athletes or in those with increased stimulation such as intake of caffeine, alcohol, and/or nicotine. In adults without structural heart disease, PVCs induced during exercise and recovery phases were associated with increased risk of mortality (Frolkis et al. 2003). PVCs also occur in those with surgically-corrected congenital heart disease, myocarditis, right-ventricular dysfunction, congestive heart failure, cardiomyopathy, ventricular hypertrophy, myocardial infarction, ventricular non-compaction and iatrogenic causes (Chandar et al. 1990; Vaksmann et al. 1990; Espinola-Zavaleta et al. 2006; Sestito et al. 2007).

3.2.5 *Clinical presentation*: PVCs are the most common cause of irregular heart beats in children. They are usually detected incidentally and occasionally produce symptoms. Single PVCs are generally well-tolerated by children. Symptoms secondary to PVCs include palpitations, lightheadedness, fatigue, chest pain, and shortness of breath.

3.2.6 *ECG*: To be classified as PVC, four criteria should be met: 1) premature QRS without a premature P wave, 2) difference in QRS morphology between PVC and regular QRS complex, 3) prolonged QRS duration for age, and 4) different QRS and T wave vectors. Unifocal PVCs have a fixed morphology, as opposed to PACs with aberrant conduction. Multifocal PVCs have different morphologies due to the different locations of onset and electrical instability of the ventricle (Silka and Garson 1999). There is a compensatory pause after PVC, i.e., R-R interval produced by SA node initiated QRS complexes on either side of the PVC is equal to twice the normal R-R interval (figure 3). PVCs may present as isolated, couplets, bigeminy or trigeminy pattern. If the PVC originates in the right ventricle, the QRS morphology appears as a left bundle branch block pattern and if the PVC originates in the left ventricle, the QRS morphology appears as a right bundle branch block pattern.

3.2.7 *Differential diagnoses*: 1) Premature atrial complex with aberrant conduction, 2) premature junctional complex with aberrant conduction, and 3) anterograde conduction over an accessory pathway with pre-excitation.

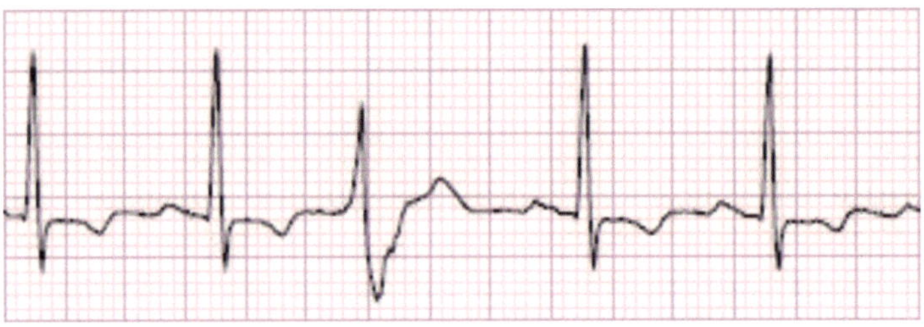

Fig. 3. Premature ventricular complex with a compensatory pause

3.2.8 *Work-up*: A detailed history of episodes is necessary. A history of congenital heart disease with subsequent surgical correction should be obtained. In addition to an ECG and 24-hour Holter monitoring, an exercise test is important in determining whether the frequency of PVCs or symptoms worsen with activity (Paridon 2006; Zipes 2006). Multifocal PVCs in structural heart disease require further workup. Echocardiography and electrophysiology studies may be warranted in surgically corrected patients or those with structural heart disease if there are PVCs and malignant ventricular arrhythmias (Case 1999).

3.2.9 *Management and Prognosis*: Management of PVCs depends on two factors: 1) a history of structural heart disease or surgically corrected congenital heart disease, and 2) the symptoms experienced by the patient. In children, PVCs are considered to be benign if they disappear with exercise (Attina et al. 1987). The majority of children with normal hearts presenting with asymptomatic single PVC, bigeminy, or trigeminy do not require treatment. Given that surgically-corrected congenital heart disease is associated with increased predisposition to non-sustained ventricular tachycardia and sudden cardiac death, children may require treatment with anti-arrhythmics under the supervision of a pediatric cardiologist. Beta-blockers can assist in suppressing PVCs in symptomatic patients (Alexander 2001a). If symptoms are not medically controlled, catheter ablation is an option (Zhu et al. 1995). Prognosis depends on whether there is underlying structural and metabolic heart disease. PVCs inducible during exercise can be ominous in patients with structural heart disease and are of higher significance (Silka and Garson 1999). Athletes with structural heart disease in high-risk groups with PVCs should be restricted to low-intensity sports (Zipes and Garson 1994).

3.3 Premature junctional complexes

3.3.1 *Definition*: A premature junctional complex (PJC) or beat (PJB) is a premature discharge that originates in the AV junction either at the level of the AV node or the bundle of His, in the absence of a preceding atrial discharge.

3.3.2 *Incidence*: PJCs can occur in structurally normal or abnormal hearts and in all age groups. The incidence and prevalence are not well known. Among 16-19 year old males, 0.21% had premature junctional complexes on 12-lead ECG and similar in other age groups (Hiss and Lamb 1962).

3.3.3 *Mechanism*: PJCs arise due to increased automaticity or triggered activity due to after depolarizations within the AV junction (Hoffman and Cranefield 1964; Rosen et al. 1980). PJCs may predispose the patient to ventricular tachycardia. Potential causes include normal variants, use of stimulants or alcohol, hypokalemia, hypoxemia, ischemia, and digitalis toxicity (Sherron et al. 1985).

3.3.4 *Clinical presentation*: It may be incidentally detected or may produce symptoms like palpitations, syncope, or dizziness.

3.3.5 *ECG*: ECG shows QRS complex morphology similar to sinus node originated activation, without preceding P-wave. A PJC conducting to the ventricle with aberrancy has a QRS complex comparable to PVC. A retrograde P-wave may appear before, during, or after the QRS complex (Sherron et al. 1985) (Figure 4).

3.3.6 *Work-up*: Depending on the frequency of the PJCs, an ECG can identify the premature complexes. If unsuccessful, a 24-hour Holter monitor may be used. An electrophysiology study maybe needed to identify the location of the origin of the PJCs; origin distal to the AV node can initiate ventricular tachycardia (Sherron et al. 1985).

3.3.7 *Management and Prognosis*: Patients with PJCs are usually left untreated. The management of underlying causes is essential to decrease symptomatic PJCs. If symptoms are severe, medical management and pacing may be warranted to increase the heart rate.

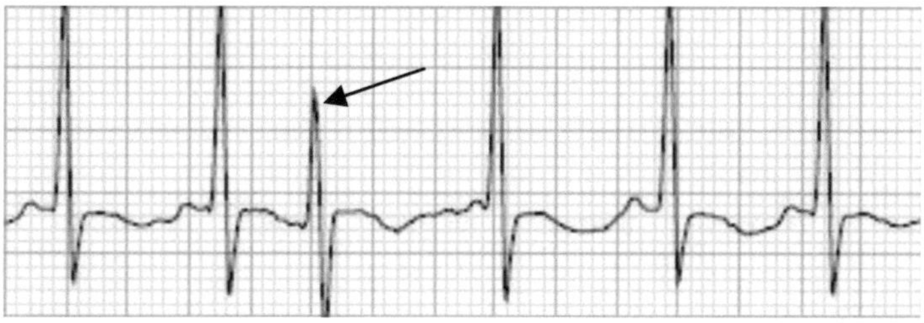

Fig. 4. Premature junctional complex

4. Bradyarrhythmias

4.1 Sinus node dysfunction (SND)

4.1.1 *Definition*: The inability of the sino-atrial (SA) node to discharge/activate (sinus pause/arrest) or inappropriately activate (tachycardia-bradycardia syndrome) the atrial tissue.

4.1.2 *Incidence*: SND is relatively uncommon in children with normal cardiac anatomy and the exact incidence is unknown. However, it is a common problem in those who have had surgery for congenital heart disease (CHD), especially in patients with Mustard, Senning, and Fontan procedures (Fishberger 2001). Approximately 2/3 of all immediate post-transplant patients have SND (Jacquet et al. 1990).

4.1.3 *Mechanism*: In sinus node pause/arrest, there is a lack of discharge from the SA node; causing no activation of the atria. With sinus node exit block, the activation may be delayed significantly or blocked completely at the nodal region, without activation of the atria. In tachycardia-bradycardia syndrome, severe sinus bradycardia is followed by tachycardia in the form of atrial flutter in the pediatric population and atrial fibrillation/flutter in adults with repaired congenital heart disease (Duster et al. 1985; Gelatt et al. 1994).

4.1.4 *Natural history*: Sinus node dysfunction may present as severe sinus bradycardia, sinus pause or arrest, periods of junctional rhythm, and/or alternating tachycardia-bradycardia periods. Sinus node dysfunction increases in frequency with age of the patient and time from surgery.

4.1.5 *Clinical presentation*: It depends on the age, underlying cardiac conduction abnormality, and hemodynamic status. Although majority of children with structurally normal hearts remain asymptomatic; fatigue, exercise intolerance, palpitations, chest pain, dizziness, and syncope may occur (Fishberger 2001). These symptoms are more frequent in those with corrected congenital heart disease. Infants present with poor feeding, lethargy or heart failure. Sudden death is an uncommon presentation.

4.1.6 *ECG*: ECG may show severe sinus bradycardia, sinus pause, junctional rhythm, and/or atrial fibrillation/flutter. Due to the short duration, significant episodes can be missed.

4.1.7 *Work-up*: Non-invasive testing includes a 12-lead ECG, a Holter monitor, an event monitor and exercise stress test. Depending on the frequency of the symptoms and the age group, a 24-hour Holter monitor can be employed. In an older age group with less frequent symptoms, an event recorder can be used to record rhythm abnormalities. In patients who are able to exercise, a treadmill stress test will show lower heart rate response to maximal exercise and rapid decrease in heart rate during recovery time immediately after the test (Martin and Kugler 1999; Fishberger 2001). Intrinsic heart rate (IHR) is the heart rate with complete blockade of autonomic activity with atropine and propranolol (Jose AD and Collison D, 1970). Normal value of IHR is defined as 118.1 – (0.57 x age). The intrinsic heart rate decreases with age in complete autonomic blockade but decreases at a faster rate in patients with SND (Benditt et al. 1984). In invasive testing, an electrophysiology study is undertaken to evaluate sinus node automaticity, and conduction time. Sino-atrial conduction time (SACT) and sinus node recovery time (SNRT) are assessed with premature atrial stimulation and atrial overdrive pacing, respectively. The length of SNRT evaluates the sinus node automaticity; prolongation of SNRT indicates suppression of sinus node automatic function.

4.1.8 *Management and Prognosis*: Medical treatment is dependent on the type of sinus node dysfunction and the presence of associated symptoms. Choice of medications should be selected cautiously and the patient should be monitored closely.

1. Sinus bradycardia and pause/arrest < 3 sec: no further management; pause/arrest > 3 sec requires evaluation. In severe sinus bradycardia with hemodynamic instability, sympathomimetic drugs such as atropine and isoproterenol or transcutaneous pacing are used.

2. Tachycardia-Bradycardia syndrome management is difficult. Drugs used to manage tachycardia may worsen sinus bradycardia and should be used judiciously and may necessitate cardiac pacing.

With failed medical therapy and the need for long-term anti-arrhythmic medications, pacemaker implantation is indicated. According to the 2002 ACC guidelines for pacemaker implantation (Gregaratos 2002), documented symptomatic bradycardia (Class I), symptomatic chronotropic incompetence (Class I), syncope of unknown etiology with electrophysiologic studies suggestive of SND (Class IIa), and chronic awake heart rate < 40 (Class IIb) are primary indicators for permanent pacing. Permanent pacing is indicated in bradycardia-tachycardia (Class IIa). In refractory or symptomatic SND patients who have failed medical therapy, permanent pacemaker implantation improves clinical status. Pacemaker implantation can provide anti-bradycardia pacing in severe bradycardia; in tachycardia-bradycardia syndrome, pacemaker can provide anti-tachycardia and anti-bradycardia pacing.

4.2 First-degree atrio-ventricular heart block

4.2.1 *Definition*: Delay in atrio-ventricular conduction at the level of the atrial tissue, AV node, and/or the His-Purkinje system.

4.2.2 *Incidence*: First degree AV block has been detected in 6% of neonates (Ferrer 1977). Among 10-13 year old males, 8.5% had first degree heart block (Scott et al. 1980).

4.2.3 *Mechanism*: Common mechanism in pediatric patients is hypervagotonia. However, other causes include medications which prolong AV-node refractory period, electrolyte abnormalities, hypothermia, hypothyroidism, rheumatic fever, myocarditis, Lyme disease, congenital heart disease that stretches the atria at the AV node area, cardiac surgery, and myopathies (Weindling 2001). Four sites for first degree AV block with a normal QRS include: atrium (3-20%) (Sherron et al. 1985), AV node (35-90%) (Sherron et al. 1985), Bundle of His (15%) (Sherron et al. 1985) and infra-Hisian conduction system. It is more common in endocardial cushion defects and Ebstein's anomaly of the tricuspid valve due to intraatrial conduction delay (Sherron et al. 1985). Increased vagal tone, calcium-channel blockers, digoxin, and beta-blockers are common causes of AV nodal delay. Quinidine, procainamide, and disopyramide impair phase 0 depolarization and cause delay in bundle of His conduction. Finally, prolongation of conduction in the infra-Hisian region can be caused by sodium-channel blockers as above. With first degree AV block with a wide QRS complex, conduction in the AV node or the bundle of His is delayed; bilateral bundle branch conduction is slowed in most cases; two levels of conduction delay can also be seen (Peuch et al. 1976).

4.2.4 *Natural history*: First degree heart block has the potential, although rarely, to progress to higher-degree heart blocks in myocarditis, and adults with ischemic heart disease. In a 30-year follow up of adult males with moderate P-R interval prolongation, first degree heart block was benign (Mymin et al. 1986).

4.2.5 *Clinical presentation*: Patients with first degree AV block are asymptomatic unless associated with significant left ventricular (LV) dysfunction. Marked prolongation of the PR interval can cause symptoms mimicking pacemaker-like syndrome.

4.2.6 *ECG*: There is prolongation of PR interval beyond the normal ranges for age. Normal P-R interval naturally varies with age in the pediatric population and prolongation of the P-R interval should be viewed in this context (Figure 5).

4.2.7 *Work-up*: An ECG can detect first degree block with or without infranodal disease based on QRS pattern. Atropine and exercise stress testing decrease the vagal tone and enhance AV nodal conduction, thereby shortening the PR interval. If the delay is due to infranodal disease, the conduction delay is worsened. Electrophysiology study can be used to determine the site of conduction delay.

4.2.8 *Management and Prognosis*: Family history of rhythm or connective tissue disease should be obtained. Repeat ECGs are indicated in those with suspected progression to higher grade blocks. Indications for a pacemaker include first degree block with symptoms suggestive of a pacemaker-like syndrome (Class IIa), and presence of first degree block in neuromuscular diseases and LV dysfunction (Class IIb) (Gregaratos 2002).

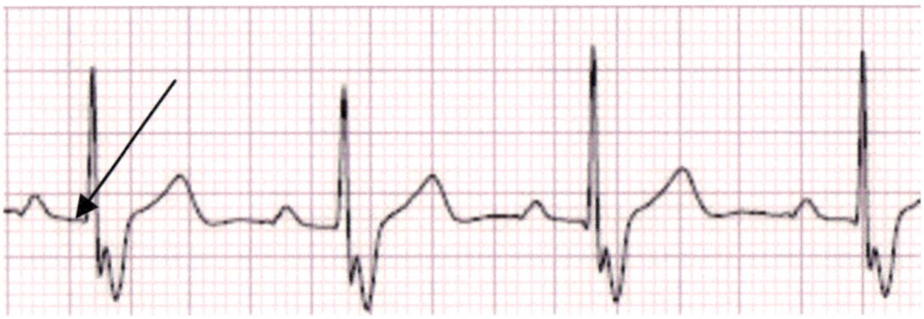

Fig. 5. First degree AV block

4.3 Second-degree atrio-ventricular heart block

4.3.1 *Definition*: Second-degree heart block is atrio-ventricular block in which some atrial discharges are not conducted to the ventricles. It is classified as Mobitz type I (Wenckebach phenomena), Mobitz type II and high grade.

4.3.2 *Incidence*: Wenckebach phenomena was detected in 2% of infants, 7% of toddlers and 6% of children at rest (von Bernuth et al. 1989).

4.3.3 *Mechanism*: Mobitz type I (Wenckebach) block occurs at the AV node and His-Purkinje system in a ratio of 3:1, respectively (Peuch et al. 1976). Wenckebach phenomenon results from hypervagotonia in athletes and young subjects (Stein et al. 2002). Previous cardiac surgery and ischemic heart disease in adulthood are associated with Wenckebach phenomena. Mobitz type II block occurs infra-nodally in most cases (Dhingra et al. 1974).

4.3.4 *Natural history*: Mobitz type I block is usually benign. However, in pediatric population without heart disease, Mobitz type I block may serve as intermediary prior to development of idiopathic complete heart block (Young et al. 1977). In adults, second degree AV-nodal block proximal to the His bundle has a benign course in those without heart disease; but is associated with poor prognosis in those with underlying heart disease (Strasberg et al. 1981). Mobitz type II can progress to symptomatic complete heart block and is associated with Stokes-Adams attacks and sudden death (Dhingra et al. 1974).

4.3.5 *Clinical presentation*: Mobitz type I block is usually well tolerated; but may present with significant bradycardia. Patients with Mobitz type II block may be asymptomatic; but can present with bradycardia, exercise intolerance, syncope, postural hypotension, and sudden death.

4.3.6 *ECG*: Mobitz type I shows progressive prolongation of PR interval followed by a non-conducted atrial discharge (Figure 6a). Mobitz type II is characterized by stable PR interval with intermittent failed conduction (Figure 6b). PR interval can be normal or prolonged.

4.3.7 *Work-up*: ECG is diagnostic. If ECG is inconclusive, a 24-hour monitor is suggested. If there is one conducted beat in a cycle as in a 2:1 block, it is difficult to differentiate between Mobitz types I and II blocks; atropine can be used to elicit a 3:2 conduction in Mobitz type I block. Response to atropine suggests the block to be at or proximal to the AV node. If exercise initiates or exacerbates Mobitz type I block, infranodal location of the block is suspected. An electrophysiology study is indicated if there is unexplained syncope, and AV block distal to the AV node, to identify the location of the block (Zipes et al. 1995). In complete or high grade second degree AV block, an echocardiogram is indicated (Cheitlin et al. 2003).

4.3.8 *Management*: Medical management of Mobitz type I includes identification and treatment of underlying causes. Sympathomimetic agents such as scopolamine, theophylline, or glycopyrrolate can be used in symptomatic bradycardia secondary to increased vagal tone. In patients with Mobitz type II, syncope is a poor prognostic factor (Dhingra et al. 1974). Symptomatic chronic bradycardia in Mobitz type I and type II (Class I), Mobitz type II with bifascicular or trifascicular block (Class I), Mobitz type II with wide QRS (Class I), asymptomatic Mobitz type II (Class IIa), and neuromuscular disease with AV block (Class IIb) are all indications for permanent pacemaker implantation (Gregaratos 2002).

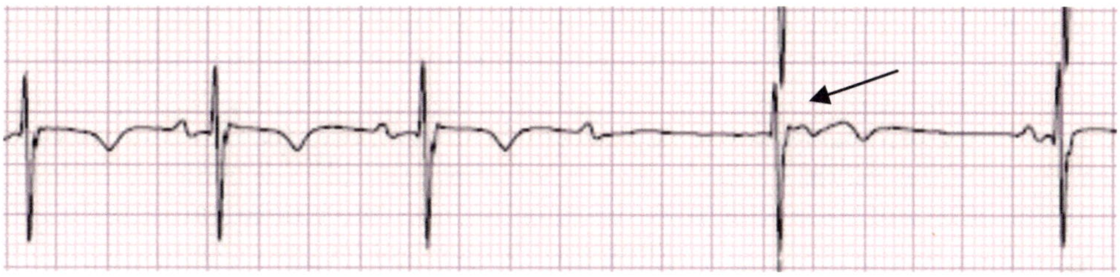

Fig. 6.a Second degree Type I AV block (Wenckebach)

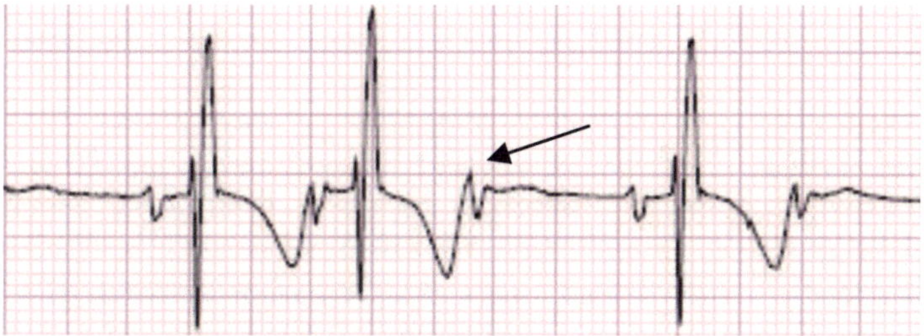

Fig. 6.b Second degree Type II (Mobitz) AV block

4.4 Third-degree (Complete) Atrio-Ventricular Heart Block

4.4.1 *Definition*: Complete failure of conduction of atrial impulses to the ventricles.

4.4.2 *Incidence*: Complete heart block may be acquired or congenital. The most common cause of acquired complete heart block in pediatric patients is surgery for left ventricular outflow tract obstruction, repair of corrected transposition of the great arteries (L-TGA), ventricular septal defects and TOF. Acquired complete AV block is also seen in Lyme carditis, myocarditis, myopathies, and metabolic diseases. Congenital complete heart block occurs 1 per 15,000 to 1 per 22,000 live births and is often associated with maternal connective tissue disease, in particular systemic lupus erythematosis (Michaelsson and Engle 1972). Spontaneous complete heart block is seen in left atrial isomerism, endocardial cushion defects and in 20% of patients with L-TGA (Huhta et al. 1983; Lundstrom et al. 1990).

4.4.3 *Mechanism*: Possible mechanisms include abnormal development of the conduction system and the AV node, or acquired most commonly after cardiac surgery. The escape rhythms below the AV node take over when the atrial discharge is not conducted to the ventricles. The rate of the escape rhythm correlates with the level of the block, with the proximal sites having a higher rate.

4.4.4 *Natural history*: Complete heart block is associated with L-TGA and septal defects, as well as sequelae of maternal connective tissue. Mortality is highest during the neonatal period (Roberts and Gillette 1977). Congenital complete heart block in structurally normal heart, when uncorrected, leads to cardiac enlargement with impaired ventricular systolic function (Beaufort-Krol et al. 2007). There is a significant correlation between persistent heart rate of 50 or less and incidence of syncope, pre-syncope, and/or sudden death (Karpawich et al. 1981; Dewey et al. 1987).

4.4.5 *Clinical presentation*: Many patients are asymptomatic in early life. Symptoms range from none to palpitations, chest pain, weakness, syncope, exercise intolerance, dizziness, and congestive heart failure in congenital complete heart block. Symptoms are usually dependent on ventricular rate, frequency of premature ventricular beats, and atrio-ventricular synchrony.

4.4.6 *ECG*: Complete heart block is depicted by atrio-ventricular conduction blockade. In patients with normal hearts, the QRS complex is narrow if the block is at the AV node or His bundle; the QRS complex is wide if the block occurs after the bifurcation of the bundle of His (Weindling 2001). An ECG should be used to differentiate complete heart block from accelerated junctional rhythm or severe sinus bradycardia with appropriate junctional escape rate (Weindling 2001). Complete heart block is associated with a prior lesser-degree block (25%) and accompanied or preceded by bundle branch block (Levine et al. 1956). Associated prolongation of QT interval is seen in about 18% of congenital complete heart block (Figure 7).

4.4.7 *Work-up*: A 12-lead ECG establishes the diagnosis. In symptomatic patients treated with a pacemaker and with a suspicion of another arrhythmia (Class I), and patients with premature, concealed junctional depolarizations as in pseudo-AV block (Class II), an electrophysiology study is indicated (Zipes et al. 1995). In patients with complete AV block or advanced second-degree AV block, an echocardiogram is used to visualize cardiac function, size, structure, and valvular regurgitation (Cheitlin et al. 2003; Beaufort-Krol et al. 2007). Exercise stress testing in asymptomatic patients with congenital complete heart block is used to determine degree of exercise tolerance and arrhythmias associated with exercise (Gibbons et al. 2002).

4.4.8 *Management and Prognosis*: Primary mode of management of patients with complete heart block is pacemaker implantation. The time of pacemaker implantation is controversial. Third degree AV block with symptomatic bradycardia, post-operative complete heart block that does not resolve in 7-10 days, and congenital complete heart block with wide QRS escape rhythm and ventricular dysfunction, and congenital complete heart block with rate <50 bpm are Class I indications for pacemaker implantation (Gregaratos 2002). Prognosis for neonates and infants post pacemaker implantation is very good (Aellig et al. 2007).

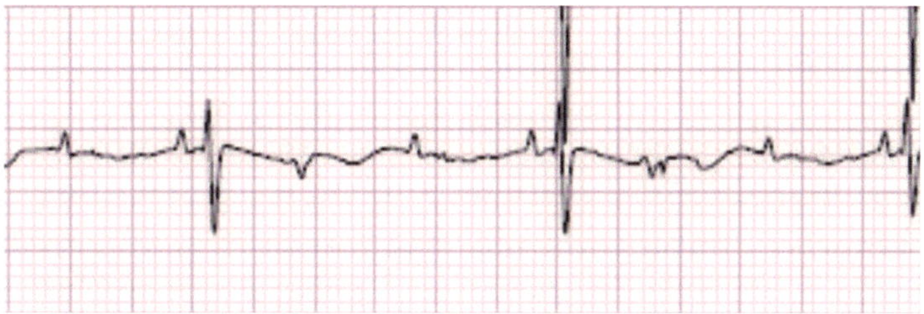

Fig. 7. Third degree (complete) AV block

4.5 Atrial escape rhythm

4.5.1 *Definition*: Atrial escape rhythm arises from ectopic atrial foci during periods of severe sinus bradycardia or significant sinus node dysfunction. These atrial ectopic foci have slower spontaneous rates and are unstable. The exact incidence of atrial escape rhythm is not known

4.5.2 *Mechanism*: The automaticity of an ectopic atrial focus generates a faster rate than the dysfunctional sinus node by escaping overdrive suppression of the SA node. Atrial escape rhythm rate is between 60-80 beats per minute (Dubin 2000).

4.5.3 *Natural history*: Atrial escape rhythm occurs in sinus node dysfunction and severe sinus bradycardia. Resolution or treatment of a slow underlying sinus rhythm resolves the atrial escape rhythm. Automaticity in ectopic foci are more responsive to autonomic control compared to the SA node (Randall et al. 1981).

4.5.4 *Clinical presentation*: Most symptoms are secondary to underlying rhythm abnormalities such as sinus node dysfunction with severe sinus bradycardia, sinus pause and/or sinus arrest. These include dizziness, exercise intolerance, and possible syncope.

4.5.5 *ECG*: The P-wave morphology differs from the sinus P-wave. The P-wave is smaller and shorter in duration with the P-wave axis dependent on the location of the ectopic focus. The PR interval may be shorter than the normal PR interval due to the proximity of the ectopic atrial focus to the AV node. The atrial escape rhythm is slower than the normal sinus rate.

4.5.6 *Work-up*: Work-up is focused on identifying the underlying abnormality leading to increased automaticity or suppression of the sinus node.

4.5.7 *Management and Prognosis*: In symptomatic patients, slow sinus rhythm is managed with sympathomimetic agents. If unresponsive to medical treatment, pacemaker implantation may be necessary for management of sinus node dysfunction or severe sinus bradycardia.

4.6 Atrio-ventricular junctional escape rhythm

4.6.1 *Definition*: AV junctional escape rhythm is defined as an ectopic rhythm starting in the AV junction due to failure of the atrial impulse to conduct. The ectopic rhythm may originate between the AV node and the bundle of His.

4.6.2 *Incidence*: Episodes of junctional escape rhythm were reported in 19% of full-term neonates (Southall et al; Southall et al. 1980).

4.6.3 *Mechanism*: AV junctional escape rhythm occurs due to enhanced automaticity or a reentry mechanism. The ectopic focus can occur below the AV node and at or above the bundle of His, in the absence or suppression of an SA node or atrial impulse (Gamble et al. 2007). Due to the lack of overdrive suppression from the higher pacemakers, the AV junction has its intrinsic automaticity. The junctional escape rate ranges between 40-60 beats per minute (Dubin 2000).

4.6.4 *Natural history*: The junctional pacemaker can exist in the region of the distal AV node or the proximal portion of the His-bundle near the AV-node (Alison et al. 1995). Nodal escape rhythm is associated with apnea (Valimaki and Tarlo 1971). The rate of AV junctional escape rhythm varies with underlying conditions, such as sick sinus syndrome, complete heart block, ablation of AV node, congenital heart surgery, hypertrophic cardiomyopathy, and ischemia (Kleinfeld and Boal 1978; Alison et al. 1995; Shepard et al. 1998). Inflammation, hypoxia, metabolic, drugs, or electrolyte disturbances are implicated in the etiology of junctional rhythms (Fisch and Knoebel 1970).

4.6.5 *Clinical presentation*: Symptoms pertaining to AV junctional escape rhythm are related to suppression of the sino-atrial tissues and or failure to conduct to the junction. Symptoms include dizziness, exercise intolerance, near syncope or syncope.

4.6.6 *ECG*: In AV junctional escape rhythm, there are no P-waves before the QRS complexes; they may occur simultaneously or follow the QRS complexes. The QRS complex is narrow if the focus is closer to the AV node or wide if proximal to the His bundle bifurcation. In the case of complete AV block, P-waves of sinus origin are dissociated from the QRS complexes.

4.6.7 *Work-up*: ECG may identify the rhythm; if unsuccessful, a Holter monitor can help identify the rhythm abnormality. Workup should also include identifying the causes listed above.

4.6.8 *Management and Prognosis*: Pacemaker implantation may be needed in symptomatic bradycardia due to junctional escape rhythm.

4.7 Idioventricular escape rhythm

4.7.1 *Definition*: Ventricular escape (idioventricular) rhythm arises below the bifurcation of the His bundle. The ventricular escape results when the higher pacemaker systems are unable to generate and/or conduct an impulse to the ventricles. It is rare and incidence is not known.

4.7.2 *Mechanism*: The automaticity of the ventricular myocardium is pronounced in the absence of supraventricular impulses. The overdrive suppression from higher pacemaker centers is absent, leading to the automaticity of the ventricular focus to conduct to the ventricles. Idioventricular rate ranges from 20-40 beats per minute (Dubin 2000).

4.7.3 *Natural history*: Idioventricular rhythm is seen with hypothermia, drugs, and ischemia (Talbot and Greaves 1976).

4.7.4 *Clinical presentation*: Stokes-Adams syncopal attacks are more prevalent in ventricular escape rhythm than atrial or junctional escape rhythms. This is also accompanied by dizziness and exercise intolerance.

4.7.5 *ECG*: The ECG shows wide QRS complexes with a rate of 20-40 beats per minute. If P-waves exist, they occur independently and are dissociated from the ventricular beats.

4.7.6 *Work-up*: ECG is the first step in diagnosing ventricular escape rhythm. Holter and event recorders are alternatives when ECG is not diagnostic. Electrophysiology study is indicated (class IIA) in patients with suspected bradyarrhythmias with syncope (Zipes 2006). An EP study can establish the level of the AV block.

4.7.7 *Management and Prognosis*: Symptomatic relief is important in patients with ventricular escape rhythm. Pacemaker implantation with ventricular pacing is essential to avoid Stokes-Adams attacks.

5. Tachy-arrhythmias

5.1 Atrial tachy-arrhythmias

5.1.1 Physiologic (appropriate) sinus tachycardia

5.1.1.1 *Definition*: Sinus tachycardia is an automatic rhythm characterized by rapid discharge from the sinus node due to physiologic influences (Walsh 2001b; Blomstrom-Lundqvist et al. 2003; Blomstrom-Lundqvist 2003). The rate of sinus tachycardia is dependent on age.

5.1.1.2 *Incidence*: Dependent on the body's increased sympathetic response to physiologic phenomena, such as fever, dehydration, anxiety, pain, medications, anemia, hyperthyroidism and heart failure.

5.1.1.3 *Mechanism*: Occurs due to increased automaticity with rate variability associated with increased sympathetic response or vagal withdrawal.

5.1.1.4 *Natural history*: Decreasing the underlying enhanced sympathetic tone or increasing the vagal tone will decrease the sinus tachycardia.

5.1.1.5 *Clinical presentation*: The inciting factor for sympathetic response or vagal withdrawal is the usual presenting symptom. Very high rate of sinus tachycardia can compromise cardiac output by decreasing the ventricular filling time.

5.1.1.6 *ECG*: There is a normal P-wave axis and a P-wave precedes each QRS complex (Van Hare 1999). P-waves may have larger amplitude and become peaked (Blomstrom-Lundqvist 2003).

5.1.1.7 *Work-up*: Identify the extrinsic factors causing the tachycardia and treat them. It is also necessary to rule out inappropriate sinus tachycardia (see below).

5.1.1.8 *Management and Prognosis*: Prognosis depends on the nature of the underlying cause. No specific treatment is required for physiologic sinus tachycardia except treatment of the underlying causes. Beta-adrenergic receptor blockers may occasionally be used for treatment of physiologic symptomatic sinus tachycardia (Blomstrom-Lundqvist 2003).

5.1.2 Inappropriate Sinus Tachycardia (IST)

5.1.2.1 *Definition*: Elevated resting heart rate for the physiological state and/or an exaggerated heart rate response to exercise or stress (Krahn et al. 1995; Blomstrom-Lundqvist 2003).

5.1.2.2 *Incidence*: IST often follows a viral illness or physical trauma, usually in women (90%) who are generally healthy physically and emotionally (Fogoros 2006).

5.1.2.3 *Mechanism*: Etiology is not known. The mechanism may involve a primary sino-atrial (SA) node disorder with increased automaticity, a dysautonomia with increased sympathetic tone, decreased parasympathetic tone, and/or increased SA node beta-adrenergic sensitivity, or impaired baroreflex control (Krahn et al. 1995; Fogoros 2006; Morillo and Guzman 2007). Another mechanism is stimulation of the beta-adrenergic receptors by anti-beta adrenergic autoantibodies (Chiale et al. 2006).

5.1.2.4 *Natural history*: IST is more common in women in the 20s and 30s, who are otherwise healthy. It is likely to improve over time (Fogoros 2006).

5.1.2.5 *Clinical presentation*: Palpitations, lightheadedness, exercise intolerance, and fatigue are common symptoms. Patients may also have orthostatic intolerance, chest pain, anxiety, depression, headache and myalgia, gastro-intestinal disturbances, and diaphoresis (Shen 2005; Fogoros 2006). Only consistent finding on physical exam is tachycardia (Shen 2005; Fogoros 2006).

5.1.2.6 *ECG*: P-wave morphology and axis is similar to that of normal sinus rhythm (Shen 2005). There is tachycardia at rest on ECG.

5.1.2.7 *Diagnosis*: Criteria for diagnosis include: a) persistent sinus tachycardia during the day with increased rate in response to activity and normalization during sleep per 24-hour Holter recording, b) non-paroxysmal tachycardia and symptoms, c) P-wave morphology and activation similar to sinus rhythm, and d) exclusion of secondary causes of sinus tachycardia (Blomstrom-Lundqvist 2003).

5.1.2.8 *Work-up*: In addition to the ECG, a 24-holter monitor will document elevated mean heart rates above normal for age, elevated daytime heart rates, and/or exaggerated elevation in sinus rate from supine to upright position (Shen 2005). A diagnostic electrophysiology (EP) study should be considered if the etiology of the tachycardia is unclear (to rule out sinus node re-entry tachycardia). EP study consistent with IST would include slow warm up and cool down phases suggesting sinus node involvement, surface P-wave similar to that of normal sinus rhythm, and earliest activation arising near the sinus node area along the crista terminalis during mapping. IST is not initiated with programmed stimulation of the atria (Lin and Callans 2004). In addition to electrophysiology testing, there is also a need for autonomic dysregulation testing. Neurologic, cardiovascular rehabilitation, and psychiatric consultations are often necessary because IST is a diagnosis of exclusion (Shen 2005).

5.1.2.9 *Management and Prognosis*: Treatment involves a multidisciplinary approach. Medications including beta blockers, calcium channel blockers and class IC anti-arrhythmic agents decrease SA node automaticity (Chiale et al. 2006). However in patients with IST secondary to autonomic dysregulation, control of heart rate does not always lead to resolution of symptoms. In patients with no evidence of autonomic dysregulation if biofeedback, meditation, and medical therapy fail, superolateral crista terminalis ablation could be considered (Shen 2005; Fogoros 2006). Risks of RF ablation include SVC syndrome, diaphragmatic paralysis and persistent junctional rhythm. The prognosis of IST is benign over a mean follow-up of 6 years (Still et al. 2005).

5.1.3 Sinus Node Re-entry Tachycardia

5.1.3.1 *Definition*: Sino-atrial node re-entry tachycardia (SNRT) is a paroxysmal arrhythmia characterized by a re-entry mechanism that is located entirely within the SA node or the perisinus atrial tissue (Lin and Callans 2004).

5.1.3.2 *Incidence*: Incidence of SNRT is underestimated due to lack of symptoms very often. In patients undergoing electrophysiology study for supraventricular tachycardia, incidence ranges from 1.8%-16.9% (Blomstrom-Lundqvist 2003). Incidence of SNRT is higher (10%) in those with underlying organic heart disease (Garson Jr. and Gillette 1981).

5.1.3.3 Mechanism: A re-entry mechanism is present but it is not known whether the entire circuit is within the SA node or involves perisinus atrial tissue.

5.1.3.4 *Clinical presentation*: Patients are often asymptomatic. Symptoms include palpitations, lightheadedness, presyncope, and rarely syncope (Gomes et al. 1985).

5.1.3.5 *ECG*: SNRT heart rate ranges from 80-200 beats/min. P-wave axis and morphology are similar to that of normal sinus rhythm. P-R interval is shorter than R-P interval. An atrio-ventricular (AV) nodal Wenckebach block may be present (Olgin and Zipes 2005a).

5.1.3.6 *Diagnosis*: Criteria for diagnosis include: a) paroxysmal tachycardia, b) P-wave morphology and endocardial atrial activation similar to that of normal sinus rhythm, c) inducibility with programmed premature atrial stimuli irrespective of the location of stimulation or the AV junction, d) the ability to terminate the arrhythmia with atrial premature beat or atrial pacing, and e) termination with vagal maneuvers or adenosine (Narula 1974; Blomstrom-Lundqvist 2003).

5.1.3.7 *Work-up*: Electrophysiology study is indicated in patients with frequent and poorly-tolerated episodes of tachycardia, unclear mechanism of tachycardia, and refractoriness to medications.

5.1.3.8 *Management and Prognosis*: Vagal maneuvers or adenosine may interrupt the tachycardia. Acutely, atrial pacing is effective. Beta blockers, calcium channel blockers, amiodarone, and digitalis can benefit patients with increased frequency of symptoms. However, prophylactic treatment of SNRT is not recommended. In patients undergoing an electrophysiology study, catheter ablation can be successful (Goya et al. 1999).

5.1.4 Ectopic (focal) Atrial Tachycardia

5.1.4.1 *Definition*: Ectopic or focal atrial tachycardia (EAT) is a tachycardia mediated by inappropriate atrial impulse generation from a single atrial focus outside of the SA node (Walsh 2001a).

5.1.4.2 *Incidence*: EAT is commonly found in children and teenagers and makes up approximately 15% of all newly diagnosed supraventricular tachycardias across all ages (Walsh 2001a). Both genders are equally affected. Prevalence of EAT is 0.34% in asymptomatic male patients and 0.46% in symptomatic male patients (Poutiainen et al. 1999).

5.1.4.3 *Mechanism*: EAT can be due to three mechanisms: a) enhanced automaticity, b) triggered activity, and c) microreentry (Roberts-Thomson et al. 2006). The tachycardia cannot be initiated or terminated with programmed stimuli (Walsh 2001a). However, the exact mechanism is difficult to ascertain.

5.1.4.4 *Natural history*: In the majority of patients, the course is benign. Persistent incessant EAT can lead to ventricular dysfunction, congestive heart failure and low cardiac output states, termed tachycardia-mediated cardiomyopathy. However, termination of the rhythm can lead to improvement in ventricular function (Packer et al. 1986; Naheed et al. 1995). There is slowing of heart rate with time, with reversion to sinus rhythm or change in P-wave morphology (Poutiainen et al. 1999).

5.1.4.5 *Clinical presentation*: Young patients are often asymptomatic until onset of left ventricular dysfunction. Patients may also have palpitations, lightheadedness, and exercise intolerance even with normal LV function (Walsh 2001a).

5.1.4.6 *ECG*: ECG shows a supraventricular tachycardia with rates within normal range to 300 beats per minute. ECG criteria for diagnosis include: a) the P-wave morphology and axis different than that of normal sinus rhythm, b) acceleration after initiation and deceleration before termination, c) unaffected by presence of an atrio-ventricular block, and d) an initial P-wave of the tachycardia similar to the subsequent P-waves (Olgin and Zipes 2005a). The QRS complex is similar to that of sinus rhythm.

5.1.4.7 *Work-up*: The location of the ectopic focus can be determined by noting P-wave frontal plane axis. "Warm-up" and "cool-down" patterns can be appreciated and suggestive of an automatic mechanism. AV-block (Mobitz 1) can be appreciated episodically during sleep. Adenosine administration will demonstrate AV-block with continuous marching of P-waves (Figure 8). When the ectopic focus is close to the sinus node and/or there is poor ventricular function, electrophysiology testing is necessary to differentiate between sinus tachycardia, atrial flutter, and ectopic atrial tachycardia. Difficulty to terminate tachycardia with pacing maneuvers and external cardioversion are suggestive of EAT (Walsh 2001a). Echocardiography at the time of diagnosis is important to document the ventricular function (Naheed et al. 1995).

5.1.4.8 *Management and Prognosis*: Paroxysmal and incessant atrial tachycardia are difficult to treat medically (Blomstrom-Lundqvist 2003). Acute therapy includes IV verapamil and IV beta blockers. There is no termination of tachycardia with atrial pacing, except for mild slowing of the heart rate. DC cardioversion is usually not effective but may be effective in those with micro-re-entry mechanism. Class IA (e.g. quinidine) and IC (e.g. flecainide, propafenone) anti-arrhythmics are indicated for those without cardiac failure and Class III (amiodarone) is recommended in those with poor ventricular function (Blomstrom-Lundqvist 2003). Chronic therapy includes calcium channel blockers, Classes IA, IC, and III anti-arrhythmics; Class IC is not indicated in those with coronary artery disease. Intravenous amiodarone or oral sotalol can reduce rates and restore sinus rhythm (Skinner and Sharland 2008). Catheter ablation is successful in 86-90% with recurrence rate of 8% (Walsh 2001a; Hsieh and Chen 2002). In children, 75% had restoration of normal sinus rhythm after medical therapy (Naheed et al. 1995). In patients with drug refractory EAT or incessant AT with tachycardia-induced cardiomyopathy, best option is ablation of the focus (Blomstrom-Lundqvist 2003). Because digitalis toxicity can elicit atrial tachycardia, check digitalis levels and avoid hypokalemia.

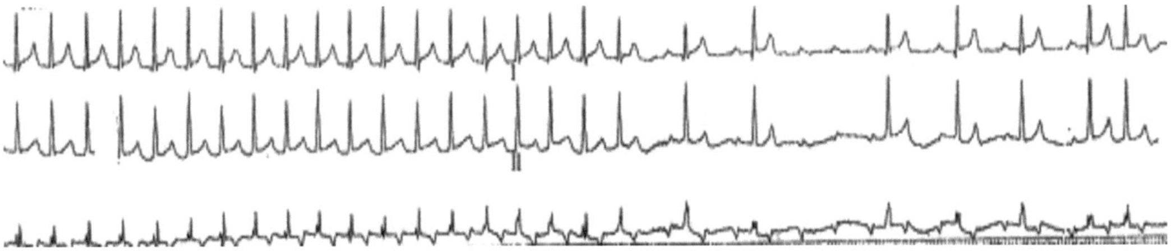

Fig. 8. Ectopic atrial tachycardia with effect of adenosine

5.1.5 Multifocal (chaotic) Atrial Tachycardia

5.1.5.1 *Definition*: Tachycardia characterized by electrocardiographic finding of multiple (at least three) distinct P-wave morphologies with irregular P-P intervals, isoelectric baseline between P-waves and ventricular rate >100 beats/min (Blomstrom-Lundqvist 2003).

5.1.5.2 *Incidence*: MAT is a rare entity. In the pediatric age group, it is reported exclusively in neonates and infants, mostly associated with a normal heart (Kastor 1990). It is also associated with post-operative congenital heart disease, hypertrophic and dilated cardiomyopathies, and unrepaired atrial septal defects (Walsh 2001a). Incidence is 0.2% among infants presenting with new onset arrhythmias (Salim et al. 1995). It is associated with significant respiratory disease in adults. It is also associated with hypoxemia, glucose intolerance, hypokalemia, digitalis, and chronic renal failure (Kones et al. 1974).

5.1.5.3 *Mechanism*: Exact mechanism of MAT is unclear; however, automaticity versus triggered activity is postulated (Walsh 2001a).

5.1.5.4 *Natural history*: Spontaneous resolution may occur in 50-80% of patients with MAT by 12-18 months of age (Sokoloski 1999). There is no recurrence of MAT in infants with normal cardiac structure (Walsh 2001a).

5.1.5.6 *Clinical presentation*: Most patients are asymptomatic at the time of detection. If tachycardia is persistent, cardiomyopathy develops and symptoms consistent with cardiomyopathy arise.

5.1.5.7 *ECG*: Diagnostic criteria include: 1) irregular atrial rates, 2) at least three different P-wave configurations, 3) isoelectric baseline between discrete P waves, 4) irregular P-P, P-R, and R-R intervals, and 5) absence of a dominant atrial pacemaker (Sokoloski 1999). Atrial rate may range from 150-500 beats/minute.
5.1.5.8 *Work-up*: Meeting ECG criteria is sufficient for diagnosis of MAT (figure 9).
5.1.5.9 *Management and Prognosis*: It is usually not responsive to DC cardioversion, vagal maneuvers, or IV antiarrhythmics. However, digoxin, beta blockers, amiodarone, and flecainide are options to consider. Calcium channel blockers are not indicated in neonates and infants less than one year of age. When drug therapy is successful, it should be continued for 6-12 months. In rare cases with medication refractory MAT, multiple foci ablation is required. In refractory cases, AV node ablation with ventricular pacemaker implantation may be necessary (Walsh 2001a).

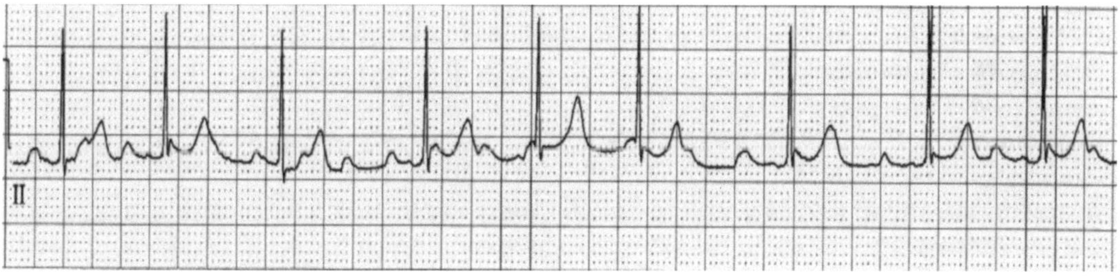

Fig. 9. Multifocal atrial tachycardia

5.1.6 Atrial flutter

5.1.6.1 *Definition*: Atrial flutter is a regular atrial tachycardia due to a macro-reentrant rhythm confined to the atrium. There are two types of atrial flutter: 1) typical or Type I and 2) atypical or Type II. Typical atrial flutter is the most common, cavo-tricuspid isthmus-dependent, terminated by rapid atrial pacing and is further divided into counter-clockwise and clockwise circuits. Atypical atrial flutter has a faster rate (>350 beats/minute), and is not cavo-tricuspid isthmus-dependent (Saoudi et al. 2001; Waldo 2004). Left atrial flutter is also considered to be atypical (Garan 2008).
5.1.6.2 *Incidence*: In a study of 380 patients with first flutter episode between 1 and 25 years of life, 81% had congenital heart disease, and 8% had normal hearts (Garson Jr. et al. 1985). Among adults, the incidence of atrial flutter overall was 88 per 100,000 person-years with male predominance (4:1) and is noted in patients with heart failure, pulmonary disease, thyrotoxicosis, post repair of congenital heart defects, and mitral valve disease (Granada et al. 2000; Waldo 2004). The incidence of atypical atrial flutter is rare in patients without prior cardiac surgery. Atypical right atrial flutter occurs in 8% of patients with atrial flutter (Yang et al. 2001). Persistent or recurrent atrial flutter is common in patients post-cardiac surgery (Waldo 2004).
5.1.6.3 *Mechanism*: The mechanism of atrial flutter is re-entry with an excitable gap, within the atrium, right more than left (Waldo 2004). The flutter circuit requires an initially activated region to repolarize as the action potential travels through the slow conduction tissue and reactivates the initial part, thereby creating a re-entry circuit. The atrial activation along the circuit proceeds from the coronary sinus superiorly to the high right atrium area and craniocaudally along the free wall and medially to the isthmus between the tricuspid valve and the inferior vena cava in a counter-clockwise manner. There is an area of slow

conduction in the posteroinferior aspect of the circuit. The clockwise or reverse typical circuit proceeds in the opposite direction (Sokoloski 1999).

5.1.6.4 *Natural history*: In patients less than one year of age and with no previous cardiac surgery, atrial flutter spontaneously converts in 26%. Congestive heart failure was more prevalent in those with atrial flutter of long duration. Of the infants with decreased ventricular function, all recovered normal function after conversion to sinus rhythm. If patients had additional arrhythmia, recurrence of atrial flutter was more likely (Texter et al. 2006). Atrial flutter persisting over a long period of time can evolve into atrial fibrillation (Waldo 2004).

5.1.6.5 *Clinical presentation*: In neonates, 80% are asymptomatic and 20% may present with congestive heart failure (Texter et al. 2006). Older patients can experience palpitations, dizziness, chest tightness, chest pain, shortness of breath, and fatigue. Hypotension, poor exercise tolerance, congestive heart failure and impaired cardiac output can also result from atrial flutter (Blomstrom-Lundqvist 2003; Andrew and Montenero 2007).

5.1.6.6 *ECG*: Counterclockwise (typical) atrial flutter has negative flutter (F) waves in the inferior leads II, III, and aVF and positive F waves in Lead V1 (figure 10). Clockwise (reverse typical) atrial flutter shows positive F waves in the inferior leads II, III, and aVF and negative F waves in lead V1 (Blomstrom-Lundqvist 2003). In typical atrial flutter, P waves are absent. The flutter rate can range from 240-340 beats/minute with no isoelectric interval between consecutive waves. Flutter rates in infants can be as high as 580 beats/minute with rapid ventricular response rates of 200 beats/minute with 2:1 AV conduction in 75% and variable block in the remainder (Texter et al. 2006). Flutter waves typically have 90-degree axis. The QRS complexes appear normal unless there is rate-dependent aberrancy or block.

5.1.6.7 *Work-up*: Echocardiogram is indicated in those with congestive heart failure to evaluate ventricular function and structure.

5.1.6.8 *Management and Prognosis*: Management of atrial flutter is accomplished through electrical cardioversion, rapid atrial pacing, pharmacological therapy, and catheter ablation. The goal of flutter management is to decrease the ventricular rate and to restore normal sinus rhythm. Chronic anti-arrhythmic therapy may not be needed in those with uncomplicated, asymptomatic atrial flutter after conversion to sinus rhythm (Texter et al. 2006; Skinner and Sharland 2008). Drugs are successful in controlling atrial flutter in about 58% of young patients. Amiodarone, digoxin, and propranolol are found to be effective (Garson Jr. et al. 1985). Atrial flutter causing hemodynamic instability should be terminated acutely with electrical cardioversion (2J/Kg) (Class 1 level of evidence) (Blomstrom-Lundqvist 2003; Texter et al. 2006). Although cardioversion is successful acutely, atrial flutter recurs frequently. Recurrences of atrial flutter can be prevented by administering Class IA, IC, and III anti-arrhythmic agents. Ventricular rate can be controlled with AV-nodal blockers such as digitalis and class II (beta blockers), III (amiodarone, sotalol), and IV (calcium channel blockers) anti-arrhythmic agents. Flecainide (Class IC anti-arrhythmic) should be administered with an AV-node blocking agent. As flecainide slows the atrial rate, it may facilitate 1:1 AV conduction, leading to clinical compromise (Skinner and Sharland 2008). Calcium channel antagonists are contraindicated in children less than one year of age. When atrial flutter is refractory to medical management, transesophageal atrial overdrive pacing (TEAP) and catheter ablation are excellent options. In a study by Ajisaka (1997), paroxysmal atrial flutter was terminated in greater than 50 percent of the adult subjects with low-output, short-duration TEAP (Ajisaka et al. 1997). In young adults with repaired congenital heart disease, 50-88% had successful ablation of recurrent atrial flutter

(Blomstrom-Lundqvist 2003). Catheter ablation is used to create a bidirectional conduction block across the cavo-tricuspid isthmus. In addition to palliating with catheter ablation, underlying causes of atrial flutter such as stimulants and sympathomimetic agents should also be eliminated.

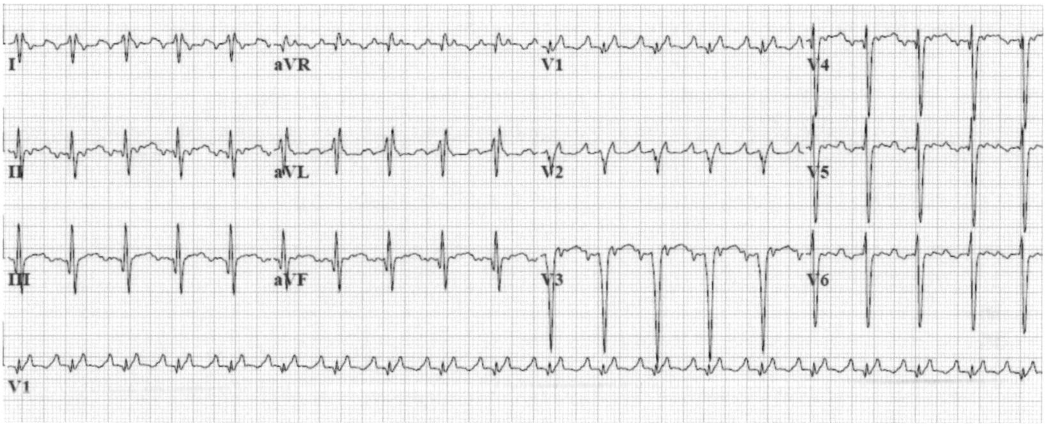

Fig. 10. Atrial flutter

5.1.7 Intra-atrial Reentry Tachycardia

5.1.7.1 *Definition*: Intra-atrial reentry tachycardia (IART) is a group of reentry tachycardia associated with repaired or unrepaired congenital heart disease (CHD). It is also known as slow atrial flutter, incisional atrial tachycardia, and macro-reentrant atrial tachycardia. It is very often a long-term complication of cardiac surgery involving the atrium (Triedman 2001). It is frequently associated with Fontan, Mustard, Senning, repaired tetralogy of Fallot, and TAPVR repairs. Risk factors for IART are older age of surgery and long-term follow-up.

5.1.7.2 *Incidence*: Incidence of IART often depends on the congenital heart disease and the surgery preceding the onset. Structural heart disease is evident in about 89% of patients with IART (Haines and DiMarco 1990).

5.1.7.3 *Mechanism*: IART has a re-entrant mechanism defined within the atrium and does not necessarily follow the atrial flutter circuit. Majority of the reentrant circuits are mainly confined to the right atrium (Triedman 2001).

5.1.7.4 *Natural history*: IART is intimately associated with atrial fibrillation and thromboembolic phenomena. Natural history is associated with increased frequency of recurrences, regardless of treatment with anti-arrhythmic medications or ablation (Triedman 2004). Intermediate follow-up post ablation of IART shows frequent recurrence with new IART configurations (Triedman et al. 1997).

5.1.7.5 *Clinical presentation*: Symptoms in patients with IART can range from being asymptomatic to congestive heart failure to significant cardiovascular compromise, including sudden cardiac death (Triedman 2004). Sinus node dysfunction with symptomatic bradycardia is a common association with IART.

5.1.7.6 *ECG*: Flutter morphology or uniform P waves are frequently noted with constant cycle length longer than typical atrial flutter (figure 11). Multiple ECG morphologies can be obtained from a single patient due to various activation mechanisms. There is often 1:1 AV conduction based on the cycle length. There is sudden onset and termination with pacing and is entrainable (Triedman 2001; Triedman 2004).

5.1.7.7 *Work-up*: In refractory atrial reentry arrhythmias, an electrophysiology study must be conducted to further elucidate the nature of the substrate responsible for IART.
5.1.7.8 *Management and Prognosis*: Acute management in cardiovascular compromise consists of direct current (DC) cardioversion. Other options in clinically stable patients include anti-arrhythmic medications, atrial overdrive pacing, and anti-tachycardia pacing with pacemakers and transesophageal pacing. For chronic therapy, sotalol and amiodarone have been reported to be effective in approximately 60% (Triedman 2001). Implanted anti-tachycardia pacemakers provide relief from symptomatic tachycardia and bradycardia associated with sinus node dysfunction. In cases refractory to medical management, catheter ablation can be attempted. Intra-operative surgical Maze procedure is reserved for patients that have failed catheter ablation or are scheduled to undergo surgery for another indication.

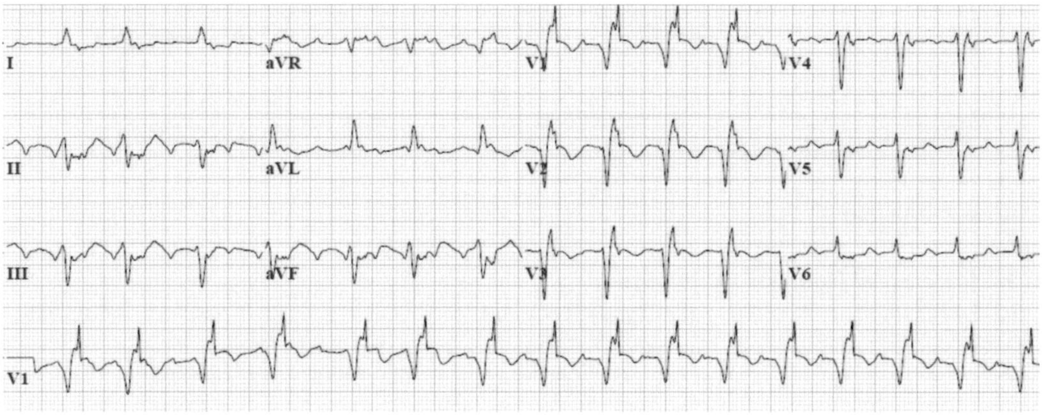

Fig. 11. Intra-atrial re-entrant tachycardia

6.1 Atrio-Ventricular Reciprocating Tachycardia

6.1.1 *Definition*: Atrio-ventricular reciprocating tachycardia (AVRT) is a re-entrant tachycardia with an accessory electrical connection between the atrial and ventricular myocardium in addition to the AV node (Blaufox and Saul 2001). The accessory pathway (AP) can be "concealed" with only retrograde conduction, "manifest" with antegrade or bidirectional conduction. The manifestation of antegrade conduction is presence of pre-excitation with short PR on the electrocardiogram during sinus rhythm suggestive of Wolff-Parkinson-White (WPW) syndrome. Orthodromic AVRT employs prograde conduction through the AV node and bundle of His with retrograde conduction through the AP. Antidromic AVRT employs AP for atrio-ventricular conduction with retrograde conduction through the bundle of His and AV node.
6.1.2 *Incidence*: AVRT is the most common cause of supraventricular tachycardia in children without prior cardiac surgery or neuromuscular disease, comprising 73 to 85 percent (Ko et al. 1992; Etheridge and Judd 1999). It is more common in infancy compared to AVNRT, the incidence of which increases in older children (Ko et al. 1992). Accessory pathways are associated with congenital heart defects in 6-26% of the children. The common heart defects associated with accessory pathways are Ebstein's anomaly of the tricuspid valve, ventricular inversion (L-TGA), hypertrophic cardiomyopathy, and mitral valve prolapse (Van Hare 1999).

6.1.3 *Mechanism*: As the name suggests, AVRT has a reentrant mechanism. The reentrant mechanism is characterized by an accessory pathway in the left or right atrio-ventricular grooves, i.e. extranodal pathway. Atriofascicular and nodofascicular (Mahaim), and atrionodal (James) AP are other variants. The left free wall is the most common site of the AP, followed by posteroseptal and right free wall AP (Calkins et al. 1999). Even in patients with manifest AP, orthodromic narrow complex reciprocating tachycardia is still the most common manifestation.

6.1.4 *Natural history*: In patients with WPW syndrome with onset less than 2 months of age, SVT disappeared in 93% and reappeared in 31% at an average age of 8 years (Perry and Garson Jr. 1990). In patients with onset after 5 years of age, seventy eight percent had persistence at 7 years of follow-up. Multiple and right-sided AP were more frequent in patients with congenital heart disease (Perry and Garson Jr. 1990). Congenital heart defects are present in 20 - 37% of patients with WPW (Deal et al. 1985; Perry and Garson Jr. 1990). Patients with WPW syndrome are also prone to develop atrial fibrillation with increased risk of sudden death (Hare 1999).

6.1.5 *Clinical presentation*: Symptoms are usually paroxysmal but may be incessant. Symptoms may occur with or without triggers, including activity and exertion. Location, rate, duration of tachycardia, and the type of AP very often determine the nature of symptoms. Infants tolerate higher rates of tachycardia compared to adolescents and adults. Patients perceive sensed tachycardia with or without associated symptoms including dizziness, lightheadedness, and mild chest discomfort. Heart failure symptoms with orthopnea, paroxysmal nocturnal dyspnea, fatigue, tachypnea, diaphoresis are often present in those with persistent tachycardia (Van Hare 1999). Sudden death is attributed to the presence of atrial fibrillation with rapid ventricular response across the accessory pathway (Van Hare 1999). In orthodromic AVRT, shortness of breath, fatigue, and dizziness are common; syncope is less common (Blaufox and Saul 2001). In antidromic AVRT, dizziness, syncope, and tendency towards unstable ventricular rhythm are more common than orthodromic AVRT (Blaufox and Saul 2001).

6.1.6 *ECG*: ECG findings are determined by presence of tachycardia, normal sinus rhythm, and type of accessory pathway. In normal sinus rhythm, WPW syndrome is evident by the presence of pre-excitation (delta wave) with short PR interval. The pre-excited complex is a fusion complex resulting from initial pre-excitation of ventricular myocardium adjacent to the AP giving rise to the delta wave, followed by fusion of depolarization of the remainder of the ventricular myocardium by normal conduction. In orthodromic AVRT, the QRS complexes are narrow due to normal prograde conduction through the AV node and bundle of His and retrograde conduction via the AP (figure 12). Orthodromic AVRT have RP interval shorter than the PR interval with a P-wave on the upstroke of the T-wave during tachycardia, which differentiates it from AVNRT (Van Hare 1999). In antidromic AVRT, the QRS complexes are wide due to antegrade conduction down the AP and retrograde conduction across the AV node or another AP. AV block terminates the tachycardia due to the role of AV node in the tachycardia. WPW is characterized by wide QRS complexes with short PR interval. Mahaim AP has pre-excitation with widened QRS complexes but normal PR interval and usually manifest as a wide complex tachycardia with left bundle branch block pattern. Though the terminology is obsolete, Lown-Ganong-Levine (LGL) syndrome has normal QRS complexes with short PR interval.

6.1.7 *Work-up*: Baseline ECG during sinus rhythm may show pre-excitation. Depending on the frequency of sensed tachycardia or other symptoms, a Holter monitor or a loop recorder can be used. Echocardiogram may be obtained to rule out structural heart defects. In patients with pre-excitation, exercise stress test to stratify the risk of sudden catastrophic event can be performed. Persistent pre-excitation at peak exercise may suggest a short refractory period of the accessory fiber with a higher risk for sudden catastrophic event (Blaufox and Saul 2001). To differentiate between narrow complex tachycardias, including concealed pathways, AVNRT, and atrial tachycardias, an EP study is required. An EP study will also assist in differentiating antidromic AVRT from other wide-complex tachycardias.

6.1.8 *Management and Prognosis*: Acute management in patients with significant hemodynamic compromise requires synchronized DC cardioversion. Adenosine administration is effective and esmolol may be used. Flecainide and procainamide are recommended in pre-excited SVT (Blomstrom-Lundqvist 2003). Digoxin and calcium channel blockers are contra-indicated in patients with WPW syndrome. In stable patients, vagal maneuvers may be effective in terminating the arrhythmia. Calcium channel blockers are contraindicated in infants. Catheter ablation is a class I indication for managing AVRT (Blomstrom-Lundqvist 2003). Left free wall AP was predictive of ablation success while right free wall, posteroseptal, septal, and multiple APs were predictive of recurrence (Calkins et al. 1999). Medical therapy includes beta blockers to block AV node conduction and decrease premature ectopic beats, and class IA, IC, and III antiarrhythmics (Triedman 2001).

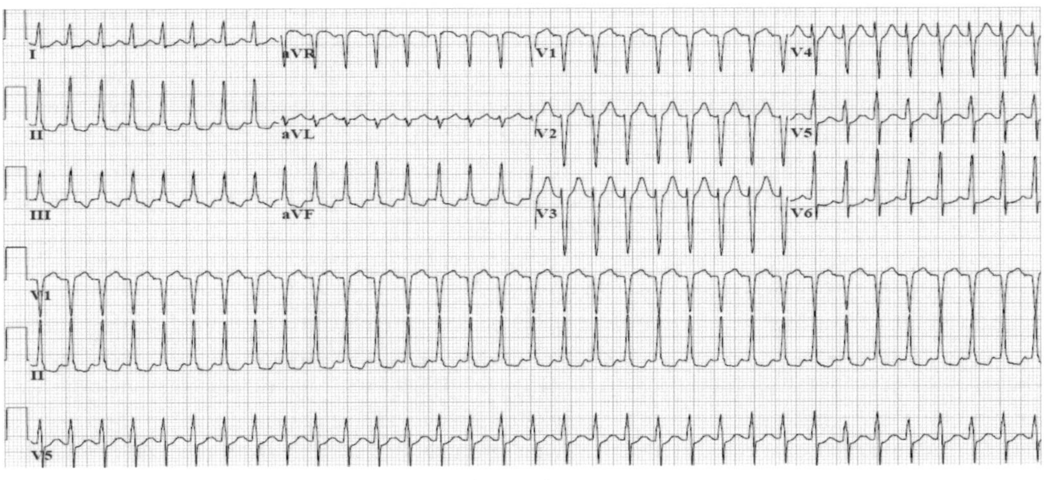

Fig. 12. Orthodromic AV reciprocating tachycardia

6.2 Atrio-Ventricular Node Reentry Tachycardia

6.2.1 *Definition*: Atrio-ventricular node reentry tachycardia (AVNRT) is a re-entry tachycardia that is dependent on existence of dual discrete pathways within or in proximity of the AV node, one with slow conduction and short effective refractory period and the other with fast conduction and long refractory period (Zimmerman 2001; Lockwood et al. 2004). The typical ventricular rate in children ranges from 120 to 280 beats/minute (Zimmerman 2001). AVNRT is often associated with an accessory pathway.

6.2.2 *Incidence*: AVNRT is the most common SVT in adults but consists of 13% of SVT in children without underlying heart disease and rarely in children under two years of age (Ko et al. 1992). In infants, 15% of SVT was due to AVNRT (Etheridge and Judd 1999).

6.2.3 *Mechanism*: Dual AV node physiology is present in 33-35% of the children without clinical or inducible AVNRT in congenital or acquired heart disease (Casta et al. 1980). The "slow-fast" or typical form of the AVNRT is the most common form. A premature atrial or junctional beat blocks the fast pathway with subsequent antegrade conduction through the slow pathway. If the fast pathway recovers as the impulse conducts through the slow pathway, the substrate for reentry is present. In the less common "fast-slow" or atypical form of AVNRT, the premature atrial impulse is blocked in the slow pathway and is conducted antegrade along the fast pathway. If the slow pathway recovers, a reentry substrate is present; antegrade conduction down the fast pathway and retrograde conduction up the slow pathway is present (Zimmerman 2001). The least common form is the "slow-slow" dual node physiology. There is retrograde atrial activation with early atrial activation in the low right atrium, followed by left and remaining right atrial activation (Olgin and Zipes 2005a).

6.2.4 *Natural history*: AVNRT is not life-threatening and patients with minimal symptoms do well without therapy. Female patients are more symptomatic and tend to present with syncope (Drago et al. 2006).

6.2.5 *Clinical presentation*: Symptoms include palpitations, chest pain, heart failure, and shock, and rarely syncope, dependent on the duration of the AVNRT. Tachycardia is paroxysmal.

6.2.6 *ECG*: AVNRT is a regular narrow QRS complex tachycardia with abrupt onset and termination. The QRS complex may appear wider in case of baseline bundle branch block or rate dependent aberrant conduction. There is no pre-excitation appreciated during normal sinus rhythm in sole AVNRT. In slow-fast AVNRT, retrograde P-waves are not appreciated and are located within the terminal part of the QRS complexes. In fast-slow AVNRT, the P waves have a superior axis with RP interval longer than PR interval.

6.2.7 *Work-up*: An electrophysiology study is indicated to definitively establish the diagnosis of AVNRT and dual AV node physiology.

6.2.8 *Management and Prognosis*: Management of AVNRT is based on the frequency and the symptoms during the episodes. In those with infrequent, asymptomatic episodes, no treatment is necessary. Paroxysmal episodes may be terminated with Valsalva maneuver or carotid sinus massage. In acute decompensation, DC synchronized cardioversion, adenosine, IV beta blockers or digoxin can be employed (Zimmerman 2001). In patients with infrequent episodes desiring complete control, ablation is recommended. Patients with recurrent AVNRT refractory to beta blockers and calcium channel blockers, flecanide and sotalol are class IIA recommendations. In recurrent, symptomatic patients with significant side effects of medications and those with poorly tolerated AVNRT, catheter ablation of the slow AV nodal pathway is suggested (Blomstrom-Lundqvist 2003).

7. Junctional Tachy-arrhythmias

7.1 Junctional Ectopic Tachycardia

7.1.1 *Definition*: Junctional ectopic tachycardia (JET), also called junctional automatic tachycardia, is an incessant tachycardia characterized by rapid heart rate with the focus of abnormal automaticity in the junction. Ventricular rates in patients with JET ranges from 140-370 beats/minute (Villain et al. 1990).

7.1.2 *Incidence*: Incidence of JET occurs in two cohorts: neonatal and post-operative patients. Congenital JET occurs in the first six months of life and a family history is usually present (Sarubbi et al. 2002). Overall, JET occurs in 1% of congenital heart repairs (Walsh 2001a). JET occurred in 22% of Tetralogy of Fallot (TOF) repairs, 10% of atrio-ventricular septal defect repairs, and 3.7% of VSD repairs (Dodge-Khatami et al. 2002). Predictors of post-operative JET were younger age (Hoffman et al. 2002), lower body weight (Rekawek et al. 2007), resection of muscle bundles, higher bypass temperatures, and relief of right ventricular outflow tract obstruction through the right atrium (Dodge-Khatami et al. 2002).

7.1.3 *Mechanism*: Although the mechanism of JET is unclear, abnormal (enhanced) automaticity of the junction has been put forth. In post-operative congenital heart disease patients, it is hypothesized that direct trauma or infiltrative hemorrhage of the conduction system leads to enhanced automaticity of the His bundle (Dodge-Khatami et al. 2002).

7.1.4 *Natural history*: Congenital JET is associated with high mortality, most of which is attributed to sudden cardiac death (Villain et al. 1990). Concurrent arrhythmias may co-exist with JET, such as complete heart block, ventricular tachycardia, and persistent junctional reciprocating tachycardia. Post-operative JET is a transient state lasting on average 36 hours (Walsh 2001a) and is associated with higher mortality and longer intensive care unit (ICU) stay (Andreasen et al. 2008).

7.1.5 *Clinical presentation*: Congenital JET presents with cardiomegaly with concomitant heart failure in more than 50 percent, death in 35 percent (Villain et al. 1990), hydrops fetalis, and echocardiographic evidence of left ventricular dysfunction. In post-operative JET, the decreased ventricular filling time leads to cardiovascular compromise.

7.1.6 *ECG*: ECG criteria include 1) QRS morphology similar to that of sinus rhythm, 2) rapid ventricular rate, and 3) dissociated sinus rhythm with atrial rate often less than ventricular rate or retrograde 1:1 conduction (Walsh 2001a). If variability exists in R-R interval, appropriately timed P-waves may conduct to the ventricular tissue (Figure 13).

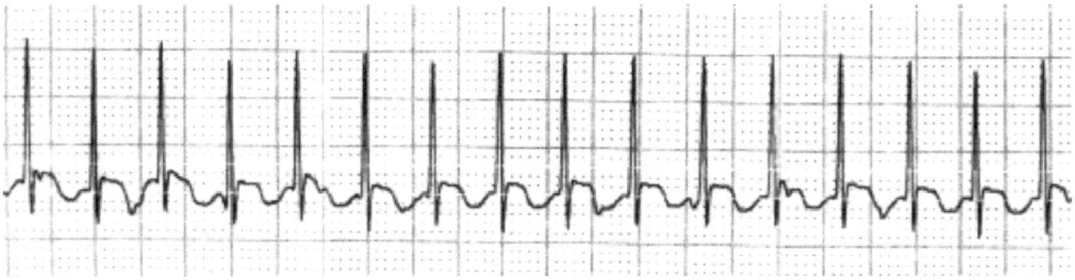

Fig. 13. Junctional ectopic tachycardia

7.1.7 *Work-up*: An electrophysiology study is generally not necessary in patients with JET, unless ablation is being considered for medication-refractory symptoms (Walsh 2001a). In cases of 1:1 retrograde conduction across the AV node, adenosine can clarify the underlying rhythm by blocking the AV node.

7.1.8 *Management and Prognosis*: Management of post-operative JET includes achievement of AV synchrony and rate control. Atrial pacing above the rate of JET may establish rate control (Walsh 2001a). Post-operative JET is generally responsive to intravenous amiodarone, a class III antiarrhythmic (Shah and Rhodes 1998). Mean length of time for termination of post-operative JET after loading and infusion of amiodarone was 4.5 hours with majority achieving control within 12 hours (Plumpton et al. 2005). Decreasing the body core temperature to 32-34 °C, decreasing the sympathomimetic catecholamine levels, optimizing volume, electrolytes and hemoglobin contribute to decreased ventricular rate by decreasing the automaticity (Cabrera et al. 2002). Magnesium supplementation has been shown to be beneficial in prevention of post-operative JET (Dorman et al. 2000). JET is unresponsive to DC cardioversion, overdrive pacing, and programmed atrial or ventricular stimulation (Sarubbi et al. 2003). Pharmacologic treatment of congenital JET with monotherapy is less successful than combined therapy with amiodarone, digoxin or class IA medication (Sarubbi et al. 2002). Patients with drug-refractory congenital JET should undergo catheter ablation with maintenance of the normal atrio-ventricular conduction (Walsh 2001a). A pacemaker is recommended in those children with evidence of impaired conduction with atrial stimulation, sinus dysfunction, or spontaneous AV block on ECG or Holter monitor (Walsh 2001a).

7.2 Persistent Junctional Reciprocating Tachycardia

7.2.1 *Definition*: Persistent or permanent junctional reciprocating tachycardia (PJRT) is an incessant tachycardia characterized by prograde conduction through the AV node and retrograde conduction through a slow accessory pathway located in the posteroseptal (74%) region with decremental conduction properties (Critelli, G. et al. 1984; Lindinger, A. et al. 1998; Vaksmann, G. et al. 2006). PJRT is a narrow complex tachycardia with rates ranging from 120-250 beats/min and infants having higher tachycardia rates than children (Dorostkar et al. 1999).

7.2.2 *Incidence*: PJRT consists of 1% to 6% of all supraventricular tachycardia (Dorostkar et al. 1999; Blaufox and Saul 2001). It can present in infancy and into early childhood.

7.2.3 *Mechanism*: PJRT has a reentrant mechanism with accessory pathways which are mostly isolated and in patients without congenital heart disease (Vaksmann, G et al. 2006).

7.2.4 *Natural history*: In a recent study by Vaksmann et al (2006), PJRT resolved spontaneously in 22 percent (Vaksmann, G et al. 2006). Long term persistence of PJRT can lead to tachycardia-mediated cardiomyopathy, which resolves with appropriate rate control (Lindinger, A et al. 1998; Noe et al. 2002). Uncontrolled PJRT may lead to death.

7.2.5 *Clinical presentation*: Patients often are asymptomatic in childhood. Symptomatic patients present with intermittent palpitations, exercise intolerance, and syncope (Dorostkar et al. 1999).

7.2.6 *ECG*: ECG shows retrograde P-wave in leads II, III, aVF, and left lateral leads, and R-P interval longer than P-R interval (Dorostkar et al. 1999). The long R-P interval is attributed to the slow retrograde conduction. In sinus rhythm, there is no delta wave and P-R interval is normal (Critelli, G et al. 1984). QRS complexes are narrow.

7.2.7 *Work-up*: PJRT is likely under-diagnosed in childhood and patients present with heart failure with associated ventricular dysfunction. An ECG and Holter monitor should be considered. An echocardiogram should be performed to assess the cardiac function and structure and serial echocardiograms are necessary in those with depressed LV function. An electrophysiology study and catheter ablation may be performed in refractory PJRT associated with decreased ventricular function (Dorostkar et al. 1999).

7.2.8 *Management and Prognosis*: Many patients with stable infrequent episodes and slow tachycardia may not require medical therapy (Lindinger, A et al. 1998). In pediatric patients, amiodarone and verapamil alone had success rates of 84-94% (Vaksmann, G et al. 2006). Digoxin alone had a success rate of 50%. Hence, medical therapy with anti-arrhythmic drugs should be advocated prior to consideration of catheter ablation (Drago et al. 2001). Pediatric and adult patients with medication-refractory incessant PJRT should undergo direct current catheter ablation, with good safety and efficacy (Aguinaga et al. 1998).

8.1 Ventricular Tachycardia

8.1.1 *Definition*: Ventricular tachycardia (VT) is a tachycardia with rates greater than 120 beats per minute and originating within the ventricles or the lower conduction system with ventriculo-atrial dissociation. Non-sustained VT is defined as a three or more consecutive beats of ventricular origin that terminate spontaneously with no hemodynamic compromise and lasting less than 30 seconds. Sustained VT persists longer than 30 seconds or requires medical or electrical intervention to terminate the tachycardia (AHA 2007).

8.1.2 *Incidence*: In healthy teenage boys, short episodes of ventricular tachycardia were present in 3% (Dickinson and Scott 1984). Incidence of VT is higher in patients with congenital heart disease. Approximately 30% of post-operative tetralogy of Fallot patients had sustained monomorphic VT and 4.4% had polymorphic VT, which contributes to 2% annual risk of sudden cardiac death (Khairy et al. 2004; Walsh, E. and Cecchin, F. 2007). VT originates in the RVOT in 60%-80% of structurally normal hearts (Lerman et al. 2004). Idiopathic VT is also associated with aortic valve disease, corrected transposition of the great arteries, Ebstein's anomaly of the tricuspid valve, Eisenmenger's syndrome, long QT syndrome, unrepaired tetralogy of Fallot, arrhythmogenic right ventricular dysplasia, and myocardial infarction (Callans, D. and Josephson, M. 2004; Fontaine et al. 2004; Walsh, E. P. and Cecchin, F. 2007).

8.1.3 *Mechanism*: Ventricular tachycardia characterized by a re-entry mechanism can be initiated and terminated with programmed stimuli (Callans, D and Josephson, ME 2004). VT may also be secondary to automaticity or triggered activity.

8.1.4 *Natural history*: Post-operative congenital heart disease patients are at high risk of VT and sudden cardiac death. In patients with normal hearts, younger children (90%) and older populations (50%-70%) have resolution of VT within 2 to 10 years (Alexander 2001b). However, symptomatic younger patients had worse prognosis (Davis et al. 1996). In patients with normal intracardiac anatomy, only 50% have an actual diagnosis such as hypertrophic cardiomyopathy, dilated cardiomyopathy, myocarditis, myocardial hamartoma, and metabolic disease (Davis et al. 1996). Ventricular tachycardia is present in 50%-60% of patients with dilated cardiomyopathy and responsible for 8%-50% of deaths (Galvin and Ruskin 2004).

8.1.5 *Clinical presentation*: Clinical presentation is variable (Davis et al. 1996). Symptoms may range from palpitations, light headedness, syncope, shortness of breath, neck fullness, and chest pain to death (Silka and Garson Jr. 1999).

8.1.6 *ECG*: Monomorphic VT is a wide complex tachycardia with same QRS morphology, which suggests a single re-entrant focus (figure 14). Polymorphic VT is a wide complex tachycardia with variable QRS morphology. Torsades de pointe is a form of polymorphic VT and associated with long QT syndrome and variable electrical activation. (Figure 15)

8.1.7 *Work-up*: Obtain a thorough personal and family history including history of sudden cardiac death. An ECG of the arrhythmia is useful but very difficult to capture very often; however, a resting ECG is a class 1 recommendation (Zipes and Camm 2006). Check electrolytes, in particular hypokalemia, hyperkalemia, and hypomagnesemia. In patients with recurrent syncope, a holter monitor or event recorder is indicated. An echocardiogram is necessary to identify structural heart disease and evaluate cardiac function in those at risk for sudden cardiac death such as dilated, hypertrophic, and arrhythmogenic RV dysplasia, myocarditis, and inherited disorders (Zipes and Camm 2006). An exercise stress test is indicated in all individuals, regardless of age, known or suspected to have exercise-induced ventricular tachycardia. An electrophysiology study is warranted in patients with congenital/structural heart disease, those with unknown etiology of VT, and those with syncope of unknown etiology with LV dysfunction (Zipes and Camm 2006).

8.1.8 *Management and Prognosis*: All wide complex tachycardias need to be treated like ventricular tachycardia unless proven otherwise. A-V dissociation, superior QRS axis and positive or negative concordance of QRS complexes in the precordial leads suggest ventricular origin. In patients with normal hearts, episodes of non-sustained VT has good prognosis. Avoid medications that prolong QT interval and correct electrolyte abnormalities. In patients with sustained VT with hemodynamic compromise, direct current (DC) cardioversion is indicated (Zipes and Camm 2006). In stable monomorphic VT, IV procainamide or amiodarone, and/or transvenous catheter pace termination maybe employed. In patients with polymorphic VT, DC cardioversion, IV amiodarone and beta blockers maybe employed. Internal cardiac defibrillator is indicated in patients with congenital heart disease who have survived cardiac arrest, patients with severely impaired ventricular function, and those on chronic optimal medical therapy with a life expectancy of at least one year (Zipes and Camm 2006).

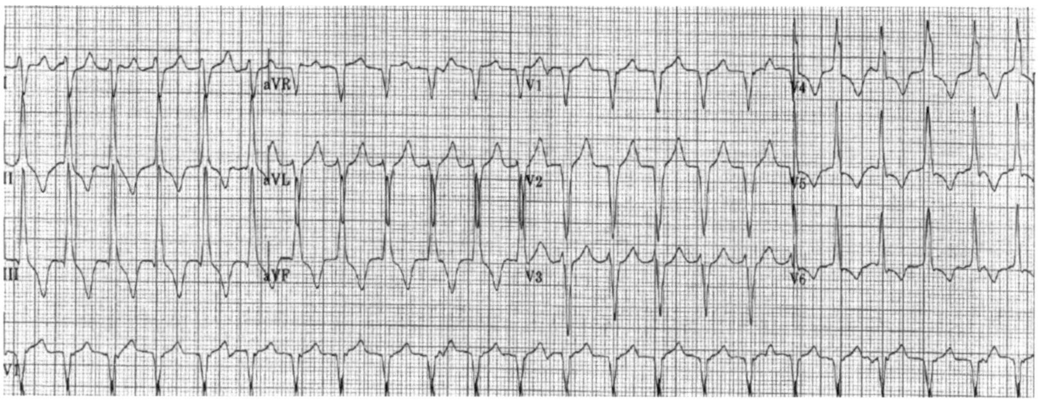

Fig. 14. Ventricular tachycardia

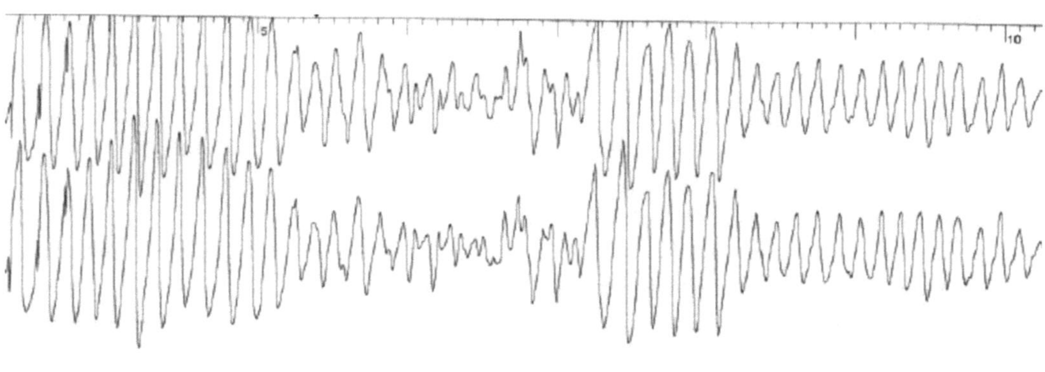

Fig. 15. Torsades de pointe

9. References

Aellig, N. C.C. Balmer, et al. (2007). "Long-term follow-up after pacemaker implantation in neonates and infants." Ann Thorac Surg 83(4): 1420-3.

Aguinaga, L.J. Primo, et al. (1998). "Long-Term Follow-Up in Patients with the Permanent Form of Junctional Reciprocating Tachycardia Treated with Radiofrequency Ablation." Pacing and Clinical Electrophysiology 21(11): 2073-2078.

Ajisaka, H.T. Hiraki, et al. (1997). "Direct Conversion of Atrial Flutter to Sinus Rhythm with Low-output, Short-duration Transesophageal Atrial Pacing." Clinical Cardiology 20(9): 762-6.

Alexander, M. (2001b). Ventricular Arrhythmias in Children and Young Adults. *Cardiac Arrhythmias in Children and Young Adults with Congenital Heart Disease*. E. Walsh, J. Saulet al. Philadelphia, PA, Lippincott Williams & Wilkins: 201-234.

Alison, J. F.J. A. Yeung-Lai-Wah, et al. (1995). "Characterization of junctional rhythm after atrioventricular node ablation." Circulation 91(1): 84-90.

Andreasen, J., S. Johnsen, et al. (2008). "Junctional Ectopic Tachycardia after Surgery for Congenital Heart Disease in Children." Intersive Care Medicine 34(5): 895-902.

Andrew, P. and A. Montenero (2007). "Atrial Flutter: A Focus on Treatment Options for a Common Supraventricular Tachyarrhythmia." Journal of Cardiovascular Medicine 8: 558-567.

Attina, D. A.F. Mori, et al. (1987). "Long-term follow-up in children without heart disease with ventricular premature beats." Eur Heart J 8 Suppl D: 21-3.

Beaufort-Krol, G. C.M. J. Schasfoort-van Leeuwen, et al. (2007). "Longitudinal echocardiographic follow-up in children with congenital complete atrioventricular block." Pacing Clin Electrophysiol 30(11): 1339-43.

Benditt, D. G.G. J. Klein, et al. (1984). "Enhanced atrioventricular nodal conduction in man: electrophysiologic effects of pharmacologic autonomic blockade." Circulation 69(6): 1088-95.

Blaufox, A. and J. Saul (2001). Accessory-Pathway-Mediated Tachycardias. *Cardiac Arrhythmias in Children and Young Adults with Congenital Heart Disease*. E. Walsh, J. Saulet al. Philadelphia, PA, Lippincott Williams & Wilkins: 173-199.

Blomstrom-Lundqvist, C.M. M. Scheinman, et al. (2003). "ACC/AHA/ESC guidelines for the management of patients with supraventricular arrhythmias--executive summary. a report of the American college of cardiology/American heart association task force on practice guidelines and the European society of cardiology committee for practice guidelines (writing committee to develop guidelines for the management of patients with supraventricular arrhythmias) developed in collaboration with NASPE-Heart Rhythm Society." J Am Coll Cardiol 42(8): 1493-531.

Brodsky, M.D. Wu, et al. (1977). "Arrhythmias documented by 24 hour continuous electrocardiographic monitoring in 50 male medical students without apparent heart disease." Am J Cardiol 39(3): 390-5.

Cabrera, D.D. Rodrigo Carbonero, et al. (2002). "The Treatment of Post-operative Junctional Ectopic Tachycardia." Anales Espanoles de Pediatria 56(6): 505-9.

Calkins, H.P. Yong, et al. (1999). "Catheter Ablation of Accessory Pathways, Atrioventricular Nodal Reentrant Tachycardia, and the Atrioventricular Junction: Final Results of a Prospective, Multicenter Clinical Trial." Circulation 99(2): 262-70.

Callans, D. and M. Josephson (2004). Ventricular tachycardia in patients with coronary artery disease. *Cardiac Electrophysiology: From cell to bedside.* D. P. Zipes and J. Jalife. Philadelphia, PA: 569-574.

Case, C. L. (1999). "Diagnosis and treatment of pediatric arrhythmias." Pediatr Clin North Am 46(2): 347-54.

Casta, A.G. Wolff, et al. (1980). "Dual Atrioventricular Nodal Pathways: A Benign Finding in Arrhythmia-free Children with Heart Disease." American Journal of Cardiology 46(6): 1013-8.

Chandar, J. S.G. S. Wolff, et al. (1990). "Ventricular arrhythmias in postoperative tetralogy of Fallot." Am J Cardiol 65(9): 655-61.

Cheitlin, M. D.W. F. Armstrong, et al. (2003). "ACC/AHA/ASE 2003 guideline update for the clinical application of echocardiography--summary article: a report of the American College of Cardiology/American Heart Association Task Force on Practice Guidelines (ACC/AHA/ASE Committee to Update the 1997 Guidelines for the Clinical Application of Echocardiography)." J Am Coll Cardiol 42(5): 954-70.

Chiale, P.H. Garro, et al. (2006). "Inappropriate Sinus Tachycardia may be Related to an Immunologic Disorder Involving Cardiac Beta Adrenergic Receptors." Heart Rhythm 3(10): 1182-6.

Chiang, B. N.L. V. Perlman, et al. (1969). "Relationship of premature systoles to coronary heart disease and sudden death in the Tecumseh epidemiologic study." Ann Intern Med 70(6): 1159-66.

Coker, R.A. Koziell, et al. (1984). "Does the sympathetic nervous system influence sinus arrhythmia in man? Evidence from combined autonomic blockade." J Physiol 356: 459-64.

Critelli, G.J. J. Gallagher, et al. (1984). "Anatomic and electrophysiologic substrate of the permanent form of junctional reciprocating tachycardia." J Am Coll Cardiol 4(3): 601-10.

Davis, A.R. Gow, et al. (1996). "Clinical Spectrum, Therapeutic Management, and Follow-up of Ventricular Tachycardia in Infants and Young Children." American Heart Journal 131: 186-91.

Deal, B.J. Keane, et al. (1985). "Wolff-Parkinson-White Syndrome and Supraventricular Tachycardia During Infancy: Management and Follow-up." Journal of The American College of Cardiology 5(1): 130-5.

Dewey, R. C., M. A. Capeless, et al. (1987). "Use of ambulatory electrocardiographic monitoring to identify high-risk patients with congenital complete heart block." N Engl J Med 316(14): 835-9.

Dhingra, R. C.P. Denes, et al. (1974). "The significance of second degree atrioventricular block and bundle branch block. Observations regarding site and type of block." Circulation 49(4): 638-46.

Dickinson, D. and O. Scott (1984). "Ambulatory Electrographic Monitoring in 100 Healthy Teenage Boys." British Heart Journal 51(2): 179-83.

Dodge-Khatami, A.O. Miller, et al. (2002). "Surgical Substrates of Postoperative Junctional Ectopic Tachycardia in Congenital Heart Defects." Journal of Thoracic and Cardiovascular Surgery 123(4): 624-630.

Dorman, B.R. Sade, et al. (2000). "Magnesium Supplementation in the Prevention of Arrhythmias in Pediatric Patients Undergoing Surgery for Congenital Heart Defects." American Heart Journal 139(3): 522-8.

Dorostkar, P.M. Silka, et al. (1999). "Clinical Course of Persistent Junctional Reciprocating Tachycardia." Journal of The American College of Cardiology 33: 366-75.

Drago, F.G. Grutter, et al. (2006). "Atrioventricular Nodal Reentrant Tachycardia in Children." Pediatric Cardiology 27(4): 454-59.

Drago, F.M. Silvetti, et al. (2001). "Permanent Juncational Reciprocating Tachycardia in Infants and Children: Effectiveness of Medical and Non-Medical Treatment." Italian Heart Journal 2(6): 456-61.

Dubin, D. (2000). Rapid Interpretation of EKGs. Fort Meyers, COVER Publishing Company, Pages.

Duster, M. C.M. T. Bink-Boelkens, et al. (1985). "Long-term follow-up of dysrhythmias following the Mustard procedure." Am Heart J 109(6): 1323-6.

Espinola-Zavaleta, N.M. E. Soto, et al. (2006). "Non-compacted cardiomyopathy: clinical-echocardiographic study." Cardiovasc Ultrasound 4: 35.

Etheridge, S. and V. Judd (1999). "Supraventricular Tachycardia in Infancy: Evaluation, Management, and Follow-up." Archives of Pediatric Adolescent Medicine 153(3): 267-71.

Ferrer, P. (1977). Arrhythmias in the neonate, infant, and child. *Arrhythmias in the Neonate*. N. Roberts and H. Gelband. New York, Appleton-Century-Crofts: 265-316.

Fisch, C. and S. B. Knoebel (1970). "Junctional rhythms." Prog Cardiovasc Dis 13(2): 141-58.

Fishberger, S. (2001). Sinus Node Dysfunction. *Cardiac Arrhythmias in Children and Young Adults with Congenital Heart Disease*. E. Walsh, J. Saulet al. Philadelphia, Lippincott Williams & Wilkins: 271-283.

Fogoros, R. (2006). The Electrophysiology Study in the Evaluation of the SA Node, AV Node, and His-Purkinje System. Malden, MA, Blackwell Publishing, Inc., Pages.

Fontaine, G.P. Forres, et al. (2004). Ventricular Tachycardia in Arrhythmogenic Right Ventricular Cardiomyopathies. *Cardiac Electrophysiology: From cell to bedside*. D. P. Zipes and J. Jallife. Philadelphia, PA, W.B.Saunders: 588-600.

Frolkis, J. P.C. E. Pothier, et al. (2003). "Frequent ventricular ectopy after exercise as a predictor of death." N Engl J Med 348(9): 781-90.

Galvin, J. and J. Ruskin, Eds. (2004). Ventricular Tachycardia in Patients with Dilated Cardiomyopathy. Philadelphia, PA, Saunders: Pages.

Gamble, Y. D., W. P. Lutin, et al. (2007). "Non-sinus bradyarrhythmias in very low birth weight infants." J Perinatol 27(1): 65-7.

Garan, H. (2008). "Atypical Atrial Flutter." Heart Rhythm 5: 618-621.

Garson Jr., A.M. Bink-Boelkens, et al. (1985). "Atrial Flutter in the Young: a Collaborative Study of 380 cases." Journal of The American College of Cardiology 6(4): 871-8.

Garson Jr., A. and P. Gillette (1981). "Electrophysiologic Studies of Supraventricular Tachycardia in Children. I. Clinical-electrophysiologic Correlations." American Heart Journal 102(2): 233-250.

Gelatt, M.R. M. Hamilton, et al. (1994). "Risk factors for atrial tachyarrhythmias after the Fontan operation." J Am Coll Cardiol 24(7): 1735-41.

Gibbons, R. J.G. J. Balady, et al. (2002). "ACC/AHA 2002 guideline update for exercise testing: summary article: a report of the American College of Cardiology/American

Heart Association Task Force on Practice Guidelines (Committee to Update the 1997 Exercise Testing Guidelines)." Circulation 106(14): 1883-92.
Gomes, A., R. Hariman, et al. (1985). "Sustained Symptomatic Sinus Node Reentrant Tachycardia: Incidence, Clinical Significance, Electrophysiologic Observations and the Effects of Antiarrhythmic Agents." Journal of The American College of Cardiology 5: 45-47.
Goya, M.Y. Iesaka, et al. (1999). "Radiofrequency Catheter Ablation for Sinoatrial Node Reentrant Tachycardia." Japanese Circulation Journal 63: 177-83.
Granada, J.W. Uribe, et al. (2000). "Incidence and Predictors of Atrial Flutter in the General Population." Journal of The American College of Cardiology 36(7): 2242-6.
Gregaratos, G. (2002). "ACC/AHA/NASPE 2002 Guideline Update for Implantation of Cardiac Pacemakers and Antiarrhythmia Devices." Circulation.
Haines, D. and J. DiMarco (1990). "Sustained intraatrial reentrant tachycardia: clinical, electrocardiographic and electrophysiologic characteristics and long-term follow-up." Journal of The American College of Cardiology 15(6): 1345-54.
Hare, G. V. (1999). Supraventicular Tachycardia. *Clinical Pediatric Arrhythmias.* P. G. A. G. Jr. Philadelphia, W.B.Saunders Company: 97-120.
Hiss, R. G. and L. E. Lamb (1962). "Electrocardiographic findings in 122,043 individuals." Circulation 25: 947-61.
Hoffman, B. F. and P. F. Cranefield (1964). "The Physiological Basis Of Cardiac Arrhythmias." Am J Med 37: 670-84.
Hoffman, T.D. Bush, et al. (2002). "Postoperative Junctional Ectopic Tachycardia in Children: Incidence, Risk Factors, and Treatment." Annals of Thoracic Surgery 74(5): 1607-11.
Hsieh, M. and S. Chen (2002). Catheter Ablation in Focal Tachycardia. *Catheter Ablation of Arrhythmias.* D. Zipes and M. Haissaguerre. Armonk, NY, Futura Publishing Co., Inc.: 185-204.
Huhta, J. C.J. D. Maloney, et al. (1983). "Complete atrioventricular block in patients with atrioventricular discordance." Circulation 67(6): 1374-7.
Jacquet, L.G. Ziady, et al. (1990). "Cardiac rhythm disturbances early after orthotopic heart transplantation: prevalence and clinical importance of the observed abnormalities." J Am Coll Cardiol 16(4): 832-7.
Jideus, L.M. Kesek, et al. (2006). "The role of premature atrial contractions as the main triggers of postoperative atrial fibrillation." J Electrocardiol 39(1): 48-54.
Karpawich, P. P.P. C. Gillette, et al. (1981). "Congenital complete atrioventricular block: clinical and electrophysiologic predictors of need for pacemaker insertion." Am J Cardiol 48(6): 1098-102.
Kastor, J. (1990). "Multifocal Atrial Tachycardia." New England Journal of Medicine 322: 1713.
Kaushal, P. and J. A. Taylor (2002). "Inter-relations among declines in arterial distensibility, baroreflex function and respiratory sinus arrhythmia." J Am Coll Cardiol 39(9): 1524-30.
Khairy, P.M. Landzberg, et al. (2004). "Value of Programmed Ventricular Stimulatino after Tetralogy of Fallot Repair: a Multicenter Study." Circulation 109(16): 1994-2000.
Kleinfeld, M. J. and B. H. Boal (1978). "Junctional escape rhythm in the sick sinus syndrome." Cardiology 63(4): 193-8.

Ko, J.B. Deal, et al. (1992). "Supraventricular Tachycardia Mechanisms and their Age Distribution in Pediatric Patients." American Journal of Cardiology 69(12): 1028-32.

Kones, R., J. Phillips, et al. (1974). "Mechanism and Management of Chaotic Atrial Mechanism." Cardiology 59: 92.

Krahn, A.R. Yee, et al. (1995). "Inappropriate sinus tachycardia: evaluation and thearpy." Journal of Cardiovascular Electrophysiology 6(12): 1124-8.

Lerman, B.K. Stein, et al., Eds. (2004). Ventricular Tachycardia in Patients with Structurally Normal Hearts. Philadelphia, PA, Saunders: Pages.

Levine, S. A., H. Miller, et al. (1956). "Some clinical features of complete heart block." Circulation 13(6): 801-24.

Lin, D. and D. Callans (2004). Clinical Arrhythmias: Mechanisms, Features, and Management. Supraventricular Arrhythmias. *Cardiac Electrophysiology From Cell to Bedside*. D. Zipes and J. Jaliffe. Philadelphia, PA, Saunders: 479-484.

Lindinger, A.A. Heisel, et al. (1998). "Permanent junctional re-entry tachycardia. A multicentre long-term follow-up study in infants, children and young adults." Eur Heart J 19(6): 936-42.

Lockwood, D.K. Otomo, et al. (2004). Electrophysiologic Characteristics of Atrioventricular Nodal Reentrant Tachycardia: Implications for the Reentrant Circuits. *Cardiac Electrophysiology From Cell to Bedside*. D. Zipes and J. Jaliffe. Philadelphia, PA, Saunders: 537-557.

Lundstrom, U.C. Bull, et al. (1990). "The natural and "unnatural" history of congenitally corrected transposition." Am J Cardiol 65(18): 1222-9.

Martin, A. and J. Kugler (1999). Sinus Node Dysfunction. *Clinical Pediatric Arrhythmias*. P. Gillette and A. Garson, Jr. Philadelphia, W.B. Saunders Company: 51-62.

Michaelsson, M. and M. A. Engle (1972). "Congenital complete heart block: an international study of the natural history." Cardiovasc Clin 4(3): 85-101.

Morillo, C. and J. Guzman (2007). "Inappropriate sinus tachycardia: an update." Rev Esp Cardiol 60(Suppl 3): 10-14.

Mymin, D.F. A. Mathewson, et al. (1986). "The natural history of primary first-degree atrioventricular heart block." N Engl J Med 315(19): 1183-7.

Naheed, Z.J. Strasburger, et al. (1995). "Natural History and Management Strategies of Automatic Atrial Tachycardia in Children." American Journal of Cardiology 75(5-6): 405-7.

Narula, O. (1974). "A Mechanism for Supraventricular Tachycardia." Circulation 50: 1114-28.

Noe, P.V. Van Driel, et al. (2002). "Rapid Recovery of Cardiac Function after Catheter Ablation of Persistent Junctional Reciprocating Tachycardia in Children." Pacing and Clinical Electrophysiology 25(2): 191-4.

Olgin, J. and D. Zipes (2005a). Specific Arrhythmias: Diagnosis and Treatment. *Braunwald's Heart Disease*. D. ZipesP. Libbyet al. Philadelphia, PA, Elsevier Saunders. 1: 803-863.

Olgin, J. and D. Zipes (2005b). Specific Arrhythmias: Diagnosis and Treatment: Premature Ventricular Complexes. *Braunwald's Heart Disease: A Textbook of Cardiovascular Medicine*. D. ZipesE. Braunwaldet al. Philadelphia, Saunders: 838-841.

Packer, D.G. Bardy, et al. (1986). "Tachycardia-induced Cardiomyopathy: A Reversible Form of Left Ventricular Dysfunction." American Journal of Cardiology 57(8): 563-570.

Paridon, S. (2006). "Clinical stress testing in the pediatric age group. A statement from the American Heart Association Council on Cardiobascular Disease in the Young,

Committee on Atherosclerosis, Hypertension, and Obesity in Youth." Circulation 113(15): 1905-20.
Perry, J. and A. Garson Jr. (1990). "Supraventricular Tachycardia due to Wolff-Parkinson-White Syndrome in Children: Early Disappearance and Late Recurrence." Journal of The American College of Cardiology 16(5): 1215-20.
Peuch, P., R. Groileau, et al. (1976). Incidence of different types of A-V block and their localization by His bundle recordings. *The Conduction System of the Heart.* H. J. Wellens, K. I. Lieet al. Leiden, Stenfert: 467.
Plumpton, K., R. Justo, et al. (2005). "Amiodarone for Post-operative Junctional Ectopic Tachycardia." Cariology in the Young 15(1): 13-8.
Poutiainen, A.M. Koistinen, et al. (1999). "Prevalence and natural course of ectopic atrial tachycardia." European Heart Journal 20(9): 694-700.
Randall, W. C., W. H. Wehrmacher, et al. (1981). "Hierarchy of supraventricular pacemakers." J Thorac Cardiovasc Surg 82(5): 797-800.
Rekawek, J.A. Kansy, et al. (2007). "Risk Factors for Cardiac Arrhythmias in Children with Congenital Heart Disease after Surgical Intervention in the Early Postoperative Period." Journal of Thoracic and Cardiovascular Surgery 133(4): 900-4.
Roberts-Thomson, K., P. Kistler, et al. (2006). "Focal Atrial Tachycardia I: Clinical Features, Diagnosis, Mechanisms, and Anatomic Location." Pacing and Clinical Electrophysiology 29(6): 643-652.
Roberts, N. K. and P. C. Gillette (1977). "Electrophysiologic study of the condition system in normal children." Pediatrics 60(6): 858-63.
Rosen, M. R.C. Fisch, et al. (1980). "Can accelerated atrioventricular junctional escape rhythms be explained by delayed afterdepolarizations?" Am J Cardiol 45(6): 1272-84.
Salim, M., C. Case, et al. (1995). "Chaotic Atrial Tachycardia in Children." American Heart Journal 129: 831-33.
Saoudi, N.F. Cosio, et al. (2001). "A Classification of Atrial Flutter and Regular Atrial Tachycardia According to Electrophysiological Mechanisms and Anatomica Bases." European Heart Journal 22: 1162-1182.
Sarubbi, B.B. Musto, et al. (2002). "Congenital Junctional Ectopic Tachycardia in Children and Adolescents: a 20 Year Experience Based Study." Heart 88: 188-190.
Sarubbi, B.P. Vergara, et al. (2003). "Congenital Junctional Ectopic Tachycardia: Presentation and Outcome." Indian Pacing and Electrophysiology Journal 3(3): 143-7.
Scott, O., G. J. Williams, et al. (1980). "Results of 24 hour ambulatory monitoring of electrocardiogram in 131 healthy boys aged 10 to 13 years." Br Heart J 44(3): 304-8.
Sestito, A.M. Pardeo, et al. (2007). "Cardiac magnetic resonance of healthy children and young adults with frequent premature ventricular complexes." J Cardiovasc Med (Hagerstown) 8(9): 692-8.
Shah, M. and L. Rhodes (1998). "Management of Postoperative Arrhythmias and Junctional Ectopic Tachycardia." Seminars in Thoracic and Cardiovascular surgery. Pediatric Cardiac Surgery Annual 1: 91-102.
Shen, W. (2005). "How to Manage Patients with Inappropriate Sinus Tachycardia." Heart Rhythm 2(9): 1015-19.

Shepard, R. K.A. Natale, et al. (1998). "Physiology of the escape rhythm after radiofrequency atrioventricular junctional ablation." Pacing Clin Electrophysiol 21(5): 1085-92.

Sherron, P.E. Torres-Arraut, et al. (1985). "Site of conduction delay and electrophysiologic significance of first-degree atrioventricular block in children with heart disease." Am J Cardiol 55(11): 1323-7.

Silka, M. and A. Garson Jr. (1999). Ventricular Arrhythmias. *Clinical Pediatric Arrhythmias*. P. Gillette and A. Garson Jr. Philadelphia, PA, WB Saunders: 121-145.

Silka, M. J. and A. Garson, Jr. (1999). Ventricular Arrhythmias. *Clinical Pediatric Arrhythmias*. P. C. Gillette and A. Garson, Jr. Philadelphia, W.B. Saunders Company: 121-145.

Skinner JR, Sharland G. Detection and management of life threatening arrhythmias in the perinatal period. Early Human Development 2008;84(3):161-172..

Sobotka, P. A.J. H. Mayer, et al. (1981). "Arrhythmias documented by 24-hour continuous ambulatory electrocardiographic monitoring in young women without apparent heart disease." Am Heart J 101(6): 753-9.

Sokoloski, M. (1999). Tachyarrhythmias Confined to the Atrium. *Clinical Pediatric Arrhythmias*. P. Gillette and A. Garson Jr. Philadelphia, PA, WB Saunders.

Southall, D. P.J. Richards, et al. (1980). "Study of cardiac rhythm in healthy newborn infants." Br Heart J 43(1): 14-20.

Stein, R.C. M. Medeiros, et al. (2002). "Intrinsic sinus and atrioventricular node electrophysiologic adaptations in endurance athletes." J Am Coll Cardiol 39(6): 1033-8.

Still, A.P. Raatikainen, et al. (2005). "Prevalence, Characteristic and Natural Course of Inappropriate Sinus Tachycardia." Europace 7: 104-12.

Strasberg, B.Y. L. F. Amat, et al. (1981). "Natural history of chronic second-degree atrioventricular nodal block." Circulation 63(5): 1043-9.

Sugimoto, T.H. Hayakawa, et al. (1986). "Clinical evaluation of bisoprolol in the treatment of extrasystoles and sinus tachycardia: an interim report." J Cardiovasc Pharmacol 8 Suppl 11: S171-4.

Talbot, S. and M. Greaves (1976). "Association of ventricular extrasystoles and ventricular tachycardia with idioventricular rhythm." Br Heart J 38(5): 457-64.

Texter, K.N. Kertesz, et al. (2006). "Atrial Flutter in Infants." Journal of The American College of Cardiology 48(5): 1040-6.

Triedman, J. (2001). Atrial Reentrant Tachycardias. *Cardiac Arrhythmias in Children and Young Adults with Congenital Heart Disease*. E. Walsh, J. Saulet al. Philadelphia, PA, Lippincott Williams & Wilkins: 137-159.

Triedman, J. (2004). Atrial Arrhythmias in Congenital Heart Disease. *Cardiac Electrophysiology From Cell to Bedside*. D. Zipes and J. Jaliffe. Philadelphia, PA: 558-568.

Triedman, J.D. Bergau, et al. (1997). "Efficacy of Radiofrequency Ablation for Control of Intraatrial Reentry Tachycardia in Patient with Congenital Heart Disease." Journal of The American College of Cardiology 30(4): 1032-38.

Vaksmann, G.C. D'Hoinne, et al. (2006). "Permanent junctional reciprocating tachycardia in children: a multicentre study on clinical profile and outcome." Heart 92(1): 101-4.

Vaksmann, G.A. Fournier, et al. (1990). "Frequency and prognosis of arrhythmias after operative "correction" of tetralogy of Fallot." Am J Cardiol 66(3): 346-9.

Valimaki, I. and P. A. Tarlo (1971). "Heart rate patterns and apnea in newborn infants." Am J Obstet Gynecol 110(3): 343-9.

Van Hare, G. (1999). Supraventricular Tachycardia. *Clinical Pediatric Arrhythmias*. P. Gillette and A. Garson Jr. Philadelphia, W.B. Saunders Company: 97-120.

Villain, E.V. Vetter, et al. (1990). "Evolving Concepts in the Management of Congenital Junctional Ectopic Tachycardia. A Multicenter Study." Circulation 81(5): 1544-9.

von Bernuth, G.R. Toussaint, et al. (1989). "[Heart rate and heart rhythm in healthy infants and children]." Klin Padiatr 201(2): 98-103.

Waldo, A. (2004). Atrial Flutter: Mechanisms, Clinical Features, and Management. *Cardiac Electrophysiology From Cell to Bedside*. D. Zipes and J. Jaliffe. Philadelphia, PA, Saunders: 490-499.

Wallace, A. G. and W. M. Daggett (1964). "Re-Excitation of the Atrium. "the Echo Phenomenon"." Am Heart J 68: 661-6.

Walsh, E. (2001a). Automatic Atrial and Junctional Tachycardias. *Cardiac Arrhythmias in Children and Young Adults with Congenital Heart Disease*. E. Walsh, J. Saulet al. Philadelphia, PA, Lippincott Williams & Wilkins: 115-135.

Walsh, E. (2001b). Diagnosis and Acute Management of Tachycardias. *Cardiac Arrhythmias in Children and Young Adults with Congenital Heart Disease*. E. Walsh, J. Saulet al. Philadelphia, Lippincott Williams & Wilkins: 95-113.

Walsh, E. P. and F. Cecchin (2007). "Arrhythmias in adult patients with congenital heart disease." Circulation 115(4): 534-45.

Weindling, S. (2001). Atrioventricular Conduction Disturbances. *Cardiac Arrhythmias in Children and Young Adults with Congenital Heart Disease*. E. Walsh, J. Saulet al. Philadelphia, Lippincott Williams & Wilkins: 285-300.

Wit, A. L. and P. F. Cranefield (1977). "Triggered and automatic activity in the canine coronary sinus." Circ Res 41(4): 434-45.

Yang, Y.J. Cheng, et al. (2001). "Atypical Right Atrial Flutters Patterns." Circulation 103(25): 3092-8.

Young, D.R. Eisenberg, et al. (1977). "Wenckebach atrioventricular block (Mobitz type I) in children and adolescents." Am J Cardiol 40(3): 393-9.

Zhu, D. W.J. D. Maloney, et al. (1995). "Radiofrequency catheter ablation for management of symptomatic ventricular ectopic activity." J Am Coll Cardiol 26(4): 843-9.

Zimmerman, F. (2001). Atrioventricular Node Reentry Tachycardia. *Cardiac Arrhythmias in Children and Young Adults with Congenital Heart Disease*. E. Walsh, J. Saulet al. Philadelphia, PA, Lippincott Williams & Wilkins: 161-172.

Zipes, D. and A. Camm (2006). "ACC/AHA/ESC 2006 guidelines for management of patients with ventricular arrhythmias and the prevention of sudden cardiac death." Journal of The American College of Cardiology 48(5): e247-346.

Zipes, D. P.J. P. DiMarco, et al. (1995). "ACC/AHA Guidelines for clinical intracardiac electrophysiological and catheter ablation procedures. A report of the American College of Cardiology/American Heart Association Task Force on Practice Guidelines (Committee on Clinical Intracardiac Electrophysiologic and Catheter Ablation Procedures), developed in collaboration with the North American Society of Pacing and Electrophysiology." J Am Coll Cardiol 26(2): 555-73.

Zipes, D. P. and A. Garson, Jr. (1994). "26th Bethesda conference: recommendations for determining eligibility for competition in athletes with cardiovascular abnormalities. Task Force 6: arrhythmias." J Am Coll Cardiol 24(4): 892-9.

5

Paced ECG Morphology – Reveals More than What It Conceals

Ajay Bahl
Department of Cardiology, Postgraduate Institute of Medical Education and Research, Chandigarh, India

1. Introduction

Ventricular paced rhythms can mask ECG changes of several conditions. This is because the paced ventricular rhythm does not follow the normal pattern of depolarization through the bundle of His and the bundle branches. Instead, depolarization initially occurs at the tip of the pacemaker lead which is usually at the apex or the septum. The depolarization then proceeds through the myocardium from one cardiomyocyte to another rather than through the conduction system of the heart. This results in abnormal depolarization and repolarization patterns. Thus the QRS complex is usually widened and the T wave is usually of opposite polarity to the QRS complex. Reaching a diagnosis from a single ECG already rendered abnormal by the paced rhythm is not easy. It is thus useful to have a baseline ECG available for comparison. Changes in the axis, QRS width and QRS complex morphology can give important clues to the diagnosis. ECG changes of acute myocardial infarction in patients with a ventricular paced rhythm are well described. There is very limited data on the usefulness of paced ECG in the diagnosis of other conditions.

2. Acute myocardial infarction

Like most other conditions, ECG finings of acute myocardial infarction can be masked by paced rhythms. Pacing leads are traditionally placed in the right ventricular apex. Most studies of ECG findings of myocardial infarction are in patients with pacing leads placed at this location. The ECG pattern of right ventricular apical pacing resembles a left bundle branch block (LBBB) and the diagnostic criteria are also similar. The increasing use of other pacing sites like the interventricular septum and outflow tract as well as biventricular pacing will result in different ECG findings but some general rules will still apply. There is lack of data on the ECG diagnosis of myocardial infarction when the pacing lead tip is placed at locations other than the apex. As these alternate pacing sites gain popularity, the criteria for myocardial infarction recognition that is discussed below may not apply.
Traditionally ECG changes in myocardial infarction in the setting of LBBB include ST segment abnormalities, abnormal Q waves and Cabrera's sign.[1] There are however some differences in the setting of LBBB and ventricular pacing. The most important difference is in value of Q waves in the diagnosis. Abnormal Q waves in leads V5 and V6 along with

increased r in lead V1 is very specific for anterior wall myocardial infarction in the setting of LBBB. In right ventricular pacing, these Q waves however could simply reflect differences in the lead tip position rather than myocardial infarction.[1,2] Thus Q in leads V5 and V6 could be normal finding in right ventricular pacing. A well positioned lead at the RV apex rarely generates a qR complex in lead I, and probably never produces a qR complex in V5 and V6 in the absence of an MI. Thus presence of Q waves in these leads, though useful should be used with the caveat that if the lead tip is not at the right ventricular apex, then Q waves may also be normally seen in these leads. Another important point is to differentiate a qR/ QR from a QS complex. This differentiation is important because a QS complex carries no diagnostic value during RV pacing in any of the leads (QS complexes can be normal in leads I, II, III, aVF, V5, and V6) whereas qR/ QR complex can have diagnostic value.[2] One cannot determine the age of the MI from the QRS complex changes.

ST segment changes are the most useful findings in diagnosing myocardial infarction in patients with paced rhythms. The GUSTO-1 trial has provided useful information in this regard. In this trial, 32 patients had ventricular paced rhythm. The only ECG criterion with a high specificity and statistical significance for the diagnosis of an acute myocardial infarction was ST segment elevation ≥5 mm in leads with a negative QRS complex.[3] Shape of the ST segment which exhibit upward convexity are useful in this context. Two other criteria with acceptable specificity were ST elevation ≥1 mm in leads with concordant QRS polarity and ST depression ≥1 mm in leads V1, V2, or V3.[3,4] It is important to remember that though these criteria are fairly specific, their sensitivity is low. The ECG criterion with the highest sensitivity for the diagnosis of an acute myocardial infarction was ST segment elevation ≥5 mm in leads with a negative QRS complex and even this criterion has a sensitivity of only around 50%.

The GUSTO-1 trial also included 131 patients with LBBB.[5] These ST segment diagnostic criteria were the similar for patients with LBBB and ventricular paced rhythms. The difference in the setting of paced rhythm as compared to LBBB was that of the 3 criteria, the one with the greatest value for the diagnosis of an acute MI in paced rhythm was ST segment elevation ≥5 mm in leads with a negative QRS complex, whereas in the setting of LBBB the criteria with the greatest value was ST elevation ≥1 mm in leads with concordant QRS polarity.

Another classical sign described is the Cabrera's sign.[1,2] Like other signs, this has also been adapted from the criteria diagnosing myocardial infarction in the setting of LBBB. Cabrera's sign is described as notching of the ascending limb of the S wave usually in leads V3 and V4, and sometimes in leads V2 and V5. The notch should be ≥ 0.03 seconds and present in 2 leads.[2] It has low sensitivity but is a very specific sign.

The diagnostic criteria described above are for anterior wall myocardial infarctions. Infarctions at other sites are usually masked by the paced rhythm. Cabrera's sign in both leads III and aVF may be of some value in diagnosing inferior wall myocardial infarction. Similarly ST elevation in lead V4R may occur in acute right ventricular infarction. This sign should however be taken with extreme caution unless accompanied by signs of inferior myocardial infarction.

There are a few important factors that could confound the diagnosis. Retrograde P waves in the terminal part of the QRS complex may mimic Cabrera's sign. Because of cardiac memory repolarization abnormalities, mostly T wave inversions may occur if the patient reverts to spontaneous rhythm. These T wave inversions are secondary to pacing per se and not related to ischemia. These can occur even after very short duration of pacing.

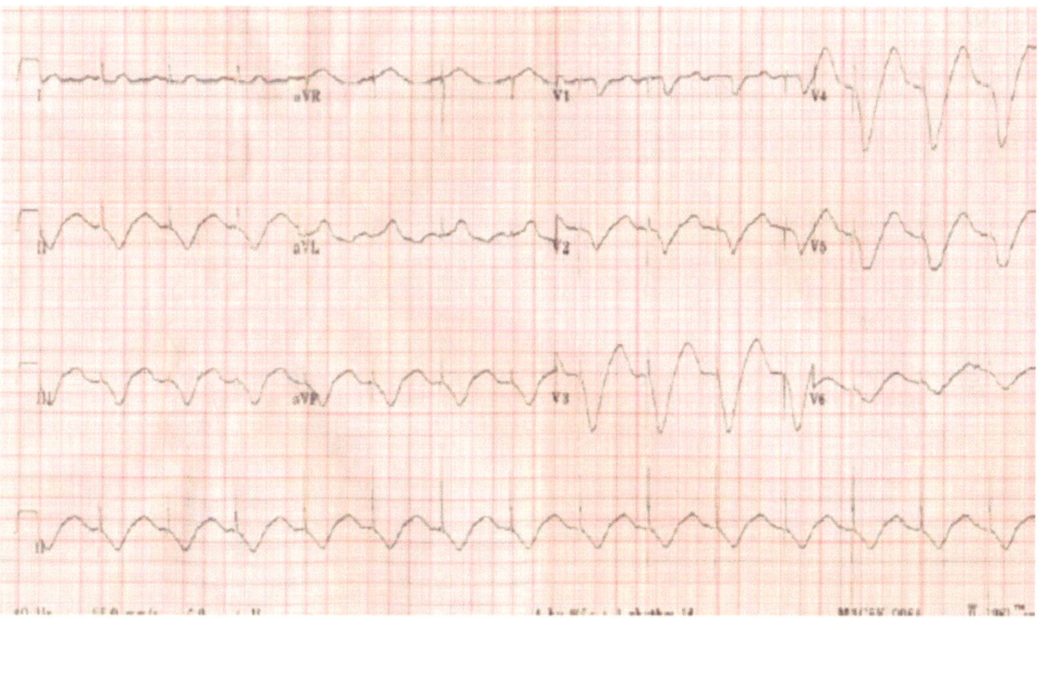

Fig. 1. ECG at presentation showing that all ventricular beats are paced. The pacing spike is followed by a wide QRS complex (QRS duration 300 milliseconds). The QRS complex is merging with T waves. No definite P waves are seen. (With permission, Bahl A et al, Indian Heart J 2009;61:93-4).

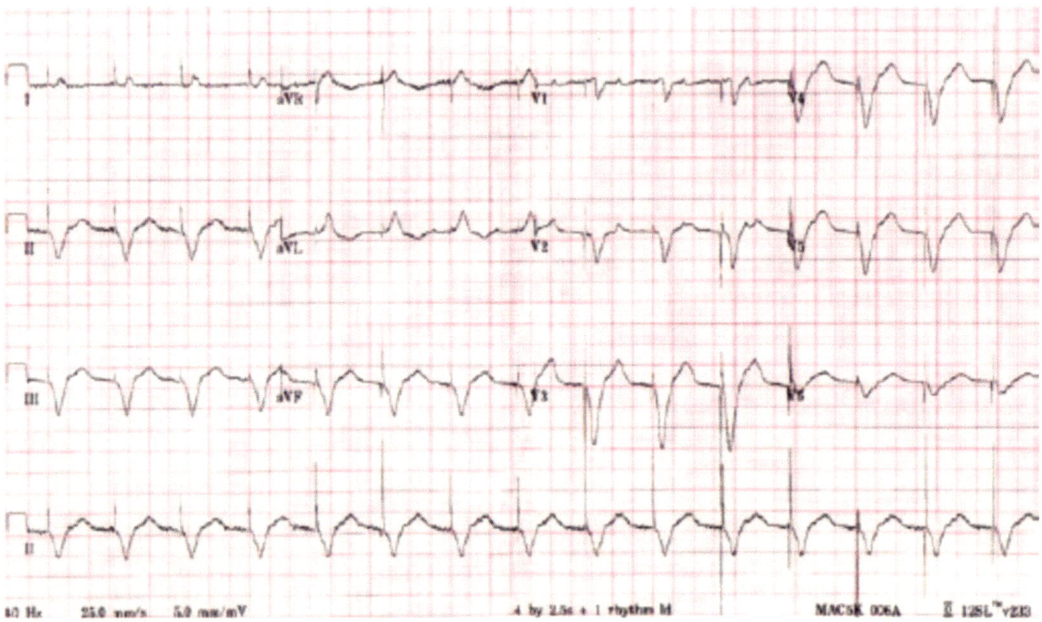

Fig. 2. ECG after correction of hyperkalemia. All ventricular beats are still paced but the QRS duration has narrowed to 190 milliseconds. The QRS complexes are greater in amplitude and the peaks are sharper in morphology. Definite P waves are seen in leads V1 and V2. (With permission, Bahl A et al, Indian Heart J 2009;61:93-4).

3. Widening of the QRS complex

Widening of the QRS complex is an important though non-specific sign in patients with paced rhythm. A baseline paced ECG is ideally required if this sign is to be used in clinical situations. QRS prolongation should trigger an alarm bell. Any observer during failed cardiopulmonary resuscitations in patients on temporary or permanent pacemakers would have noted gradual prolongation of the QRS complex with the passage of time. The QRS complex gradually becomes very wide and resembles a T wave. This is a poor prognostic sign and indicates progressive myocardial ischemia and dysfunction.

Studies using balloon inflation at time of percutaneous coronary intervention have shown that QRS prolongation could also be a marker of myocardial ischemia on the paced electrocardiogram.[6] In addition, electrolyte imbalance as in hyperkalemia could also result in QRS prolongation. Thus any change in QRS duration from baseline should be noted as it could be an important indicator of several pathologies.

4. Hyperkalemia

ECG is a useful guide in diagnosing hyperkalemia in patients in sinus rhythm. Initial change is usually a peaked T wave. This is followed by widening of QRS complexes, intraventricular conduction defects, prolongation of PR interval, absence of P wave, heart blocks, and the classical sine wave. This is because severe hyperkalemia decreases the phase 0 of the action potential resulting in widening of the QRS complex. The QRS complex continues to widen and ultimately blends with the T wave resulting in a sine wave morphology. Typical ECG changes of hyperkalemia can also be seen even during paced rhythm. These changes include QRS widening and reduction in amplitude of the QRS complex.[7,8] The QRS widening can be quite marked in some cases. These changes are especially well appreciated if an old ECG is available for comparison. Typical sine waves may also be seen on a paced ECG rhythm. These changes revert back to the baseline with correction of hyperkalemia. These ECG findings of hyperkalemia that reverted back to baseline after correction of hyperkalemia are illustrated in figures 1 and 2.

To summarize, a number of medical conditions are best diagnosed during paced rhythms when a baseline ECG is available. All patients with pacemakers should have a recorded baseline 12 lead ECG available. In case the patient with pacemaker has his own rhythm a 12 lead ECG with magnet should be kept as a taken. This would be available as a record of the paced rhythm in case the patient later becomes pacemaker dependant and has a continuously paced rhythm.

5. Acknowledgements

I thank the Honrary Editor, Indian Heart Journal for permission to use figures 1 and 2.

6. References

[1] Barold SS, Falkoff MD, Ong LS, Heinle RA. Electrocardiographic diagnosis of myocardial infarction during ventricular pacing. Cardiol Clin 1987;5:403–17.

[2] Barold SS, Herweg B, Curtis AB. Electrocardiographic diagnosis of myocardial infarction and ischemia during cardiac pacing. Cardiol Clin 2006;24:387–99.

[3] Sgarbossa EB, Pinski SL, Gates KB, Wagner GS. Early electrocardiographic diagnosis of acute myocardial infarction in the presence of ventricular paced rhythm. GUSTO-I Investigators. Am J Cardiol 1996;77:423-4.

[4] Brandt RR, Hammill SC, Higano ST. Electrocardiographic diagnosis of acute myocardial infarction during ventricular pacing. *Circulation* 1998;97:2274-5.

[5] Sgarbossa EB, Pinski SL, Barbagelata A, Underwood DA, Gates KB, Topol EJ, Califf RM, Wagner GS. Electrocardiographic diagnosis of evolving acute myocardial infarction in the presence of left bundle-branch block. GUSTO-1 (Global Utilization of Streptokinase and Tissue Plasminogen Activator for Occluded Coronary Arteries) Investigators. N Engl J Med. 1996;334:481-7.

[6] Kilic H, Atalar E, Ozer N, Ovunc K, Aksoyek S, Ozmen F, Akdemir R. Early electrocardiographic diagnosis of acute coronary ischemia on the paced electrocardiogram. International J Cardiol 2008;130:14-18.

[7] Bahl A, Swamy A, Jeevan H, Mahajan R, Talwar KK. ECG changes of hyperkalemia during paced rhythm. Indian Heart J 2009;61:93-4.

[8] Howard JA, Kosowsky BD. Electrocardiographic diagnosis of hyperkalemia in the presence of ventricular pacing and atrial fibrillation. Chest 1980;78:491-2.

6

Electrocardiograms in Acute Pericarditis

Anita Radhakrishnan and Jerome E. Granato
Department of Medicine and Division of Cardiology
West Penn Allegheny Health System, Pittsburgh
USA

1. Introduction

The pericardium surrounds the heart and consists of a visceral layer, which is contiguous with the epicardium of the heart, and a parietal layer, which forms a sac around the heart (Wann & Passen, 2008). Located between the parietal and visceral layers is a potential space called the pericardial cavity. The pericardial cavity normally contains as much as 50 mL of an ultrafiltrate of plasma. Anatomically, the pericardium isolates the heart from the rest of the mediastinum and thorax. Physiologically and under normal circumstances, the pericardium may have little if any significant role. The pericardial structure and function may be impacted by numerous pathologic conditions. Many of these conditions are listed in Table 1. A common and nonspecific condition affecting the pericardium is acute pericarditis. Acute pericarditis is a clinical syndrome that may present with chest pain, a pericardial friction rub, and gradual repolarization changes in the electrocardiogram (ECG). The diagnosis of acute pericarditis requires at least 2 of these 3 elements (Imazio et al, 2003)

2. Etiology of acute pericarditis

Infectious	Viral	Cocksacie A & B, Echovirus, Adenovirus, Mumps, Hepatitis, HIV
	Pyogenic	Pneumococcus, Streptococcus, Staphylococcus, Neisseria and Legionella
	Fungal	Histoplasmosis, Coccidiomycosis
	Other	Tuberculous, Syphilitic, Protozoal and Parasitic
Metabolic	Uremia/ Dialysis	
	Hypothyroidism	
Neoplasm	Primary or Metastatic Tumors	Primary tumors or tumors metastatic to the pericardium (lung, breast, lymphoma, and leukemia)
Trauma	Iatrogenic	Penetrating/Non-penetrating chest wall Post-irradiation, Post thoracic surgery, catheter or pacemaker perforation

Autoimmune	Sarcoidosis	
	Collagen Vascular Disorders	SLE, Rheumatoid Arthritis, Ankylosing Spondylitis, Scleroderma, Wegeners , Rheumatic Fever
Hypersensitivity	Drug Induced	Procainamide, Hydralazine, Phenytoin, INH, Minoxidil, Methysergide, Anticoagulation
Others	Acute Myocardial Infarction	Dresslers Pericarditis
	Aortic dissection	With leakage into the pericardial sac
	IBD	
	Syndromes	Loefflers Syndrome / Whipples Disease
	Familial	Familial Mediterranean Fever/Familial Pericarditis

Table 1. Causes of acute pericarditis (Zayas et al, 1995)

3. Clinical features

The chest pain associated with acute pericarditis is often described as severe, retrosternal, left sided precordial pain that is referred to the neck, arms, or the left shoulder. The pain is usually pleuritic, consequent to accompanying pleural inflammation and is characteristically, relieved by sitting up, leaning forward and may be intensified by lying supine (Troughten et al, 2004). The most specific sign of acute pericarditis is a pericardial friction rub, although it is intermittently present and often varies in intensity. It is characterized as a high-pitched scratchy sound and is heard best in end expiration and along the left sternal border with the patient leaning forward. A triple cadence is classically described, which coincides with atrial systole, ventricular systole, and rapid ventricular filling during early diastole. However, the triphasic rub occurs in only about half of patients. The origin of the sound has been attributed to the visceral and parietal layers of the pericardial sac rubbing together during different phases of the cardiac cycle (Spodick, 1975).

4. Diagnosis

4.1 Serum boimarkers

Laboratory testing for acute pericarditis is nonspecific and provides limited guidance in determining a cause. White blood cell count, erythrocyte sedimentation rate, and serum C-reactive protein level are modestly elevated in acute pericarditis regardless of the etiology. Surprisingly, a significant number of patients with pericarditis, with or without myocarditis or myocardial infarction have elevated creatinine kinase MB fraction and or troponin I values. This observation suggests that there is a significant incidence of silent myocarditis in patients who present with acute pericarditis (Imazio et al, 2003). If a particular etiology for pericarditis is suspected, the clinical presentation and associated co-morbid conditions should direct decisions for additional laboratory studies, such as rheumatoid factor, cardiac enzymes, antinuclear antibodies, or sputum samples to assess for mycobacteria.

4.2 Electrocardiography

The ECG is a rapid, inexpensive and noninvasive test that can be very useful in establishing the diagnosis of acute pericarditis. In one study, 90% of patients with the diagnosis of acute pericarditis are found to have ECG changes (Marinella, 1998). The electrocardiogaphic patterns of acute pericarditis were first reported in 1929 by Scott, Feil and Katz. They described transitory elevation of the ST segments in all three limb leads of the electrocardiogram in a case of hemopericardium and in one of purulent pericarditis (Veer and Norris 1937). Since then, the diagnosis of pericarditis is often times made with ECG changes.

In acute pericarditis, the observed electrocardiographic changes are a direct result of the inflammatory process taking place between the pericardial layers. The electrocardiogram is altered because of the extension of the inflammatory process to the sub epicardial myocardium (Bonow et al, 2008). The two classical ECG findings of acute pericarditis are ST elevation and PR depression. Elevation of the ST segment is the most sensitive and most consistent ECG finding. Typically the ST elevation is usually 1.0 - 2.0 mm and may be present in the majority of the standard ECG leads. The exception to this observation may be seen in leads AVR and V1 where the ST segment is always depressed (Koos et al, 2009). The morphology of the ST segment elevation in acute pericarditis is characteristically concave

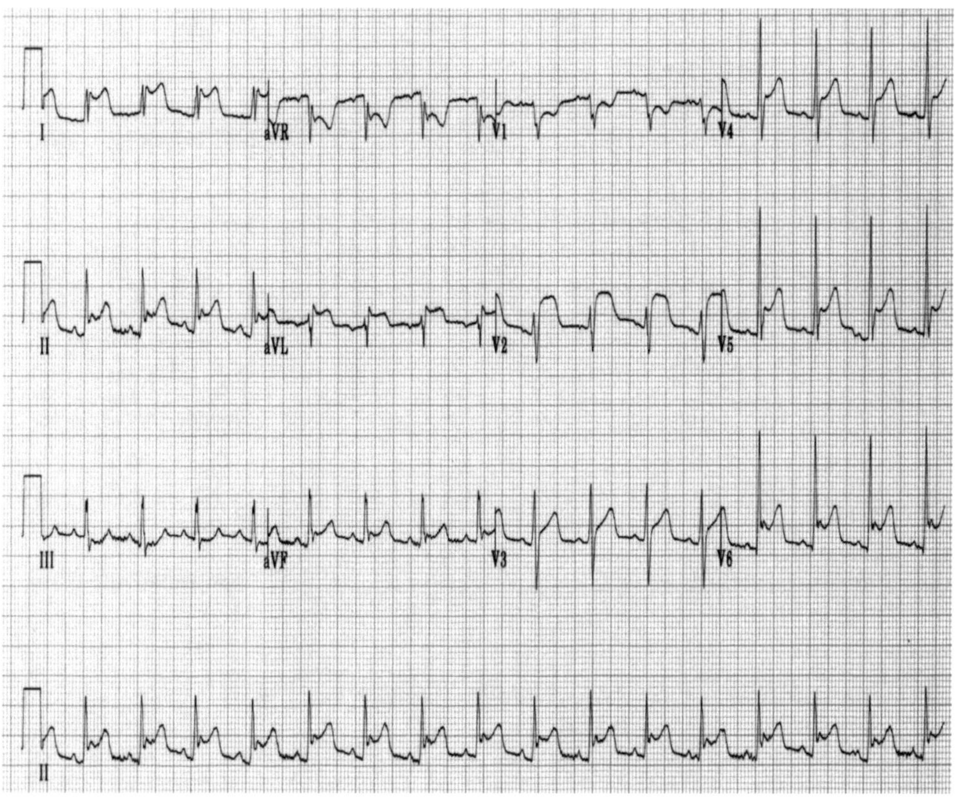

Fig. 1. An electrocardiogram in acute pericarditis showing diffuse up sloping ST segment elevations seen best here in leads II, AVL, AVF and V2 to V6. There is also subtle PR segment deviation (positive in aVR, negative in most other leads) (Hewitt el al, 2010)

and facing upwards. Some causes of pericarditis do not result in significant inflammation of the epicardium and may not be associated with the typical ECG changes. An illustration of this is uremic pericarditis, in which there is prominent fibrin deposition but little or no epicardial inflammation. As a result, the ECG usually does not exhibit the previously described ECG changes (Rutsky & Rostand, 1989). The ST segment elevations observed with acute pericarditis are often transient and are sometimes followed (after a variable time) by diffuses T wave inversions. The T wave inversions are also transient and may resolve completely with time (Maisch et al, 2004). Accordingly, there are some patients with clinical signs and symptoms of pericarditis, yet have a normal or non specific pattern on ECG. In the majority of patients, however, some electrocardiographic abnormality persists for an extended period of time. This is usually in the form of persistent T wave inversion (especially chronic pericarditis syndromes) (Maisch et al, 2004). The PR segment depression is another electrocardiographic sign of acute pericarditis. It is a very specific sign and is attributed to subepicardial atrial injury and is visible in all leads except aVR and V1. Conversely, these leads may exhibit PR-segment elevation as a manifestation of atrial wall inflammation (Hurst 2006). Thus, in acute pericarditis, the PR and ST segments typically change in opposite directions.

In acute pericarditis, the observed ECG changes typically evolve in four stages. Although all cases of pericarditis may not include each of these stages, as many as 50% do (Spodick, 2003) . The typical evolution of ECG changes in pericarditis is described below in Tables 2-5.

Stage	**Time of Onset**	**Classical ECG Findings**	**Illustration**
Stage 1	Hours to days	• Diffuse concave ST elevation with reciprocal ST depression in AVR and V1 • PR segment elevation in lead AVR • Depression of the PR segment in all other limb leads	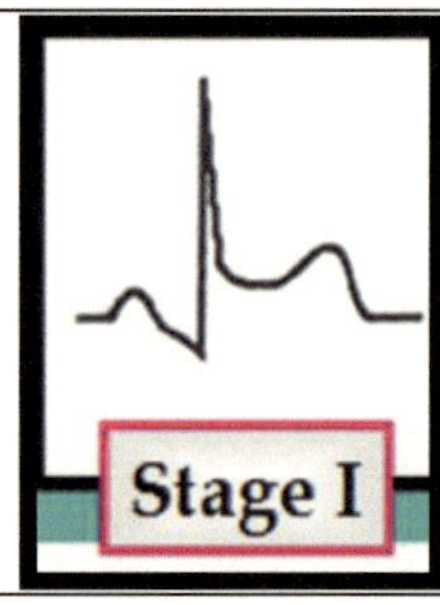

Table 2. Stage 1 of pericarditis

Stage	**Time of Onset**	**Classical ECG findings**	**Illustration**
Stage 2	Within 1st week	• Normalization of ST segments, with J point returning to normal • T wave amplitude begin to decrease	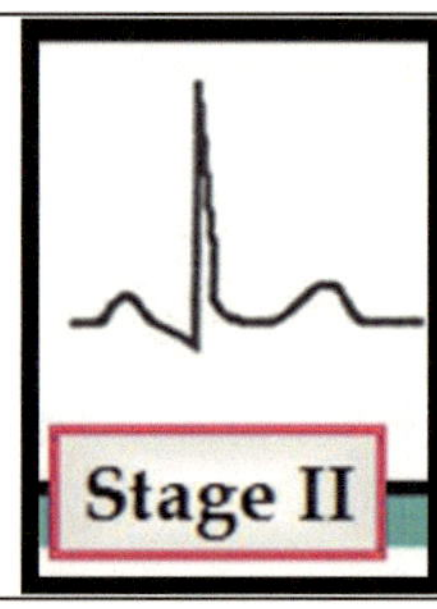

Table 3. Stage 2 of pericarditis

Stage	Time of Onset	Classic ECG Finding	Illustration
Stage 3	2-3 Weeks	• Diffuse T wave inversions, generally after the ST segments have become isoelectric	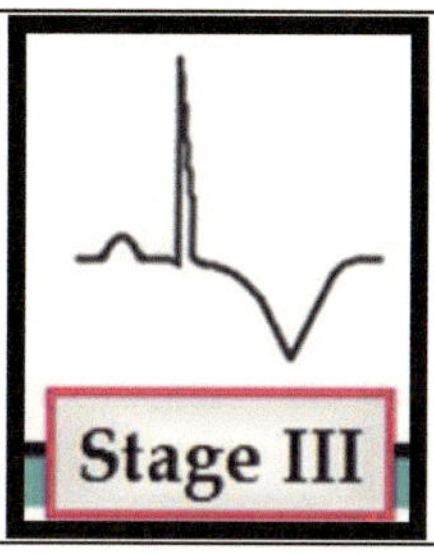

Table 4. Stage 3 of pericarditis

Stage	Time of Onset	Classic ECG Finding	Illustration
Stage 4	Up to 3 months	• Normalization of the ECG or • Indefinite persistence of T wave inversions ("chronic" pericarditis)	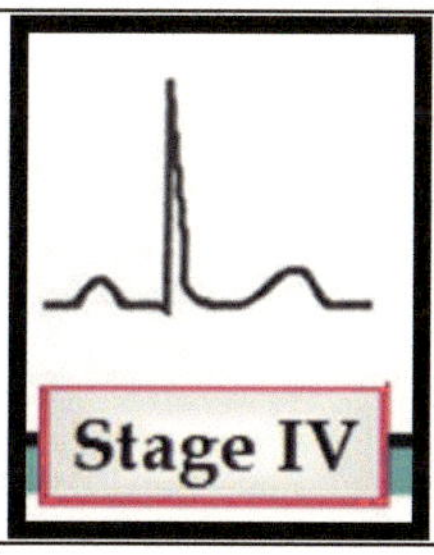

Table 5. Stage 4 of pericarditis

The ECG findings of acute pericarditis can often times be both subtle and confusing. In evaluating patients with chest discomfort and an abnormal ECG, there are other conditions that may mimic acute pericarditis and must be considered as well. These include an acute myocardial infarction and the early pattern of repolarization. Table 6 lists useful clues in differentiating acute pericarditis from these conditions.

While both acute pericarditis and acute myocardial infarction can present with chest pain and elevations in cardiac biomarkers, the electrocardiographic changes in acute pericarditis differ from those in ST elevation myocardial infarctions (STEMI) in several ways.

- Morphology – The ST segment elevation in acute pericarditis begins at the J point, which represents the junction between the end of the QRS complex and the beginning of the ST segment. The ST segment elevation rarely exceeds 5 mm, and usually retains its normal concavity. In contrast the typical finding in a STEMI presentation is convex (dome-shaped) ST elevation that may be more than 5 mm in height (Surawicz & Knilans, 2008).
- Distribution – ST segment elevations in infarction are characteristically limited to anatomical groupings of leads that correspond to the localized vascular area of the infarct (anteroseptal and anterior leads V1 to V4; lateral leads I, aVL, V5, V6; inferior leads II, III, aVF). The pericardium envelops the heart therefore the ST changes are more generalized and typically are present in most leads in pericarditis.
- Reciprocal changes – STEMI is often associated with reciprocal ST segment changes, which are not seen with pericarditis except in leads aVR and V1.

ECG Findings	Acute Pericarditis	Myocardial Infarction	Early Repolarization
ST Segment Change	Concave upward	Convex upward	Concave upward
Q waves	Absent	Present	Absent
Reciprocal ST changes	Absent	Present	Absent
Location of ST elevation	Limb and precordial leads	Area of involved artery	Precordial Leads
ST/T ratio in lead V6	>0.25	N/A	<0.25
Loss of R wave voltage	Absent	Present	Absent
PR segment depression	Present	Absent	Absent
Illustrative Example	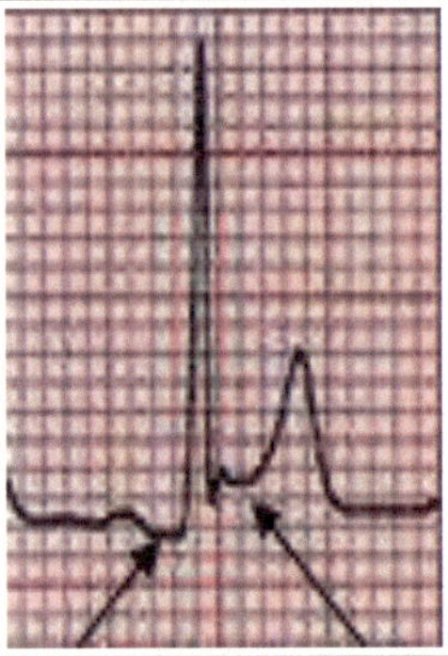	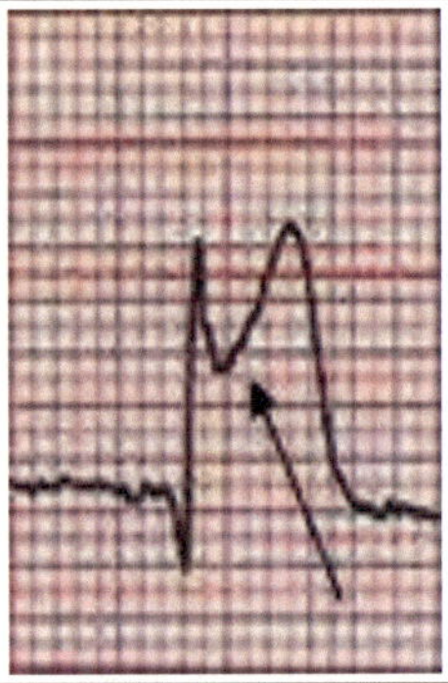	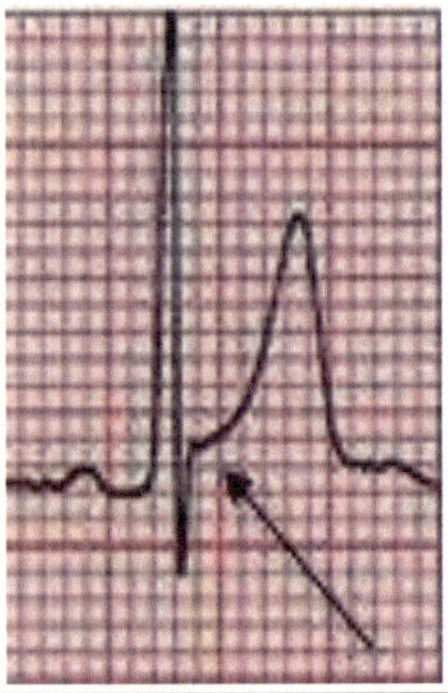

Table 6. A comparison of ECG's in acute pericarditis, acute myocardial infarction and early repolarization.

- Concurrent ST and T wave changes – ST segment elevation and T wave inversions do not generally occur simultaneously in pericarditis, while they commonly coexist in a STEMI. Peaked T waves (>10mm high in precordial leads, >5 mm high in limb leads), can be seen in STEMI but are not typical of pericarditis (Surawicz & Knilans, 2008).
- Q waves – Pathologic Q waves, which may occur with extensive injury in STEMI, are generally not seen in pericarditis. The abnormal Q waves in MI reflect the loss of positive depolarization voltages because of transmural myocardial necrosis. Pericarditis, on the other hand, generally causes only superficial inflammation. Abnormal Q waves are not seen unless there is concomitant myocarditis or preexisting cardiomyopathy or myocardial infarction (Imazio, 2011).
- PR segment – PR elevation in aVR with PR depression in other leads due to a concomitant atrial current of injury is frequently seen in acute pericarditis but rarely seen in acute STEMI.
- QT prolongation – Prolongation of the QT interval with regional T wave inversion (in the absence of drug effects or relevant metabolic disorders) favors the diagnosis of myocardial ischemia (or myopericarditis) over pericarditis alone (Marinella, 2008).

The early repolarization variant seen on an ECG may be present in as many as 30% of young adults and is often confused with acute pericarditis (Klatskey et al, 2003). The following electrocardiographic features can be helpful in distinguishing acute pericarditis from early repolarization:

- ST elevations occur in both the limb and precordial leads in most cases of acute pericarditis (47 of 48 in one study), whereas about one-half of subjects with early repolarization have no ST deviations in the limb leads . In early repolarization, ST elevation is most often present in the anterior and lateral chest leads (V3-V6), although other leads can be involved (Spodick, 1976).
- PR deviation and evolution of the ST and T changes strongly favor pericarditis, as neither is seen in early repolarization(Ginzton & Laks, 1972)

While uncommon, one of the most feared seqealae of acute pericarditis is the progression to cardiac tamponade. Cardiac tamponade is the result of the accumulation of fluid in the pericardial space to the point that it causes obstruction to the inflow of blood to the heart. This condition, if not recognized and treated promptly, is often fatal. The most common ECG sign of a large pericardial effusion is low voltage of the QRS complexes. This finding is most likely due to the attenuation of cardiac potentials caused by the fluid surrounding the heart as well as inflammatory mechanisms affecting the pericardium and myocardium (Brusch et al, 2001). Low voltage on the ECG (Figure 2) is said to be present when the cumulative amplitude of the QRS complexes in each of the six limb leads is 5 mm (0.5 mV) or less (Luenn et al, 2006). Another ECG pattern that may be observed in patients with a large pericardial effusion is total electrical alternans (Figure 3). The pattern of electrical alternans is characterized by a cyclic beat-to-beat variation in the QRS axis in the limb and precordial leads. This is a direct result of the beat to beat movement of the heart, both to and fro, that can occur in the presence of a large pericardial effusion (Billakanty and Bashir , 2006). The observations of electrical alternans with low QRS voltage and sinus tachycardia is a highly specific sign of pericardial effusion. Unfortunately, this triad of observations is only modestly sensitive in that there may be situation where larger pericardial effusion is present and some or all of these findings are absent.

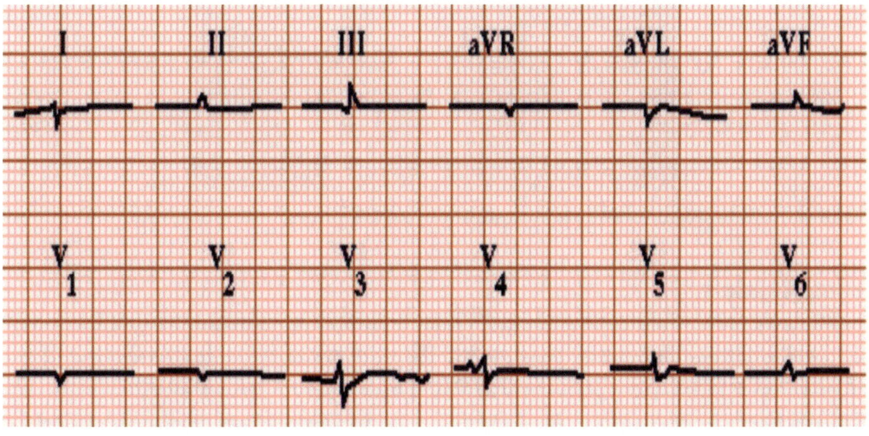

Fig. 2. An ECG in a patient with a large pericardial effusion. Note the presence of low voltage QRS in all leads.

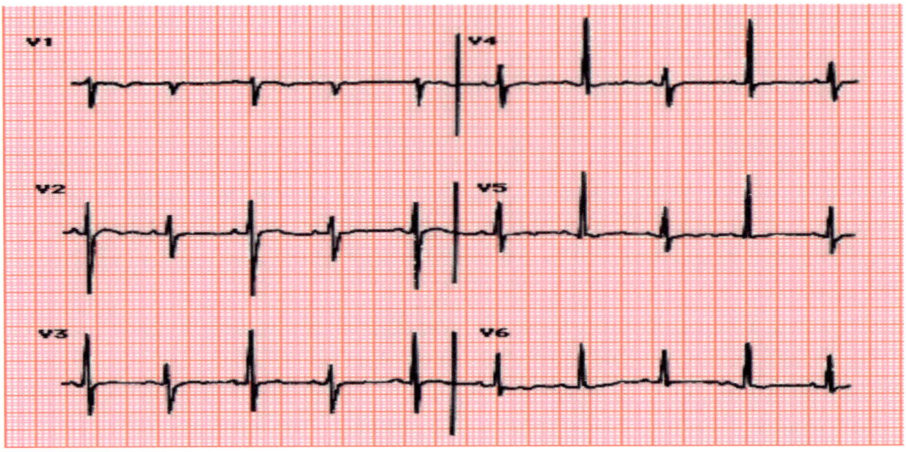

Fig. 3. An ECG in a patient with a large pericardial effusion. Note the alternating QRS axis in all precordial leads.

4.3 Chest radiograph

The chest radiograph is usually normal in uncomplicated acute idiopathic pericarditis. It is frequently useful to exclude pathology in the mediastinum or lung fields that may be the cause of pericarditis, such as thoracic malignancy or infection. A pericardial effusion should be suspected when cardiomegaly is observed and the cardiac silhouette takes on a symmetric "flask like" appearance, shown in Figure 4. (Spodick, 2003).

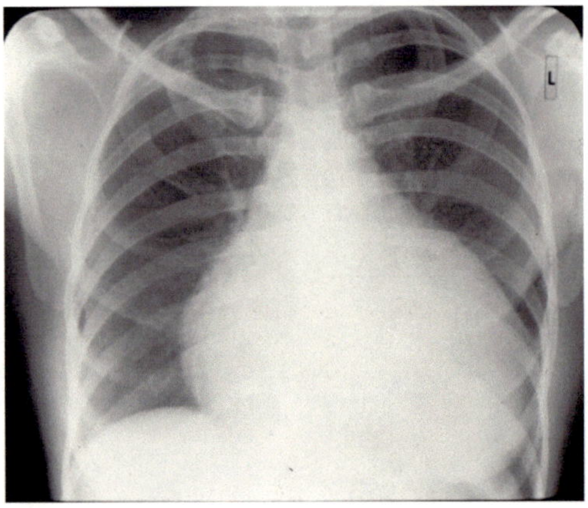

Fig. 4. Chest X ray suggestive of a large pericardial effusion.

4.4 Echocardiography

The transthoracic echocardiography (TTE) is frequently normal in patients with acute idiopathic pericarditis. The main reason for its performance is for assessing the size and nature of any associated pericardial effusion. The observation of fibrin strand within the pericardial effusion is indicative of a pericardial inflammatory response (Verhaert et al, 2010). Transthoracic echocardiography is also essential in evaluating for presence or absence cardiac tamponade. This physiologic condition may be recognized by collapse of the right atrium or right ventricle during diastole or marked variation in the transmitral and transpulmonary valve velocity profiled with respiration (Fowler 1993). In one series of 300 consecutive patients with acute pericarditis, pericardial effusion was present in 180 patients (60%). In most cases the effusion was small or moderate in size without hemodynamic consequences. Cardiac tamponade was present in only 5% of patients (Imazio et al, 2004). TTE is not needed in every patient with pericarditis, it is recommended in patients with clinical features that would suggest the presence of a systemic disorder. These might include prolonged fever, an immunocompromised state, recent trauma, elevation of cardiac enzymes greater than 2 weeks, and abnormal chest x-ray or clinical signs of cardiac tamponade. (Imazio et al, 2004, 2007)

4.5 CT/MRI

The presence of pericardial fluid or thickening may be confirmed by a CT or MRI scan. These techniques may be superior to echocardiography in detecting loculated pericardial effusions, pericardial thickening presence of pericardial masses or any associated intrathoracic pathology (Verhaert et al, 2010). Neither CT nor MRI scanning however is needed to establish the diagnosis of pericarditis. Rather, these studies are generally reserved the evaluation of other pathologic conditions which may be the cause of pericarditis.

5. Treatment

The foundation of treatment for pericarditis is to reduce and ultimately eliminate the inflammatory process that exists between the pericardial layers. For patients with idiopathic pericarditis, nonsteroidal anti-inflammatory drugs (NSAIDs) should be used with the goal of relieving chest pain, inflammation, and fever. Aspirin, ibuprofen, and indomethacin are the most commonly prescribed NSAIDs. Ibuprofen may be preferred given its reportedly lower incidence of side effects compared to the other medications. (Zayas et al, 1995) Indomethacin is an acceptable alternative, but it should be avoided in patients with coronary artery disease because of its adverse effects on coronary blood flow and blood pressure (Maisch et al, 2004). Aspirin is favored in patients with a recent history of myocardial infarction since other NSAIDs tend to impede scar formation (Hammerman et al, 1984). The use of NSAIDs in the setting of acute myocardial infarction has been associated with an increased incidence of ventricular aneurysm formation and cardiac rupture (Imazio et al, 2004). Patients who respond slowly or inadequately to NSAIDS may require supplementary narcotic analgesics and or a brief course of colchicine or steroids. In cases where the etiology of pericarditis has been identified, treatment should be focused on the underlying cause. For patients who have chronic kidney failure, increasing the frequency of dialysis usually results in improvement in the signs and symptoms of uremic pericarditis. Patients who have cancer may show some response to chemotherapy or radiation therapy. For purulent pericarditis related to a bacterial or fungal process, treatment consists of antimicrobials and surgical drainage of purulent material from the pericardium space. For patients with pericardial effusion causing a tamponade, drainage of the effusion is indicated. Needle pericardiocentesis, via a sub xiphoid approach, is effective in most medical patients with cardiac tamponade when the effusion is circumferential and moderately large (Imazio et al, 2007).

6. Follow-up

Most cases of acute pericarditis subside within 2 weeks. In approximately 15%of cases, symptoms may recur (Marinella, 1998). This is particularly true if the pericarditis is related to an ongoing and underlying illness such as an autoimmune disease or uremia. Typically, physicians should schedule a follow-up visit with these patients two weeks after the onset of their illness unless additional symptoms or medication related problems intervene. An ECG should also be considered at four weeks, bearing in mind that residual T-wave inversion may be present for several weeks during stage III of acute pericarditis.

7. Conclusion

In conclusion, acute pericarditis can be caused by many underlying conditions. Acute pericarditis can be diagnosed clinically with when associated with chest pain, pericardial friction rub and typical ECG changes. The ECG changes associated with acute pericarditis have been described as evolving through four stages including PR segment depression, ST segment elevation, T wave inversion and eventual normalization. Certain features of the ECG can help in differentiate the diagnosis of pericarditis from acute myocardial infarction or early repolarization, though this differentiation may be difficult. Treatment should be focused on the relief of symptoms and specific to any underlying cause. For patients with idiopathic pericarditis, NSAIDs are typically most effective. The prognosis associated with acute pericarditis is very good. Prompt recognition and treatment of this condition may prevent its progression to more serious complications.

8. Acknowledgments

Words alone cannot express the thanks I owe to Chocku Radhakrishnan, my husband and Mrs. Valli Radhakrishnan, my mother-in-law for their encouragement, patience and support while I wrote this paper. I would like to express gratitude to my father Mr. Ramanathan Vairavan who has encouraged me to work hard and efficiently and has always had a special interest in my personal growth. And last but not least I would like to thank my mother, Mrs. Alagu Vairavan for reminding me everyday that her love is absolutely unconditional.

9. References

Billakanty Sreedhar, MD; Riyaz Bashir, MD Echocardiographic Demonstration of Electrical Alternans *JAMA. 1976;235(1):39-41.*

Bonow Robert, Mann Douglas, Libby Peter, and Zipes Douglas.(2008)

Braunwald's Heart Disease: A Textbook of Cardiovascular Medicine. Sunders 8th ed. 2008. Pages 1076-1078

Borys Surawicz, MD, MACC and Timothy Knilans, MD, (2008) Chou's Electrocardiography in Clinical Practice, 6th Edition, 2008 pages 235-236

Bruch C, Schmermund A, Dagres N, et al. Changes in QRS voltage in cardiac tamponade and pericardial effusion: reversibility after pericardiocentesis and after anti-inflammatory drug treatment. J Am Coll Cardiol 2001; 38:219.

Fowler No. Cardiac tamponade. (1993)A clinical or an echocardiographic diagnosis? Circulation, Vol 87, 1738-1741

Ginzton LE, Laks MM. The differential diagnosis of acute pericarditis from the normal variant: new electrocardiographic criteria. Circulation 1982; 65:1004.

Hammerman H, Alker KJ, Schoen FJ, Kloner RA. Morphologic and functional effects of piroxicam on myocardial scar formation after coronary occlusion in dogs. Am J Cardiol 1984; 53:604.

Hurst J. Willis, MD, MACP. (2006) The Interpretation of Electrocardiograms: Pretense or a Well-Developed Skill? Cardiol Clin 24 (2006) 305–307

Imazio M, Demichelis B, Cecchi E, et al.(2003) Cardiac troponin I in acute pericarditis. J Am Coll Cardiol 2003; 42:2144.

Imazio M, Cecchi E, Demichelis B, et al. Indicators of poor prognosis of acute pericarditis. Circulation 2007; 115:2739.

Klatsky AL, Oehm R, Cooper RA, et al. The early repolarization normal variant electrocardiogram: correlates and consequences. Am J Med 2003; 115:171.

Koos R, Schröder J, Kühl HP. (2009)Acute viral pericarditis without typical electrocardiographic changes assessed by cardiac magnetic resonance imaging. Eur Heart J. 2009 Dec; 30(23):2844.

Luen James Yip Wei, MBBS, MRCP, Lim Yean Teng, MBBS, MRCP, Tan Huay Cheem, MBBS, M MED, Chia Boon Lock, MBBS, FRACPDiscordant Limb-Lead and Precordial-Lead QRS Voltages in Inferior Myocardial Infarction

Circulation. 2006;113:e866-e868.

Maisch B, Seferovic PM, Ristic AD, Erbel R, Rienmüller R, Adler Y, Tomkowski WZ, Thiene G, Yacoub MH. Guidelines on the diagnosis and management of pericardial diseases executive summary; the Task Force on the Diagnosis and Management of Pericardial Diseases of the European Society of Cardiology. Eur Heart J 2004; 25:587.

Marinella Mark, M.D,(1998) Electrocardiographic Manifestations and Differential Diagnosis of Acute Pericarditis American Family Physician Volume 14, Issue 1, July 1998, Pages 31-50

Rutsky, EA, Rostand, SG.(1989) Pericarditis in end-stage renal disease: Clinical characteristics and management. Semin Dialysis 1989; 2:25

Spodick DH. (1975) Pericardial rub. Prospective, Multiple observer investigation of pericardial friction in 100 patients. Am J Cardiol 1975; 35:357.

Spodick DH. Acute pericarditis: current concepts and practice. JAMA 2003; 289:1150.

Spodick DH. Differential characteristics of the electrocardiogram in early repolarization and acute pericarditis. N Engl J Med 1976; 295:523.

Troughton RW, Asher CR, Klein AL. (2004) Pericarditis. Lancet 2004; 363:717.

Veer, Joseph B. Vander M.D., Robert F. Norris M.D. (1937) The electrocardiographic changes in acute pericarditis: A clinical and pathological study. American Heart Journal. Volume 14, Issue 1, July 1937, Pages 31-50

Verhaert David, MD, Ruvin S. Gabriel, MBChB, The Role of Multimodality Imaging in the Management of Pericardial Disease Circulation: Cardiovascular Imaging. 2010; 3: 333-343

Wann Samuel, Edward Passen. (2008) Echocardiography in Pericardial Disease. Journal of the American Society of Echocardiography. Volume 21, Issue 1, Pages 7-13.

Zayas R, Anguita M, Torres F, et al. (1993) Incidence of specific etiology and role of methods for specific etiologic diagnosis of primary acute pericarditis. Am J Cardiol 1995; 75:378.

7

The Remodeling of Connexins Localized at Pulmonary Vein – Left Atria in Triggering and Maintenance of Atrial Fibrillation

Guo-qiang Zhong[1], Ri-xin Xiong, Hong-xing Song,
Yun Ling, Jing-chang Zhang and Zhe Wei
The Department of Cardiology, The First Affiliated Hospital of Guangxi Medical University,
[1]The Department of Cardiology, The People's Hospital of Guangxi Zhuang Autonomous Region,
China

1. Introduction

Atrial fibrillation is the most common sustained arrhythmia and the major cardiac cause of stroke (Sellers & Newby, 2011). Recent studies in patients and animals with paroxysmal atrial fibrillation had shown that the arrhythmia was triggered by focal sources from muscular sleeves originated in the left atria extending into pulmonary veins (Date et al.,2007; Chen et al.,2001; Patterson et al., 2007; Honjo et al., 2003). What is more, the autonomic nervous system has a crucial role in the genesis, maintenance and abruption of atrial fibrillation (Duffy& Wit, 2008; Sandres et al.,2004), and there is a fat pad localized in superior vena cava and the root of aorta as the origin of cardiac nerve, being called SVC-Ao fat pad (Kapa et al.,2010; Volders ,2010; Ji et al.,2010). The mechanism of atrial fibrillation involves multiple effects (Chiou et al.,1997; Tsuboi et al.,2000; Hoffmann et al., 2006; Haissaguerre et al.1998; Wit & Boyden,2007), the expression of connexins is changed and is associated with increased propensity for arrhythmias (Kanagaratnam et al., 2002, Herve et al., 2007, Stergiopoulos et al., 1999, Verheule S et al., 2002, Kanagaratnam et al., 2007; Valiunas et al.,2001; Valiunas et al.,2000; Cottrell et al.,2002; Elenes et al.,1999). Pulmonary veins and left atria are the primary structure of genesis, persistence of atrial fibrillation. Vagus nerve plays a key role in the initiation and maintenance of atrial fibrillation, it can mediate the electrical remodeling of atria and pulmonary vein, enhance the maintenance and stability of atrial fibrillation,. However, these effects can be inhibited by avianizing vagus nerve.

2. Overview of gap junction structure

The name "gap junction" was cioned from their appearance in electron micrographs in the 60s (Revel & Karnovsky, 1967). They are specialized at cell-cell contact regions that contain tens to thousands of intercellular channels that link two apposed cells. These channels facilitate a form of intercellular communication by permitting the regulated passage of ions and small molecules from one cell to another (Bennett & Goodenough, 1978). The gap junction

membrane channel is composed of macular aggregations of intercellular channels permitting the direct intercellular transfer of ions and small molecules. Each intercellular channel is formed by the apposition of two hexameric transmembrane channels (connexons), one from each cell (Yeager & Gilula, 1992). Each intercellular channel is composed of two oligomers with each of two adjacent tissue cells contributing one oligomer. Each connexon is built from six copies of one or more members of a protein family called the connexins (Unger et al., 1999; Perkins et al., 1998). The functional cell-cell channel is formed by the end-to-end docking of the extracellular domains of the two connexons. Therefore, the gap junction membrane channel can be thought of as a dimmer of two hexamers joined together in the gap region. In this manner, the membrane channel extends across both cell membranes.
Vertebrate gap junction channels are assembled to form multimers of one or more different proteins from a multigene family of homologous protein, which are composed of an entirely different gene family but the sequences predict a similar folding pattern. Up to now, more than 20 different connexin genes have been identified in the mouse genome and at least 6 others have been identified in other vertebrates. Connexins are highly homologous proteins with 50%-80% identity between amino acid sequences and display considerable amino acid sequences conservation between species. The distribution and developmental regulation of connexins are tissue specific. The predicted molecular mass of the connexin protein family ranges from ~26 to ~60KDa, and the proteins are named "connexin" followed by their predicted molecular mass. The connexin family can be subdivided into two classifications called α and β based on similarities in certain regions of the primary sequence. The x-ray diffraction analysis by Tibbitts etal. (1990) indicated that there was more α-helical content that could be accounted for by four transmembrane helices. The El and E2 loops are thought to be as rigid as the transmembrane domain (Hoh et al., 1993; Sosinsky, 1992). Hence, the extracellular region is visible with the crystallographic averaging used. Each extracellular protrusion may therefore include an extension of the intramembrane α-helical structure (Tibbitts et al., 1990). Mutagenesis studies have suggested that the extracellular loops contain disulfide-bonded β-sheet conformation (Foote & Nicholson, 1997), which would be expected to act as a rigid domain, for instance, connexin43 (isolated from heart tissue, Yeager & Gilula, 1992), connexin32 and connexin 26 (isolated from liver tissue, Fallon & Goodenough, 1981; Hertzberg, 1984) would be seen for the same structure . In the human heart, 4 main isoforms are expressed. Connexin43 is expressed in all chambers of the heart, but predominantly in the ventricles. Connexin45 is found in the conduction system of the heart and at low levels in the atrial and ventricular working myocardium and connexin37 is located in the endothelial gap junctions in many vessels. Finally, connexin40 is expressed mainly in the atrial working myocardium, the conduction system, and the vasculature. Connexin40 was first described in a range of animal species and subsequently mapped to human chromosome. It became apparent that connexin40 was expressed in the atrioventricular conduction system and abundantly expressed in the atrial but not in the ventricular gap junctions. Recently, a new connexin was described in the mouse heart, i.e. connexin30.2 (the human equivalent is connexin31.9), which in mice seems responsible for slowing of impulse conduction in the atrioventricular node. However, the role of connexin31.9 in the human heart is unclear, for it is not detectable in the human cardiac conduction system. Connexons formed the functional intercellular channel, which is defined as homotypic when the connexin composition of the contributing connexons is identical or heterotypic when different. The ability of connexins to form homomeric/ heterotypic channels has been examined in the Xenopus oocyte and HeLa

cell expression systems as well as in other settings. Connexin43 and connexin40 are co-expressed in several tissues, including cardiac atrial and ventricular myocytes and vascular smooth muscle. It has been shown that these connexins form functional homomeric/homotypic channels with distinct permeability and gating properties.

3. Connexon and the heart development

In the certebrate embryo, a single outflow vessel initially develops from the common ventricules undergo septation to form the four-chamber heart (Kirby & Waldo, 1995). The four-chambered heart develops from a single straight tube composed of three layers: an inner endocardium and outer myocardium separated by a thick extracellular matrix called cardiac jelly. The growing tube loops, with the convexity of the loop demarcating a functional inflow from an outflow portion of the looped tube. This original convexity forms the two ventricles by expansion and septation, and as the ventricular septum forms, the inflow and outflow must be redefined. Initially, all of the inflow is through the atrioventricular canal connecting a common atrium to the presumptive left ventricle; the entire outflow is from the presumptive right ventricle into the aortic sac via the conotruncus. Several septa are formed simultaneously, making a rearrangement of inflow and outflow critical. The atrioventricular canal is divided into left and right channels, the nascent right and left ventricles are separated by the ventricular septum, the conotruncus is converted into aortic vestibule and semilunar valve continuous with the left ventricle, and the pulmonary infundibulum and semilunar valve originating from the right ventricle (see Fig1.). Concomitantly, the outflow tract septates and rotates to generate the pulmonary and

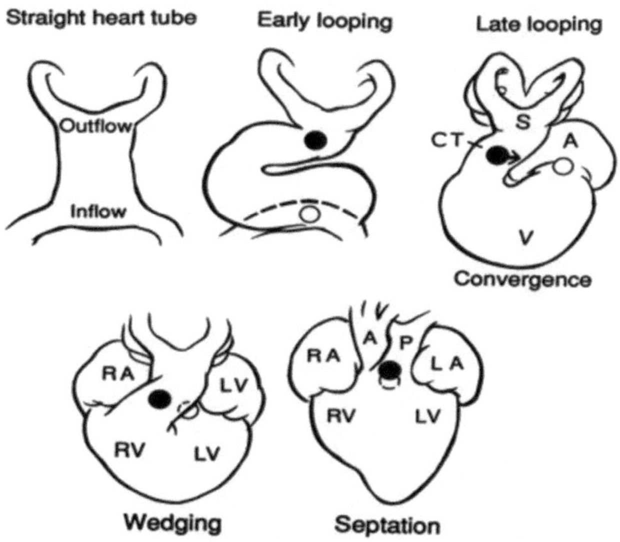

Fig. 1. Major events in development of the heart from a single straight tube. Early looping is probably a function of the myocardium. Convergence of the outflow and inflow tracts occurs during late looping and is critical for normal wedging. Wedging produces alignment of the three components that complete outflow septation. A, aorta; V, ventricle; P, pulmonary trunk; RA, right atrium; LA, left atrium; RV, right ventricle; LV, left ventricle.

aortic outflow tracts, becoming connected to the right and left ventricular chambers, respectively. This morphogenetic sequence is significantly affected by the activity of neural crest cells. With the development of heart, the co-expression of multiple connexins in diverse tissues support the idea that communication between cells does not depend on just one type of connexin, which results in forming heterotypic channels with properties different from those homotypic parental connexons.

Pluripotent mammalian embryonic stem cells, which are derived from the inner cell mass of preimplantation blastocysts, have the capacity to differentiate into cells of all three germ layers. Under suitable conditions, embryonic stem cells remain pluripotent through repeated rounds of cell division in culture. The recent isolation of human embryonic stem cells has spurred great interest in their potential use for therapeutic tissue repair because appropriate manipulation of the culture environment can induce both mouse and human embryonic stem cells to differentiate in vitro into specific somatic cell types, and the result shows human embryonic stem cells express RNA encoding most of the known human connexin genes. The mRNA of Cx25, Cx26, Cx30.3, Cx31, Cx31.1, Cx31.9, Cx37, Cx40, Cx43, Cx45, and Cx46 for all of the undifferentiated human embryonic stem cultures that were detected. The remaining connexins (Cx30, Cx30.2, Cx32, Cx36, Cx47, Cx59, and Cx62) were also reliably detected (Rackauskas et al., 2010).

4. Cardiac electrical properties of connexins and the methods for detection

For effective cardiac output, it is essential that electrical excitation spread rapidly throughout the atria and ventricles. This is effected by electrical coupling through gap junction channels at contact sites between myocytes (Danik te al., 2008; Harris, 2001; Söhl & Willecke, 2004; Moreno, 2004). These channels form a low-resistance pathway between adjacent myocytes and consist of connexin proteins. The connexin family is a large multigene family, and the channels formed by different members of this family have distinct electrical and regulatory properties (Reisner et al., 2009; Gros & Jongsma, 1996; Verheijck et al., 2001; Valiunas et al., 2002). Voltage sensitivity is particularly important in regulating the intercellular coupling between excitable cells. Cx43 channels are relatively insensitive to changes in transjunctional voltage compared with channels composed of Cx45 (Rackauskas et al., 2007; Bruzzone et al., 1993; Haubrich et al., 1996). Each gap junction composing hemichannel contains two Vj sensitive gates. The fast gate is located at the cytoplasmic entrance of hemichannels and operates from open to residual state. The slow, or "loop" gate is located toward extracellular ends of hemichannels and exhibits slow gating transition to the fully closed state. Cx26, Cx30, Cx50 close at positive voltages, and Cx31, Cx32, Cx37, Cx40, Cx43, Cx45, Cx57 at negative. Interestingly, Cx46 hemichannels close at both, positive and negative voltages. Besides, each type of connexon has a certain sensitivity to H^+, it is showed the order of decreasing sensitivity to PH: Cx50>Cx46>Cx45>Cx26>Cx37>Cx43>Cx40>Cx32, anyway, it is not completely clear whether H^+ acts directly on GJ channels. Cytoplasmic C-tail of connexins contains multiple serine, threonine, and tyrosine residues that may be phosphorylated by various protein kinases (Valiunas et al., 2000; Haubrich et al., 1996). Phosphorylation modifies electrical and metabolic communication between contiguous cells by changing channel molecular structure that affects channel unitary conductance, mean open time, or open probability. Moreover, phosphorylation alters the net charge of C-terminus that in turn may modulate voltage or pH sensitivity of the connexins(Kirchhoff et al.,2000,1998; Bukauskas et al., 2004).

From the gene level to protein expression, noval methods of detection of gap junctions can lead us to realize the therapeutic potential, including morphological diversities, ultrastructure and spatial heterogeneity. The authors induced rapid persistent atrial pacing dogs and did a comparison between removal and retention of cardiac vagus nerve in dogs (superior vena cava and aorta root fat pad, SVC-Ao fat pad), then recorded the effective refractory period and the dispersion of effective refractory period, analyzed the expression of atrial and pulmonary vein connexin40, connexin43 and the heterogeneity of its spatial distribution and the changs of atrial collagen volume fraction, tried to illuminate the correlation of atrial fibrillation with connexin40, connexin43 remodeling and the function of vagus nerve. There was obvious shortness of effective refractory period in atrial fibrillation animal models, while the removal of vagus nerve could attenuate this effect, meanwhile, the quantity and distribution of connexin40 and connexin43 changed at different locations and the deposit of collagen fibers, which might explain the mechanism of electrical heterogeneity and the structural remodeling originated from the pulmanory vein and left atria for the atrial fibrillation.

5. The distribution of connexins in heart and the relationship with arrhythmia

Gap junction remodeling is a common response to many forms of heart disease (Strom et al.,2010; Burstein et al.,2009; Kieken et al.,2009; Qu et al., 2009; Yamada et al.,2008). Previous studies have demonstrated that loss of cell-cell coupling is highly arrhythmic (Chaldoupi et al., 2009), however, a detailed understanding of arrhythmia dynamics has been lacking. With respect to mechanistically link a primary perturbation of gap junction function with arrhythmia, conduction properties, arrhythmia dynamics, and cellular electrophysiological characteristics have been detected (Zhou et al., 2008; Severs et al., 2008; Gutstein et al., 2001). Accumulative evidences showed that ventricular gap junctions contain at least 20 times more connexin43 than connexin40, while atrial gap junctions contain much more connexin40 than connexin43 (Kontogeorgis et al., 2008; Lin et al., 2010). In the ventricle, the heterogeneous loss of connexin43 gap junctions in a murine conditional cardiac connexin43 knockout model best exemplified how the focal loss of cardiac gap junctions lead to significant dispersion of conduction, increased incidence of spontaneous arrhythmias, and loss of ventricular systolic function with only minor reductions in overall connexin43 expression. The gating of connexin43-containing ventricular gap junctions during the action potential is also proposed to promote cardiac arrhythmias via inactivation and recovery that depends on transjunctional voltage (Vj) and contributes to conduction slowing or block and the formation of reentrant arrhythmias. In the atria, targeted gene deletion of connexin40 in mice produced multiple aberrations: P wave and PQ interval prolongation, prolonged sinus-node-recovery time, prolonged Wenckebach period, burst-pacing induced atrial tachyarrhythmias, reduced atrial, A-V node, and left bundle branch conduction velocity, right bundle branch block, and reduced interatrial conduction heterogeneity(Leaf et al., 2008; Gutstein et al., 2005). There are close correlation between electrical properties and the anatomy of pulmonary veins and left atria. In animal studies, data showed that segmental muscle disconnection and differential muscle narrowing at pulmonary vein and left atria junctions and complex fiber orientations within the pulmonary vein provide robust anatomical bases for conduction disturbance at the pulmonary vein and left atria junction and complex intra pulmonary vein conduction patterns (Date et al., 2007).

6. The anatomy and electrical activation in pulmonary vein and left atria

Catheter radiofrequency ablation of triggers originated from the pulmonary veins may successfully terminate paroxysmal atrial fibrillation (Jais et al., 1994). Because ablation within the pulmonary veins may result in stenosis of the pulmonary veins, the junctions between the pulmonary veins and the left atria have become new ablation targets for achieving electrical pulmonary vein isolation (Haissaguerre et al., 1998, 2000). Segmental ablation can successfully isolate the pulmonary vein by placing radiofrequency lesions in only 21% to 59% of the circumference of the pulmonary veins ostia (Pappone et al., 2000; Oral et al., 2002). Previous studies showed that ectopic beats originated from the pulmonary vein propagated to the left atria with characteristically long conduction time, often with conduction delay or block within the pulmonary vein or at the pulmonary vein and left atria junction (Nathan & Eliakim, 1966). The complex arrangement of myocardial fibers in the pulmonary vein and/or in the pulmonary vein and left atria junction is a possible reason for conduction delay or block in the pulmonary vein and left atria junction and within the pulmonary vein (Saito et al., 2000). Ho et al reported that a differential thickness of muscle sleeves could also account for a variable safety factor of propagation across the pulmonary vein and left atria junction (Ho et al., 2001). Hocini reported that zones of activation delay were observed in canine pulmonary veins and correlated with abrupt changes in fascicle orientation (Hocini et al., 2002). Hamabe identified that segmental muscle disconnection and differential muscle narrowing at pulmonary vein and left atria junctions and complex fiber orientations within the pulmonary vein provide robust anatomical bases for conduction disturbance at the pulmonary vein and left atria junction and complex intra pulmonary vein conduction patterns (Hamabe et al., 2003, see Fig2. and Fig3).

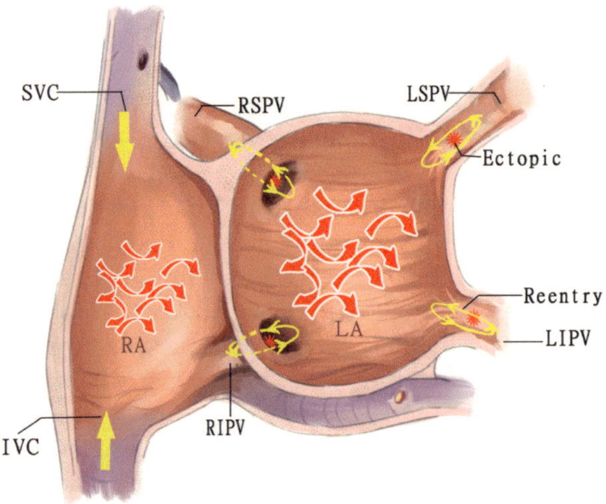

Fig. 2. Ectopic excitement exsiting in pulmanory veins and left atria conjunction, propagating into atria and forming reentry, which is so called"Atrial firbrillation begets Atrial fibrillation". SVC, superior vena cava; IVC, inferior vena cava; LIPV, left inferior pulmanory vein; RIPV, right inferior pulmanory vein; LSPV: left superior pulmanory vein; RSPV: right superior pulmanory vein. LA: left atria; RA: right atria.

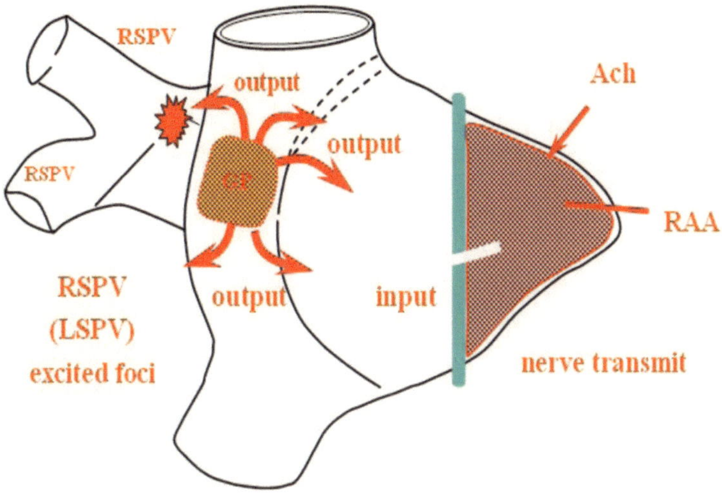

Fig. 3. Electrical remodeling of atria, Acetylcholine injecting at RAA activates ganglion to output impulse and effects on the excited foci in pulmanory veins, therefore, the arrhythmia perpetuates. Ach, acetylcholine; RAA: right atrial appendage; RSPV: right superior pulmanory vein; LSPV: left superior pulmanory vein. (Lu et al. 2008)

The autopsied heart showed that myocardial cells were localized to pulmonary vein between 9 and 38 mm from the pulmonary vein and left atria junction (Roux et al., 2004). The sleeve was composed of circularly and longitudinally oriented bundles of cardiomyocytes. The peripheral end of the myocardial sleeve was irregular. The longest myocardial sleeves were found in the superior veins and were longitudinally oriented. At the pulmonary vein and left atria junction, the circular bundles were not often circumferential. Pulmonary vein myocardial architecture confirmed the possibility of initiating atrial fibrillation. Tan (Tan et al., 2006) examined 192 sections in 32 veins obtained from 8 healthy human heart, each segment included between 7 and 20 mm of the adjoining left atria, and found 1) pulmonary vein and left atria muscular discontinuities and abrupt 90° changes in myofiber orientation were present in the pulmonary vein and left atria junction in over half of all segments examined; 2) These anisotropic features were found more frequently in the anterosuperior than posteroinferior junctions; 3) Adrenergic and cholinergic nerve densities were highest in the left atria within 5 mm from the pulmonary vein and left atria junction, higher in the superior aspect of left superior pulmanory vein, anterosuperior aspect of right superior pulmanory vein, and inferior aspects of the both inferior pulmanory veins than diametrically opposite, and higher in the epicardial than endocardial half of the tissue; 4) adrenergic and cholinergic nerves were highly co-located at tissue and cellular levels of spatial organization. Tan suggest that: 1) the pulmonary vein and left atria junction contains anatomical substrates (muscular discontinuities and abrupt fiber orientation changes) to support reentry; 2) there are no good empiric targets for segmental pulmonary vein isolation because of the widespread distributions of pulmonary vein and left atria muscular discontinuities; 3) the left atria region close to the pulmonary vein and left atria junction rather than farther away in the left atria or pulmonary vein would be the most appropriate target for autonomic modulation procedures; 4) it is not possible to selectively ablate either adrenergic or cholinergic nerves in this location because both nerve types are highly co-located in this region. Steiner found that pulmanory vein myocardial sleeves frequently harbour pathological lesions, particularly senile atrial amyloid, and scarring in atrial fibrillation (Steiner et al., 2005). The degree of scarring of the sleeves did not correlate with the degree of coronary atherosclerosis, and inferred the genesis of the scarring is not post necrotic but degenerative, due to diffuse hypoxia of the sleeve myocardium. Amyloidosis and particularly scarring of pulmanory vein myocardial sleeves appear generally in the elderly population as an arrhythmogenic substrate for atrial fibrillation.

In animal studies, pacing had different effects on connexin40 and connexin43 gap junctions, collagen content increased as well (Yeh et al., 2006). They found there was a 98% increase in connexin43 in pacing 2 weeks, and a 74% increase in pacing 6-8weeks animals. In contrast, connexin40 decreased 47% in pacing 2 weeks but increased 44% in pacing 6-8weeks animals. Our studies also found the moderate to severe deposit of collagen fibers in canine atria after persistent rapid atrial pacing (XIONG et al., 2010, see Fig4. and Fig5.), connexin40 mRNA expression decreased in left atria and right atria, but increased in left atria appendage, right atria appendage and atrial septum; connexin43 mRNA expression was reduced in left atria, right atria, left atrial appendage and right atrial appendage while increased in atiral septum (see Fig6., Fig7. and Fig8.). The pacing induced collagen remodeling and modulation on connexin40 mRNA and connexin43 mRNA expressions could be partially attenuated by removing SVC-Ao fat pad suggesting vagal nervation plays a key role in the initiation and preservation of atrial fibrillation ·

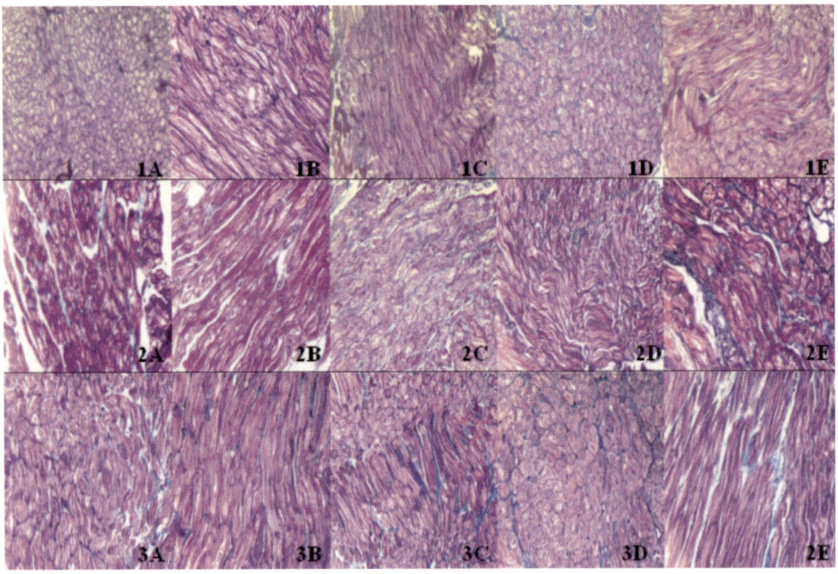

Fig. 4. Different degree of collagen fibers deposits at intercellular substance.1A to 1E: normal distribution of collagen fibers in the whole atria; 2A to 2E: severe degree of collagen fibers deposits at different locations of atria after persistent atrial pacing; 3A to 3E: moderate degree of collagen fibers deposits at different locations of atria after persistent atrial pacing without SVC-Ao fat pad.A: left atria; B: right atria; C: left atrial appendage; D: right atrial appendage; E: atrial septum; SVC-Ao fat pad: superior vena cava and aorto root fat pad.

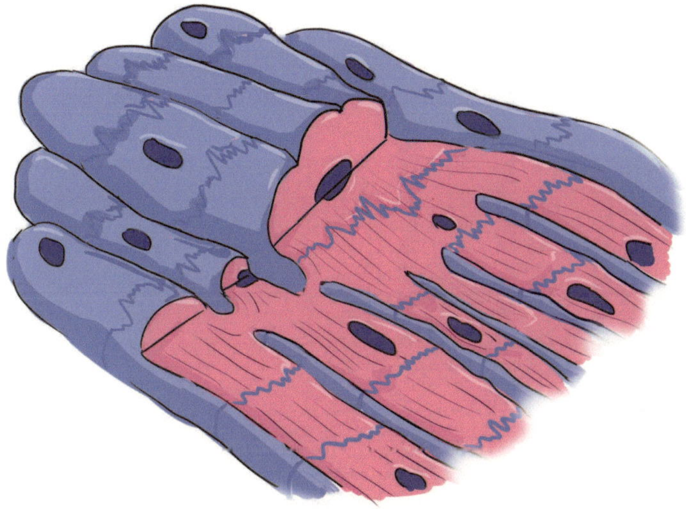

Fig. 5. Collagen fibers wrap the cardiac muscle cells and interrupt the normal intercellular electrical and signal conduction.

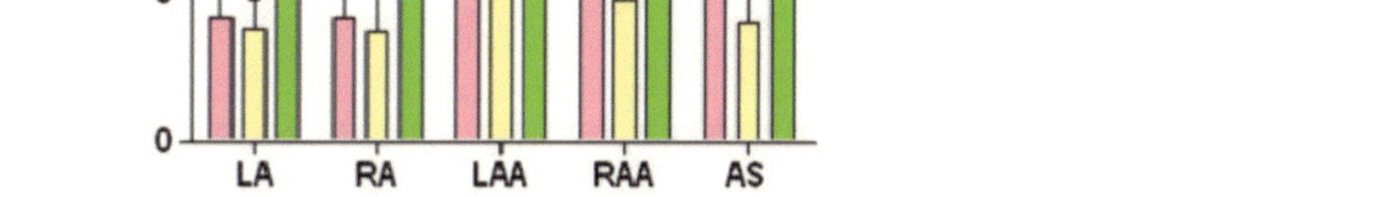

Fig. 6. Collagen Volume Fraction compared among three different groups. There was no significant spatial difference on collagen distribution in sham operated group and SVC-Ao fat pad removal group, while significant spatial difference on collagen distribution in SVC-Ao fat pad reserved group. CVF: collagen volume fraction; SVC-Ao fat pad: superior vena cava and aorto root fat pad; LA: left atria; RA: right atria; LAA: left atrial appendage; RAA: right atrial appendage; AS: atrial septum.

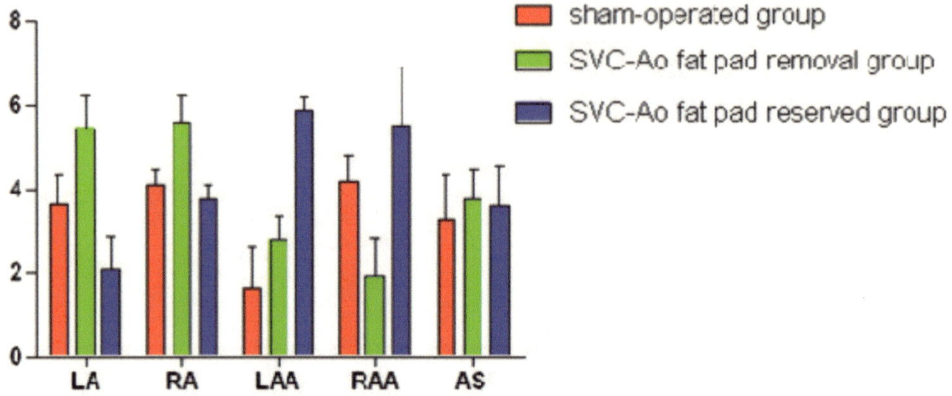

Fig. 7. Expression of Cx40 mRNA compared among three different groups. There was significant difference of increased Cx40 mRNA expression after persistent atrial pacing, the expression at atria in SVC-Ao fat pad removal group but that at atrial appendage in SVC-Ao fat pad reserved group are the significant difference. SVC-Ao fat pad: superior vena cava and aorto root fat pad; LA: left atria; RA: right atria; LAA: left atrial appendage; RAA: right atrial appendage; AS: atrial septum; Cx40: connexin 40.

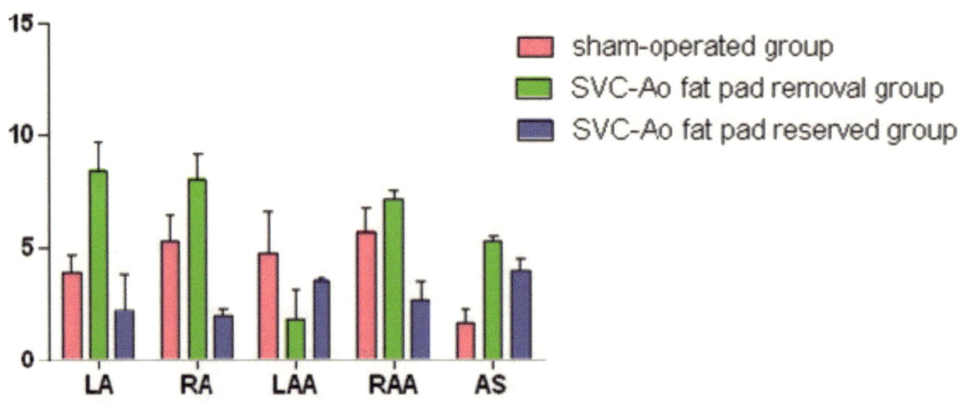

Fig. 8. Expression of Cx43 mRNA compared among three different groups. There was significant difference of increased Cx43 mRNA expression in SVC-Ao fat pad removal group but decreased Cx43 mRNA expression in SVC-Ao fat pad reserved group. The most interesting locations are left and right atria. SVC-Ao fat pad: superior vena cava and aorto root fat pad; LA: left atria; RA: right atria; LAA: left atrial appendage; RAA: right atrial appendage; AS: atrial septum; Cx43: connexin 43.

7. Acknowledgment

This work was supported by grants from the Science Foundation for Returnees of Guangxi Zhuang Autonomous Region of China (No. 0575014) and the Key Scientific Research Subject of Medical Treatment and Public Health of Guangxi Zhuang Autonomous Region of China (No. 200633).

8. References

Bennett, MV., Goodenough, DA. (1978). Gap junctions, electrotonic coupling, and intercellular communication. *Neurosci Res Program Bull,* Vol.6, No.3, pp.1-486, ISSN

Bruzzone, R., Haefliger, JA., Gimlich, RL. (1993). Connexin40, a component of gap junctions in vascular endothelium, is restricted in its ability to interact with other connexins. *Mol Biol Cell,* Vo4, No.1, pp.7-20, ISSN 1059-1524

Bukauskas, FF., Verselis, VK.(2004) . Gap junction channel gating. *Biochim Biophys Acta,* Vol.1662, No.1-2, pp.42-60, ISSN 1388-1981

Burstein, B., Comtois, P., Michael, G., Nishida, K., Villeneuve, L., Yeh, YH., Nattel, S.(2009). Changes in connexin expression and the atrial fibrillation substrate in congestive heart failure. *Circ Res,* Vol.105, No.12, pp.1213-1222, ISSN 0009-7330

Chiou, CW., Eble, JN., Zipes, DP.(1997). Efferent vagal innervation of the canine atria and sinus and atrioventricular nodes. The third fat pad. *Circulation,* Vol.95, No.11, pp.2573-2584, ISSN 0009-7322

Chen, YJ., Chen, SA., Chen, YC., Yeh, HI., Chan, P., Chang, MS., Lin, CI.(2001). Effects of Rapid Atrial Pacing on the Arrhythmogenic Activity of Single Cardiomyocytes From Pulmonary Veins: Implication in Initiation of Atrial Fibrillation. *Circulation,* Vol.104, No.11, pp.2849-2854, ISSN 0009-7322

Cottrell, GT., Wu, Y., Burt, JM.(2002). Cx40 and Cx43 expression ratio influences heteromeric/heterotypic gap junction channel properties. *Am J Physiol Cell Physiol,* Vol.282, No.6, pp. C1469–C1482, ISSN 0363-6143

Chaldoupi, SM., Loh, P., Hauer, RN.(2009). The role of connexin40 in atrial fibrillation. *Cardiovasc Res,* Vol.84, No.1, pp. 15-23, ISSN 0008-6363

Date, T., Yamane, T., Inada, K. (2007). The effects of pulmonary vein isolation on the morphology of p waves: the contribution of pulmonary vein muscle excitation to the formation of p waves. *Pacing Clin Electrophysiol,* Vol.30, No.1, pp. 93-101, ISSN 0147-8389

Duffy, HS., Wit, AL.(2008). Is there a role for remodeled connexins in AF? No simple answers. *J Mol Cell Cardiol,* Vol.44, No.1, pp.4-13, ISSN 0022-2828

Danik, SB., Rosner, G., Lader, J.(2008). Electrical remodeling contributes to complex tachyarrhythmias in connexin43-deficient mouse hearts. *FASEB J,* Vol.22, No.4, pp. 1204-1212, ISSN 0892-6638

Date, T., Yamane, T., Inada, K.()2007). The effects of pulmonary vein isolation on the morphology of p waves: the contribution of pulmonary vein muscle excitation to the formation of p waves. *Pacing Clin Electrophysiol,* Vol.30, No.1, pp. 93-101, ISSN 0147-8389

Elenes, S., Rubart, M., Moreno AP.(1999). Junctional communication between isolated pairs of canine atrial cells is mediated by homoheneous and heterogeneous gap junction channels. *J Cardiovasc Electrophysiol,* Vol.10, No.7, pp. 990–1004, ISSN 1045-3873

Gros, DB., Jongsma, HJ. (1996). Connexins in mammalian heart function. *Bioessays,* Vol.18, No.9, pp. 719-730, ISSN 0265-9247

Gutstein, DE., Danik, SB., Lewitton, S.(2005). Focal gap junction uncoupling and spontaneous ventricular ectopy. *Am J Physiol Heart Circ Physiol,* Vol.289, No.3, pp. H1091-H1098, ISSN 0363-6135

Gutstein, DE., Morley, GE., Vaidya, D.(2001). Heterogeneous expression of Gap junction channels in the heart leads to conduction defects and ventricular dysfunction. *Circulation,* Vol.104, No.10, pp. 1194-1199, ISSN 0009-7322

Hoffmann, E., Sulke, N., Edvardsson, N.(2006). on behalf of the Atrial Fibrillation Therapy (AFT) Trial Investigators Initiation of AF; New Insights Into the Initiation of Atrial Fibrillation:A Detailed Intraindividual and Interindividual Analysis of the Spontaneous Onset of Atrial Fibrillation Using New Diagnostic Pacemaker Features. *Circulation,* Vol.113, No.16, pp. 1933–1941, ISSN 0009-7322

Haissaguerre, M., Jais, P., Shah, DC.(1998). Spontaneous Initiation of Atrial Fibrillation by Ectopic Beats Originating in the Pulmonary Veins. *N Engl J Med,* Vol.339, No.10, pp. 659–666, ISSN 0028-4793

Honjo, H., Boyett, MR., Niwa, R.(2003). Pacing-Induced Spontaneous Activity in Myocardial Sleeves of Pulmonary Veins After Treatment With Ryanodine. *Circulation,* Vol.107, No.14, pp. 1937–1943, ISSN 0009-7322

Herve, JC., Bourmeyster, N., Sarrouilhe, D.(2007). Gap junctional complexes:From partners to functions. *Prog Biophys Mol Biol,* Vol.94, No.1-2, pp. 29–65, ISSN 0079-6107

Harris, AL. (2001).Emerging issues of connexin channels: biophysics fills the gap. *Q Rev Biophys,* Vol.34, No.3, pp. 325-472, ISSN 0033-5835

Haubrich, S., Schwarz, HJ., Bukauskas, F.(1996). Incompatibility of connexin 40 and 43 Hemichannels in gap junctions between mammalian cells is determined by intracellular domains. *Mol Biol Cell,* Vol.7, No.12, pp. 1995-2006, ISSN 1059-1524

Haissaguerre, M., Shah, DC., Jais, P.(2000). Electrophysiological breakthroughs from the left atrium to the pulmonary veins. *Circulation,* Vol.102, No.20, pp. 2463–2465, ISSN 0009-7322

Ho, SY., Cabrera, JA., Tran, VH.(2001). Architecture of the pulmonary veins: relevance to radiofrequency ablation. *Heart,* Vol.86, No.3, pp. 265–270, ISSN 1355-6037

Hocini, M., Ho, SY., Kawara, T.(2002). Electrical conduction in canine pulmonary veins: electrophysiological and anatomic correlation. *Circulation,* Vol.105, No.20, pp. 2442–2448, ISSN 0009-7322

Hamabe, A., Okuyama, Y., Miyauchi, Y.(2003). Correlation between anatomy and electrical activation in canine pulmonary veins. *Circulation,* Vol.107, No.11, pp. 1550-1555, ISSN 0009-7322

Ji, S., Gupta, N., Weiss, JN.(2010). The heart and its nerves: a nervous bond. *Heart Rhythm,* Vol.7, No.4, pp. 504-505, ISSN 1547-5271

Jais, P., Haissaguerre, M., Shah, DC.(1997). A focal source of atrial fibrillation treated by discrete radiofrequency ablation. *Circulation,* Vol.95, No.3, pp. 572–576, ISSN 0009-7322

Kapa, S., Venkatachalam, KL., Asirvatham, SJ.(2010). The autonomic nervous system in cardiac electrophysiology: an elegant interaction and emerging concepts. *Cardiol Rev,* Vol.18, No.6, pp. 275-284, ISSN 1061-5377

Kanagaratnam, P., Rothery, SR., Patel, P.(2002). Relative Expression of Immunolocalized Connexins 40 and 43 Correlates With Human Atrial Conduction Properties. *J Am Coll Cardiol,* Vol.39, No.1, pp. 116–123, ISSN 0735-1097

Kanagaratnam, P., Cherian, A., Stanbridge, RDL.(2004). Relationship between connexins and atrial activation during human atrial fibrillation. *J Cardiovasc Electrophys,* Vol.15, No.2, pp. 206–213, ISSN 1045-3873

Kirby, ML., Waldo, KL.(1995). Neural crest and cardiovascular patterning. *Circ Res,* Vol.77, No.2, pp. 211-215, ISSN 0009-7330

Kirchhoff, S., Kim, JS., Hagendorff, A.(2000). Abnormal cardiac conduction and morphogenesis in connexin40 and connexin43 double-deficient mice. *Circ Res,* Vol.87, No.5, pp. 399-405, ISSN 0009-7330

Kirchhoff, S., Nelles, E., Hagendorff, A.(1998). Reduced cardiac conduction velocity and predisposition to arrhythmias in connexin40-deficient mice. *Curr Biol,* Vol.8, No.5, pp. 299-302, ISSN 0960-9822

Kieken, F., Mutsaers, N., Dolmatova, E.(2009). Structural and molecular mechanisms of gap junction remodeling in epicardial border zone myocytes following myocardial infarction. *Circ Res,* Vol.104, No.9, pp. 1103-1112, ISSN 0009-7330

Kontogeorgis, A., Kaba, RA., Kang, E.(2008). Short-term pacing in the mouse alters cardiac expression of connexin43. *BMC Physiol,* Vol.8, p. 8,

Lin, X., Gemel, J., Glass, A.(2010). Connexin40 and connexin43 determine gating properties of atrial gap junction channels. *J Mol Cell Cardiol,* Vol.48, No.1, pp. 238-245, ISSN 0022-2828

Leaf, DE., Feig, JE., Vasquez, C.(2008). Connexin40 imparts conduction heterogeneity to atrial tissue. *Circ Res,* Vol.103, No.9, pp. 1001-1008, ISSN 0009-7330

Lu Z, Scherlag BJ, Lin J, Niu G, Ghias M, Jackman WM, Lazzara R, Jiang H, Po SS.(2008). Autonomic mechanism for complex fractionated atrial electrograms: evidence by fast fourier transform analysis. *J Cardiovasc Electrophysiol,* Vol.19, No.8, pp. 835-842, ISSN 1045-3873

Moreno, AP.(2004). Biophysical properties of homomeric and heteromultimeric channels formed by cardiac connexins. *Cardiovasc Res,* Vol.62, No.2, pp. 276-286, ISSN 0008-6363

Nathan, H., Eliakim, M.(1966). The junction between the left atrium and the pulmonary veins: an anatomic study of human hearts. *Circulation,* Vol.34, No.3, pp. 412- 422, ISSN 0009-7322

Oral, H., Knight, BP., Tada, H.(2002). Pulmonary vein isolation for paroxysmal and persistent atrial fibrillation. *Circulation,* Vol.105, No.9, pp. 1077–1081, ISSN 0009-7322

Patterson, E., Lazzara, R., Szabo, B.(2006). Sodium-Calcium Exchange Initiated by the Ca2+ Transient: An Arrhythmia Trigger Within Pulmonary Veins. *Journal of the American College of Cardiology,* Vol.47, No.6, pp. 1196–1206, ISSN 0735-1097

Page, RL., Wilkinson, WE., Clair, WK.(1994). Asymptomatic arrhythmias in patients with symptomatic paroxysmal atrial fibrillation and paroxysmal supraventricular tachycardia. *Circulation,* Vol.89, No.1, pp. 224–227, ISSN 0009-7322

Perkins, GA., Goodenough, DA., Sosinsky, GE.(1998). Formation of the gap junction intercellular channel requires a 30 degree rotation for interdigitating two apposing connexons. *J Mol Biol,* Vol.277, No.2, pp. 171–177, ISSN 0022-2836

Pappone, C., Rosanio, S., Oreto, G.(2000). Circumferential radiofrequency ablation of pulmonary vein ostia: a new anatomic approach for curing atrial fibrillation. *Circulation,* Vol.102, No.21, pp. 2619–2628, ISSN 0009-7322

Qu, J., Volpicelli, FM., Garcia, LI.(2009). Gap junction remodeling and spironolactone-dependent reverse remodeling in the hypertrophied heart. *Circ Res,* Vol.104, No.3, pp. 365-371, ISSN 0009-7330

Revel, JP., Karnovsky, MJ.(1967). Hexagonal array of subunits in intercellular junctions of the mouse heart and liver. *J Cell Biol,* Vol.33, No.3, pp. C7-C12, ISSN 0021-9525

Rackauskas, M., Neverauskas, V., Skeberdis, VA.(2010). Diversity and properties of connexin gap junction channels. *Medicina,* Vol.46, No.1, pp. 1-12, ISSN 1010-660X

Reisner, Y., Meiry, G., Levin, ZN.(2009). Impulse conduction and gap junctional remodelling by endothelin-1 in cultured neonatal rat ventricular myocytes. *J Cell Mol Med,* Vol.13, No.3, pp. 562-573, ISSN 1582-1838

Rackauskas, M., Kreuzberg, MM., Pranevicius, M.(2007). Gating properties of heterotypic gap junction channels formed of connexins 40, 43, and 45. *Biophys J,* Vol.92, No.6, pp. 1952-1965, ISSN 0006-3495

Roux, N., Havet, E., Mertl, P. The myocardial sleeves of thepulmonary veins: potential implications for atrial fibrillation. *Surg Radiol Anat,* Vol.26, No.4, pp. 285-289, ISSN 0930-1038

Sellers, MB., Newby, LK.(2011). Atrial fibrillation, anticoagulation, fall risk, and outcomes in elderly patients. *Am Heart J,* Vol.161, No.2, pp. 241-246, ISSN 0002-8703

Sandres, P., Jais, P., Hocini, M. Electrical disconnection of the coronary sinus by radiofrequency catheter ablation to isolate a trigger of atrial fibrillation. *J Cardiovasc Electr,* Vol.15, No.3, pp. 364–368, ISSN 1045-3873

Stergiopoulos, K., Alvarado, JL., Mastroianni, M.(1999). Heterodomain interactions as a mechanism for the regulation of connexin channels. *Circ Res,* Vol.84, No.10, pp. 1144–1155, ISSN 0009-7330

Söhl, G., Willecke, K. Gap junctions and the connexin protein family. *Cardiovasc Res,* Vol.62, No.2, pp. 228-232, ISSN 0008-6363

Strom, M., Wan, X., Poelzing, S.(2010). Gap junction heterogeneity as mechanism for electrophysiologically distinct properties across the ventricular wall. *Am J Physiol Heart Circ Physiol,* Vol.298, No.3, pp. H787-H794, ISSN 0363-6135

Severs, NJ., Bruce, AF., Dupont, E.(2008). Remodelling of gap junctions and connexin expression in diseased myocardium. *Cardiovasc Res,* Vol.80, No.1, pp. 9-19, ISSN 0008-6363

Saito, T., Waki, K., Becker, AE.(2000). Left atrial myocardial extension onto pulmonary veins in humans: anatomic observations relevant for atrial arrhythmias. *J Cardiovasc Electrophysiol,* Vol.11, No.8, pp. 888–894, ISSN 1045-3873

Steiner, I., Hájková, P., Kvasnicka, J.(2005). Pulmonary veins and atrial fibrillation: a pathological study of 100 hearts. *Cesk Patol,* Vol.41, No.4, pp. 124-131

Tsuboi, M., Furukawa, Y., Nakajima, K.(2000). Inotropic, chronotropic, and dromotropic effects mediated via parasympathetic ganglia in the dog heart. *Am J Physiol Heart Circ Physiol,* Vol.279, No.3, pp. H1201-1207, ISSN 0363-6135

Tan, AY., Li, H., Hogiu, WS.(2006). Autonomic innervation and segmental muscular disconnections at the human pulmonary vein-atrial junction: implications for catheter ablation of atrial-pulmonary vein junction. *J Am Coll Cardiol,* Vol.48, No.1, pp. 132-143, ISSN 0735-1097

Unger, VM., Kumar, NM., Gilula, NB.(1999). Three-dimensional structure of a recombinant gap junction membrane channel. *Science,* Vol.283, No.5405, pp. 1176–1180, ISSN 0036-8075

Volders, PG.(2010). Novel insights into the role of the sympathetic nervous system in cardiac arrhythmogenesis. *Heart Rhythm,* Vol.7, No.12, pp. 1900-1906, ISSN 1547-5271

Verheule, S., Wilson, EE., Arora, R.(2002). Tissue structure and connexin expression of canine pulmonary veins. *Cardiovasc Res,* Vol.55, No.4, pp. 727–738, ISSN 0008-6363

Valiunas, V., Gemel, J., Brink, PR.(2001). Gap junction channels formed by coexpressed connexin40 and connexin43. *Am J Physiol Heart Circ Physiol,* Vol.281, No.4, pp. H1675–H1689, ISSN 0363-6135

Valiunas, V., Weingart, R., Brink, PR.(2000). Formation of heterotypic gap junction channels by connexins 40 and 43. *Circ Res,* Vol.86, No.2, pp. E42–E49, ISSN 0009-7330

Verheijck, EE., Kempen, MJ., Veereschild, M.(2001). Electrophysiological features of the mouse sinoatrial node in relation to connexin distribution. *Cardiovasc Res,* Vol.52, No.1, pp. 40-50, ISSN 0008-6363

Valiunas, V., Weingart, R., Brink, PR.(2000). Formation of heterotypic gap junction channels by connexins 40 and 43. *Circ Res,* Vol.86, No.2, pp. E42-E49, ISSN 0009-7330

Valiunas, V., Beyer, EC., Brink, PR.(2002). Cardiac gap junction channels show quantitative differences in selectivity. *Circ Res,* Vol.91, No.2, pp. 104-111, ISSN 0009-7330

Valiunas, V., Polosina, YY., Miller, H.(2005). Connexin-specific cell-to-cell transfer of short interfering RNA by gap junctions. *J Physiol,* Vol.568, No.Pt2, pp. 459-468, ISSN 0022-3751

Wit, AL., Boyden, PA.(2007). Triggered activity and atrial fibrillation. *Heart Rhythm,* Vol.4, No.3, pp. S17–S23, ISSN 1547-5271

Wijffels MC, Kirchhof CJ, Dorland R, Allessie MA.(1995). Atrial fibrillation begets atrial fibrillation. A study in awake chronically instrumented goats. *Circulation,* Vol.92, No.7, pp. 1954–1968, ISSN 0009-7322

Xiong RX, Zhong GQ, Song HX, Zhang JC, Ling Y.(2010). Collagen spatial distribution in rapid atrial pacing dogs with or without superior vena cava and aortic root fat. *Zhonghua Xin Xue Guan Bing Za Zhi,* Vol.38, No.2, pp. 171-174, ISSN 0253-3758

Yeager, M., Gilula, NB.(1992). Membrane topology and quaternary structure of cardiac gap junction ion channels. *J Mol Biol,* Vol.223, No.4, pp. 929–948, ISSN 0022-2836

Yamada, KA.(2008). A change of heart: heterogeneous remodeling in heart failure. *Heart Rhythm,* Vol.5, No.8, pp. 1186-1188, ISSN 1547-5271

Yeh HI, Lai YJ, Lee SH, Chen ST, Ko YS, Chen SA, Severs NJ, Tsai CH.(2006). Remodeling of myocardial sleeve and gap junctions in canine superior vena cava after rapid pacing. *Basic Res Cardiol,* Vol.101, No.4, pp. 269-280, ISSN 0300-8428

Zhou SH, He XZ, Liu QM, Du WH, Li XP, Zhou T, Tang JQ, Li RS.(2008). Study on the spatial distribution pattern of Cx40 gap junctions in the atria of patients with coronary heart disease. *Cardiol J,* Vol.15, No.1, pp. 50-56, ISSN 1897-5593

Part 2

Myocardial Infarction

8

ECG in Acute Myocardial Infarction in the Reperfusion Era

Massimo Napodano and Catia Paganelli
University of Padova,
Italy

1. Introduction

Acute myocardial infarction can be defined from a number of different perspectives related to clinical, electrocardiographic, biochemical and pathological characteristic. The electrocardiogram (ECG) is the most important diagnostic tool in the diagnosis of ST-segment elevation myocardial infarction (STEMI), and therefore it should be accomplished immediately at hospital admission. In fact, it represents an important step not only for STEMI diagnosis, but also and more importantly for the therapeutic plan. The present article pertains to electrocadiographic findings in patients affected by persistent STEMI. Moreover, it takes into account the clinical utility of ECG in the diagnosis and therapeutic decisions of evolving STEMI, as well as the prognostic implications of the ECG evolutions in the reperfusion era.

2. Evolving ECG changes occurring in the early phase of ST-elevation myocardial infarction

Typically, the ECG in the evolving STEMI shows five abnormalities, which develop in turn: hyperacute T waves, ST-segment elevation, abnormal Q waves, T-waves inversion, normalization of the ST-segment (Figure 1).

2.1 Hyperacute T waves

The T-waves represent the period of ventricular repolarization on the surface ECG. During the first minutes of coronary arterial occlusion (Dressler et al., 1947), the earliest ECG changes are represented by an increase in the amplitude of the T-wave, the so-called "Hyperacute T-waves" (Figure 1B,C). The morphologic characteristic of hyperacute T-wave are typical of ischemic event: they are asymmetric with a broad base and generally associated with reciprocal ST segment depression. In the evolving STEMI the hyperacute T-waves turn into giant R wave (Figure 1E). Hyperacute T-waves represent the electrocardiographic expression of ischemia before the beginning of necrosis; for this reason they are considered as the most significant phase during which the reperfusion therapy may achieve the greatest benefit in term of myocardial salvage (Lee et al., 1995). Prominent T-waves, however, are also associated with other diagnoses, including hyperkalemia, early repolarization end left ventricular hypertrophy (Somers et al., 2002). Thus in the differential diagnosis, the clinicians must consider additional features related to patient, including age, comorbidity and current medical status.

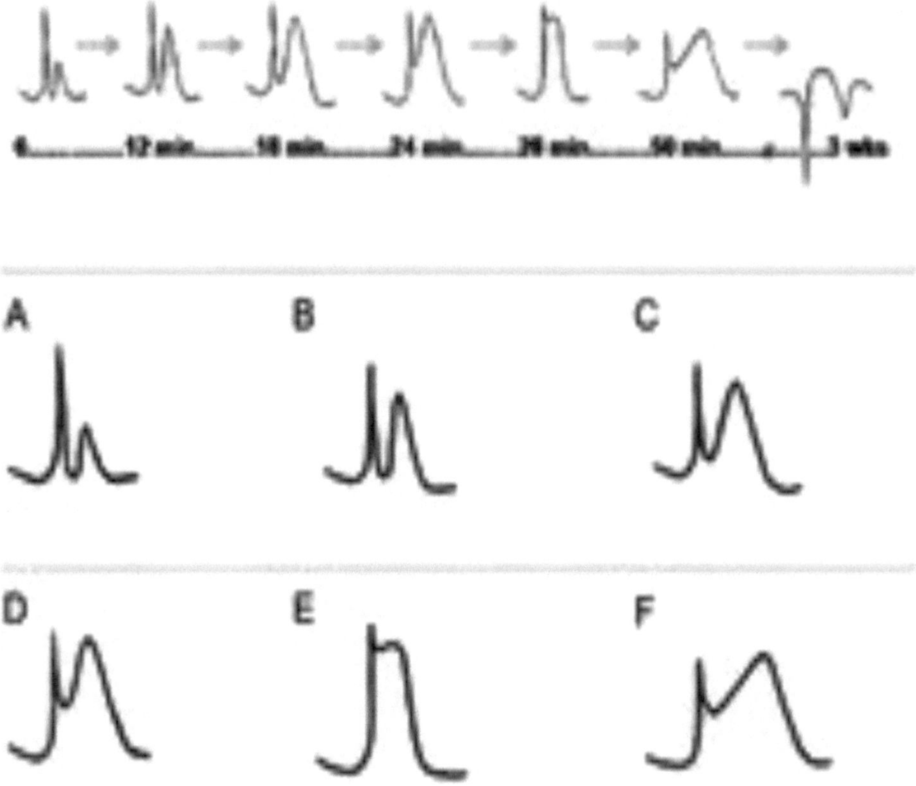

A Normal: Normal ST-segment and T-wave; **B Early, Hyper-acute T wave**: Development of Prominent T Wave; **C Hyper-acute T Wave**: Prominent T-wave with early ST-segment elevation; **D ST-segment elevation**: Progressive ST-segment elevation with persistent prominent T-wave; **E Giant R Wave**: ST - segment elevation continues with development of giant R-wave. **F ST-segment Elevation:** ST-segment elevation with oblique morphology.

Fig. 1. Evolving ECG changes occurring in the early phase of ST-elevation myocardial infarction

2.2 ST-segment elevation

The ST-segment, defined as the segment beginning at the J point and ending at the apex of the T-wave, represents the electrocardiographic period between ventricular depolarization (QRS) and repolarization (T-wave) (Figure 1A). The ST-segment changes on the standard ECG that are associated with infarction are due to flow of current across the boundary between the ischemic and nonischemic zones. ST-segment elevation generally occurs with reciprocal ST depression in ECG leads in which the axis is opposite in direction from those with ST elevation (Figure 1D). The best criteria to classify abnormally elevated ST-segment are resumed in the Minnesota code 9-2 and are defined as ST-segment elevation of 1 mm in at least 1 peripheral lead, or 2 mm elevation in at least 1 precordial lead. These criteria have 94% of specificity for STEMI with a sensitivity of 56% in STEMI diagnosis (Menown et al., 2000). The threshold values results from recognition that some elevation of the junction of the QRS complex and the ST-segment (J-point) is a normal finding. Indeed, these are dependent on gender, age, and ECG lead. Thus, the current thresholds recommended by the American Heart Association Electrocardiography and Arrhythmias, the Amrican College of Cardiology vary according to age, gender, and ECG lead (Table 1).

Men 40 years old of age and older	The threshold value for abnormal J-point elevation should be 0.2 mV (2 mm) in leads V_2 and V_3 and 0.1 mV (1 mm) in all other leads.
Men less than 40 years of age	The threshold value for abnormal J-point elevation in V_2 and V_3 should be 0.25 mV (2.5 mm).
Women of all ages	The threshold value for abnormal J-point elevation should be 0.15 mV (1.5 mm) in leads V_2 and V_3 and greater than 0.1 mV (1 mm) in all other leads.
Men and women of all ages	The threshold for abnormal J-point elevation V_3R and V_4R should be 0.05 mV (0.5 mm), except for males less than 30 years of age, for whom 0.1 mV (1 mm) is more appropriate.
Men and women of all ages	The threshold value for abnormal J-point elevation in V_7 through V_9 should be 0.05 mV (0.5 mm).
Men and women of all ages	The threshold value for abnormal J-point depression should be - 0.05 mV (-0.5 mm) in leads V_2 and V_3 and - 0.1 mV (- 1 mm) in all other leads.

Table 1. **Threshold values for ST-segment elevation according to age, gender, and ECG leads.** Adapted from AHA/ACCF/HRS (2009) Recommendations for standardization and interpretation of the electrocardiogram . *J Am Coll Cardiol*, Vol. 53, No. 11, pp. 1003-10011, ISSN 0735-1097/09/

However, ST-segment elevation can also attributed to other causes, different from acute myocardial infarction: a normal variant, frequently referred as *early repolarization,* commonly characterized by J-point elevation and rapidly upsloping or normal ST-segment; ventricular dyskinesis, often characterized by a small ST elevation; pericarditis, in which usually the ST elevation can be detected in more than one discrete region, as the inflammation involves a large portion of the epicardial surface, and reciprocal ST-depression is absent; elevated serum potassium; acute myocarditis; cardiac tumors or intra-thoracic mass. An additional ECG criteria in diagnosis of evolving STEMI is represented by the morphology of ST-segment elevation. In fact, two patterns of ST-segment morphology can be distinguish, according to the direction of the ST slope: a concave morphology and a convex morphology (Figure 2A,B). The concave morphology (Figure 2A) is hardly consistent with STEMI diagnosis, and rather related to other conditions, such as benign early repolarization, acute pericarditis. On the other hand, the convex morphology is usually associated with STEMI (Brady et al., 2001) (Figure 2B). The assessment of ST-segment elevation during STEMI is also useful to evaluate the extension of the myocardial at risk, and then the prognosis. In fact the number of leads with ST segment elevation and the sum of the total ST deviation have been related to the extension of area of myocardium at risk, defined as the extent of jeopardize ischemic myocardium, and consequently to the extent of necrotic area if reperfusion is not undertaken (Aldrich et al., 1988).

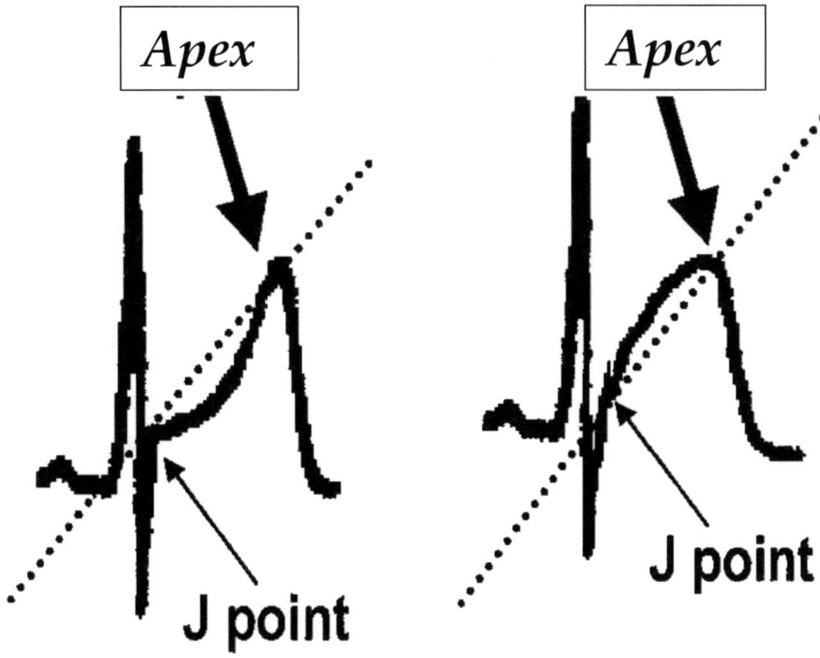

A Concave Morphology **B Convex Morphology**

A Concave Morphology: the concave morphology is characterized by downward ST slope; the ST slope remains below the virtual line drawn from the J-point to the apex of T-wave. **B Convex Morphology:** the convex morphology is characterized by upward ST-slope; the ST slope remains above the virtual line drawn from the J-point to the apex of T-wave

Fig. 2. Patterns of ST-segment elevation at ECG

Moreover , the analysis of the electrocardiographic leads revealing ST-segment elevation as well as of those showing ST depression, permits an almost accurate identification of the occluded coronary artery and also the proximal or distal location of the occlusion within that artery (Wagner et al., 2009). Anterior wall ischemia/infarction is invariably due to occlusion of the left anterior descending coronary artery and results in the spatial vector of the ST segment being directed to the left and laterally. This will be expressed as ST elevation in some or all of leads V1 through V6. The location of the occlusion within the left anterior descending coronary artery, that is, whether proximal or distal, is suggested by the chest leads in which the ST-segment elevation occurs and the presence of ST-segment elevation or depression in other leads. Occlusion of the proximal left anterior descending coronary artery above the first septal and first diagonal branches results in involvement of the basal portion of the left ventricle, as well as the anterior and lateral walls and the interventricular septum. This will result in the ST-segment spatial vector being directed superiorly and to the left and will be associated with ST-segment elevation in leads V1 through V4, I, aVL, and often aVR. It will also be associated with reciprocal ST-segment depression in the leads whose positive poles are positioned inferiorly, that is, leads II, III, aVF, and often V5 (Birnbaum et al., 1993). When the occlusion is located between the first septal and first diagonal branches, the basal interventricular septum will be spared, and the ST segment in lead V1 will not be elevated. In that situation, the ST-segment vector will be directed toward aVL, which will be elevated, and away from the positive pole of lead III, which will show depression of the ST segment. When the occlusion is located more distally, that is, below both the first septal and first diagonal branches, the basal portion of the left ventricle will not be involved, and the ST-segment vector will be oriented more inferiorly. Thus, the ST segment will not be elevated in leads V1, aVR, or aVL, and the ST segment will not be depressed in leads II, III, or aVF. Indeed, because of the inferior orientation of the ST-segment vector, elevation of the ST segment in leads II, III, and aVF may occur. In addition, ST-segment elevation may be more prominent in leads V3 through V6 and less prominent in V2than in the more proximal occlusions (Engelen et al., 1999). Inferior wall infarction that results in ST-segment elevation in only leads II, III, and aVF may be the result of occlusion of either the right coronary artery or the left circumflex coronary artery, depending on which provides the posterior descending branch, that is, which is the dominant vessel. When the right coronary artery is occluded, the spatial vector of the ST segment will usually be directed more to the right than when the left circumflex is occluded. This will result in greater ST-segment elevation in lead III than in lead II and will often be associated with ST-segment depression in leads I and aVL, leads in which the positive poles are oriented to the left and superiorly. However, recently these criteria resulted less accurate in patients with electrocardiographic small inferior myocardial infarction (Verouden et al., 2009). Indeed, when the RCA is occluded in its proximal portion, ischemia/infarction of the right ventricle may occur, which causes the spatial vector of the ST-segment shift to be directed to the right and anteriorly, as well as inferiorly. This will result in ST-segment elevation in leads placed on the right anterior chest, in positions referred to as V3R and V4R, and often in lead V1 (Correale et al., 1999). Lead V4R is the most commonly used right-sided chest lead. It is of great value in diagnosing right ventricular involvement in the setting of an inferior wall infarction and in making the distinction between right coronary artery and left circumflex coronary artery occlusion and between proximal and distal right coronary artery occlusion. It is important to recognize that the ST elevation in the right-sided chest leads associated with right ventricular infarction persists for a much shorter period of time than the ST elevation connoting inferior wall infarction that occurs in the extremity leads. For this reason, leads V3R and V4R should be recorded as rapidly as possible after the onset of chest pain. ST-segment depression in leads V1, V2, and V3 that occurs in association with an inferior wall infarction may be caused by occlusion of either the right coronary or the left circumflex artery. This ECG pattern has been termed posterior or posterolateral ischemia since the early reports based on anatomic and pathological studies of ex vivo. However, recent in vivo imaging studies, including magnetic resonance imaging, have demonstrated that the region referred to as the posterior wall was lateral rather than posterior since the oblique position of the heart within the thorax: correlating the ECG patterns of healed myocardial infarctions to their anatomic location as determined by magnetic resonance imaging, the most frequent cause of abnormally tall and broad R waves in leads V1 and V2 was involvement of the lateral and not the posterior wall of the left ventricle (Bayes de Luna et al., 2006a). On these basis it has been proposed that the term posterior be replaced by the designation lateral (Cerqueira et al., 2002). Therefore, the terms posterior ischemia and posterior infarction be replaced by the terms lateral, inferolateral, or basal-lateral depending on the associated changes in II, III, aVF, V1, V5, and V6. Such terminology has been endorsed by the International Society for Holter and Noninvasive Electrocardiography (Bayes de Luna A et al., 2006b). It is not possible to determine whether the right coronary artery or left circumflex vessel is occluded when changes of inferior wall ischemia/infarction are accompanied by depression of the ST-segment in leads V1, V2, and V3; however, the absence of such changes is more suggestive of right coronary than left circumflex artery occlusion. When the left circumflex is occluded, the spatial vector of the ST-segment in the frontal plane is more likely to be directed to the left. For this reason, the ST-segment may be elevated to a greater extent in lead II than in lead III and may be isoelectric or elevated in leads I and aVL (Bairey et al., 1987). Conversely, when a dominant right coronary artery is occluded proximally, left posterolateral and right ventricular wall involvement will be present, and the posteriorly directed ST-segment vector associated with this involvement may cancel the ST-segment elevation in lead V1 anticipated by right ventricular involvement and vice versa. The American College of Cardiology (ACC)/American Heart Association (AHA) guidelines for the management for patients with acute myocardial infarction (ACC/AHA, 2009) note the presence of electrocardiographic ST-segment elevation of greater than 0.1 mV in two anatomically contiguous leads; they suggest that such a finding is a Class I indication for urgent reperfusion therapy in the patient presumed to have STEMI. However, in few patients the presence of a left bundle branch block make the ECG less specific for the diagnosis of STEMI, because LBBB resembles STEMI changes. In this setting, the presence of suggestive symptoms and/or the certainty of the new-onset of conduction disorders may be helpful in diagnosis. Nevertheless, when these are not conclusive for diagnosis, the presence of some ECG criteria, pertaining the ST shift in relation to QRS vectors, may still indicate the diagnosis. To this regard, the ECG should be interpreted using the "rule of appropriate discordance", described by Sgarabossa and colleagues (Sgarbossa, 1996, 1998). They identified three independent electrocardiographic criteria suggesting for STEMI diagnosis in presence of LBBB: ST-segment elevation of at least 1mm that is concordant with the QRS complex; ST-segment depression of at least 1mm in leads V_2 and V_3; and ST-segment elevation of at least 5 mm that is discordant with the QRS complex. The Sgarbossa criteria provide a simple and practical diagnostic approach to identify STEMI in presence of LBBB, contributing to better address risk stratification and to optimize the risk-benefit ratio of reperfusion therapy in this challenging and high-risk population. In fact, the presence of LBBB in patients with acute myocardial infarction is usually related to large necrosis and consequently to high risk of complications and death. In fact, the new onset LBBB is related to the occlusion of the proximal left anterior descending artery and a large amount of jeopardized myocardium (Opolski et al., 1986). On the other hand, a pre-existing left bundle branch block is a powerful marker of depressed left ventricular systolic function, and any additional loss of myocardium is likely to result in large infarction and cardiogenic shock (Hamby et al., 1983)

2.3 Abnormal Q-wave

Q-wave are commonly present in normal ECG. Abnormal Q-wave suggesting myocardial necrosis have grater negative deflection and longer duration. Pathologic Q-wave typically appear within the first 9 hours of infarction, with a wide interval, ranging from few minutes to 24 hours (Perera, 2004; Goldberger, 1991). In particular in the evolution of non-reperfused myocardial infarction, Q-wave usually appear within 9 hours from coronary occlusion (Bär et al., 1996). However, it is not infrequent to observe Q-wave early after symptom onset. Abnormal Q-wave may be related to ischemia of the conduction system (Raitt at al., 1995; Smith & Whitwam, 2006). Thus, Q-wave should not be used exclusively as a marker of late presentation of acute coronary occlusion, denying patients potentially beneficial reperfusion therapy. It is important to note that, in the Global Utilization of Streptokinase and Tissue Plasminogen Activator for Occluded Coronary Arteries (GUSTO-I) trial patients who did not develop Q-wave after fibrinolysis for STEMI had a lower mortality rate when compared to those who did develop Q wave at 30 days post infarction and 1 year post infarction (Bargelata et al., 1997). Thus, the absence of Q-wave after reperfusion therapy is a powerful marker of non-transmural necrosis and then of favorable prognosis.

2.4 T-wave inversion

In healthy patients, T-wave are normally upright in the left-sided leads (I, II, V3-V6). Within hours to days, an evolving STEMI will typically demonstrate T-wave inversion (Goldberger, 1991).The inverted T-wave appear generally in the same leads showing ST-segment elevation (Oliva et al., 1993). The morphology of inverted T-wave tends to be symmetric (Goldschlager & Goldman,1989). In the course of an evolving STEMI, T-wave inversion occurs when ischemia involves the epicardium. T-wave inversion is hypothesized by Mandel et al. to occur because of delayed depolarization in ischemic tissue (Mandel et al., 1968). In normal hearts, the epicardium is the first to depolarize, whereas the endocardium is the last. Delayed repolarization of the epicardium during ischemia reverses the direction of the ventricular repolarization current. With repolarization moving in the direction of endocardium to epicardium, the repolarization vector also reverses, causing a downward deflection of the T-wave (Smith & Whitwam, 2005). T-wave inversion occurs in approximately 3/4 of all patients with a completed myocardial necrosis (Goldschlager & Goldman,1989). Presence of T-wave inversion in precordial leads, of at least 2 mm, has a positive predictive value of 86% for left anterior descending artery stenosis (Haines et al., 1983). Indeed, a deepening T-wave soon after fibrinolysis may then determine successful reperfusion. However, normalization of T-waves may also predict a lower morbidity months after STEMI. One study by Tamura et al. found that patients with T-wave normalization within 6 months of infarction had higher left ventricular ejection fraction than those who did not, indicating that patients with normalization of inverted T waves had improved myocardial recovery (Tamura et al., 1999). The morphology of the T-wave inversion may help to differentiate between these other causes of T-wave inversion. Pacemaker T wave, in other words T wave inversion related to permanent ventricular pacemakers, tend to be broader than the narrower infarction T waves. A prolonged QTc distinguishes long QT syndrome. In mitral valve prolapse, T wave may be flattened or even inverted in inferior or lateral leads (Goldberger, 1991). In stroke, T waves tend to be very wide and the QT interval prolonged (Cropp & Manning, 1960).

2.5 Normalization of the ST segment

In not-reperfused STEMI, after a peak elevation approximately 1 hour after the onset of chest pain, the ST segment reaches a plateau at about 12 hours (Essen et al., 1979), and a complete resolution within 2 weeks in 95% of patients with inferior STEMI and 40% of patients with anterior STEMI (Mills et al., 1975). Even if the resolution of the ST-segment elevation may rarely occur from spontaneous reperfusion (Parikh & Shah, 1997), nowadays the normalization of the ST-segment can be observed in the majority of patients as result of successful reperfusion therapy. In fact, after successful fibrinolysis or mechanical reopening of infarct-related artery, abrupt changes occur in ECG as result of recovery in depolarization currents across the myocites membrane. Thus a prompt decrease in ST-segment elevation is a powerful predictor of reperfusion (Richardson et al., 1988), whereas the persistence of ST-segment elevation represent a marker of unsuccessful reperfusion therapy and is an independent determinant of major adverse cardiac event (Claeys et al., 1999). Interestingly, a decrease in ST-segment elevation by at least 50% seems to be associated with 94% positive predictive value for complete reperfusion (Krucoff et al., 1993). Indeed, studies have also found that even after a complete and sustained patency of epicardial infarct-related artery obtained by pharmacological or mechanical recanalization, about one-third of patients still show a persistent ST- segment elevation, as result of unsuccessful reperfusion of the microvasculature (De Lemos & Brunwald, 2001). This condition is known as a no-reflow phenomenon, and has been related to a higher mortality and worse clinical outcome after myocardial infarction (Poli et al., 2002). Thus it is important to remark that normalization of the ST-segment indicates adequate perfusion throughout the myocardial microvasculature rather than epicardial coronary patency.

3. Choice of reperfusion strategy

Primary percutaneous coronary intervention and thrombolysis remain therapies of choice for patients presenting with evolving STEMI. However, clinical outcome after STEMI is mainly related to complete and sustained myocardial reperfusion, but strongly influenced by delay in achieving reperfusion. In fact, the extension of necrosis is time dependent, with a wave front developing from the subendocardium and extending transmurally to the epicardium over time. For every 30 minutes duration of ischemia, there is an 8-10% increase in mortality (Pinto et al., 2006). Reperfusion therapy, with dissolution or removal of the intracoronary thrombus, provides the best chance for mortality reduction. The Focused Update gives primary percutaneous coronary intervention (P-PCI) a Class IA recommendation for reperfusion, as long as it can be accomplished with a first medical contact to balloon inflation time of 90 minutes or less (Antman et al., 2008). Fibrinolysis, which is less effective than P-PCI in head-to-head trials, is given a Class IB rating as an alternative to P-PCI, as long as P-PCI can't be accomplished within 90 minutes. Although P-PCI is commonly more effective than thrombolytic therapy (TT) for the treatment of patients with STEMI, the mortality benefit of P-PCI over TT is risk and time-dependent (Antman et al., 2008; Keeley et al., 2003; Tarantini et al., 2005; Thune et al., 2005; Cannon et al., 2000; De Luca et al., 2003). As the time delay for performing P-PCI increases, the mortality benefit of P-PCI compared with fibrinolysis decreases. The P-PCI strategy may not reduce mortality when the delay is 60 min compared with immediate administration of a fibrin-specific lytic agent (Nallamothu & Bates, 2003). However, the value of 60 min is still controversial and should not be stated so categorically; other authors, for example, found that longer P-PCI-related delays do not negate the survival benefit of PPCI even when the delay is up to 3 h (Boersma et al., 2006; Stenestrand et al., 2006; Betriu & Masotti, 2005). Moreover, a recent evaluation of registry data has shown that the acceptable P-PCI-related delay depends upon the risk of the patient (Pinto et al., 2006). It has been explored the relationship between risk and P-PCI delay, adjusted for the delay at presentation, which leads to equivalent 30-day mortality between P-PCI and fibrin-specific thrombolytic therapy. Baseline mortality risk of STEMI patients is a major determinant of the acceptable time delay to choose the most appropriate therapy. Although a longer delay lowers the survival advantage of P-PCI, a longer P-PCI-related delay could be acceptable in high-risk STEMI patients (Tarantini et al.,

2010). Generally factors which preclude "waiting for PCI" include young age, anterior MI, and early (<3 hrs of pain) presentation. Factors which make delayed P-PCI the preferred strategy include contraindications to fibrinolysis, cardiogenic shock, advanced age, inferior MI, and delayed presentation (Antman et al., 2004). Whichever reperfusion strategy is chosen, it is important to maximize the effectiveness of that therapy by applying not only prompt, but also appropriate anti-platelet and anti-thrombin adjuncts. The recommendations for these therapies differ with the reperfusion method chosen. Appropriate protocol development demands maximization of the effectiveness of anti-platelet and anti-thrombin agents with each reperfusion choice.

4. Arrhythmias and conduction disturbances in the acute phase

Ventricular tachycardia (VT), Ventricular Fibrillation (VF) and complete atrio-ventricular (BAVC) block, may be the first manifestation of ischemia and requires immediate correction, since these arrhythmias may cause sudden cardiac death. VF and VT have been reported up to 20% of patients with STEMI (Henkel et al., 2006). Often arrhythmias are the manifestation of a serious underlying disorder, such as persisting ischemia, severe pump failure, or endogenous factors such as abnormal potassium levels, autonomic imbalances, hypoxia, and acid-base disturbances, that may require corrective measures. The need for arrhythmias treatment depends mainly upon the hemodynamic impact of the rhythm disorder.

4.1 Ventricular arrhythmias

VF occurring within 48 hours of the onset of STEMI has been related to higher in-hospital mortality, but not to long-term mortality. The major determinants of risk of sudden death are related more to the severity of the cardiac disease and less to frequency of classification of ventricular arrhythmias (Huikuri et al., 2001).

4.2 Ventricular ectopic rhythms

Ventricular ectopic beats are common during the initial phase of STEMI. Irrespective of their complexity (multiform QRS complex beats, short runs of ventricular beats or the R-on-T phenomenon) their value, as predictor of VF, is questionable.

4.3 Ventricular tachycardia and Ventricular fibrillation

Either not sustained VT (lasting <30s) not accelerated idioventricular rhythm (usually a harmless consequence of reperfusion with a ventricular rate<120beats), occurring in the setting of STEMI, serve as a reliably predictive marker of early VF. Sustained and/or haemodinamically compromising VT (occurring in 3%) requires suppressive therapy, and outlined in the guidelines for ventricular arrythmias (Zipes et al., 2006). Pulsless VT and VF should be managed according to the resuscitation guidelines.

4.4 Supraventricular arrhythmias

Atrial fibrillation (AF), which complicates 10-20% of STEMI is more prevalent in older patients and in those with severe LV damage and heart failure. AF is associated with increased in-hospital mortality (Fuster et al., 2006). In many cases this arrhythmia is well tolerated and no specific treatment is required. In other instances, the high ventricular response contributes to heart failure and prompt treatment is needed.

4.5 Sinus bradycardia and heart block

Sinus bradicardya: is common (9-25%) in the first hour, particularly in inferior infarction (Goldestein et al 2005). If associated with hemodynamic compromise it should be treated. *AV block:* Data from four large, randomized trials suggest that AV block occurs in almost 7% (Meine et al., 2005) and persistent LBBB in up to 5.3% of cases of STEMI (Newby et al., 1996). Patients with peri-infarction AV block have an higher in hospital mortality than those with preserved AV conduction (Meine et al., 2005). The increased mortality seems related to the extensive myocardial damage required to develop heart block rather than to heart block itself. AV block associated with inferior wall infarction is usually transient, whereas AV block related to anterior wall infarction is more often located below the AV node and associated with an unstable, wide QRS escape rhythm due to extensive myocardial necrosis. A new LBBB usually indicated extensive anterior infarction with high probability to develop complete AV block and pump failure. The preventive placement of a temporary pacing electrode may be warranted. Raccomandations for permanent cardiac pacing for persistent conduction disturbances (>14 days) due to STEMI are outlined in the ESC Guidelines for cardiac pacing.

5. ECG in pharmacological reperfusion - implications for adjunctive therapies

As a tool to identify epicardial reperfusion all methods of ST resolution, assessed by either continuous monitoring or static ECG recording, have the limitation that ST-segment changes integrate both epicardial and myocardial reperfusion. A resolution of ST-segment elevation of more than 70% of the initial value at 60 to 90 minutes after the initiation of therapy, is a powerful predictor of successful myocardial reperfusion and is therefore associated with enhanced recovery of LV function, reduced infarct size, and improved prognosis (de Lemos et al., 2000; Zeymer et al., 2001). Thus patients with complete ST-resolution at 90 minutes after fibrinolysis have a > 90% probability of a patent infarct-related artery associated with a successful reperfusion at the microvascular level. However, approximately 50% of patients with no ST-segment resolution after fibrinolysis still show a patent epicardial infarct artery. In fact in these patients the lack of ST resolution is caused by the failure of reperfusion at the level of microvasculature rather than at epicardial vessel. Thus, ST resolution represents a powerful predictor of infarct-related artery patency, but it is less accurate for predicting the persistence of epicardial vessel occlusion after fibrinolysis (Schröder et al., 2004). Therefore, in order to judge the need for adjunctive mechanical reopening of the infarct-related artery after failed fibrinolysis, by the so called "rescue angioplasty", it is important to integrate clinical and ECG data. According to the ACC/AHA guidelines, it is reasonable to monitor the pattern of ST-segment elevation, cardiac rhythm, and clinical symptoms during the 60 to 90 minutes after the initiation of fibrinolytic therapy. Non-invasive findings suggesting for a successful reperfusion include relief of symptoms, maintenance or restoration of hemodynamic and electrical stability, and a reduction of at least 50% in the initial ST-segment elevation. In this scenario, the presence of particular arrhythmias, such as not rapid ventricular tachycardia, idioventricular rhythm or not-sustained bradycardia, early after fibrinolytic administration, represents a highly specific marker of reperfusion. Otherwise, persistence of ischemic chest pain, absence of resolution of the qualifying ST-segment elevation, and hemodynamic or electrical instability are generally predictors of failed pharmacological reperfusion, needing rescue angioplasty.

6. ECG in mechanical reperfusion - implication for prognosis

Many studies, evaluating the outcomes of primary angioplasty in STEMI, found that persistent ST-segment elevation after coronary flow restoration, is one of the independent determinant of adverse cardiac event (Schröder et al., 1994; de Lemos & Braunwald, 2001). In fact, patients with persistent ST-segment elevation, even after a successful restoration of normal antegrade coronary flow in the epicardial artery, show absent or inadequate flow at level of microvasculature (van't Hof et a., 1997). This phenomenon, known as a no-reflow phenomenon, has been described in animal and clinical studies, involving about one third of patients who underwent successful recanalization of the infarct-related artery. This condition, has been related to larger necrosis, adverse ventricular remodeling and higher morbidity/mortality at short and long-term follow-up. Otherwise, a resolution of ST-segment elevation by at least 50% is associated with a high positive predictive value for successful myocardial reperfusion. In this setting, the analysis of ST-segment evolution during and after coronary recanalization represents an useful tool to guide further pharmacological treatments, as well as more aggressive management of these patients. Different methods, cut-offs, and timing have been proposed to evaluate ST-segment resolution. In most studies, resolution of ST-segment elevation has been expressed as percentage of resolution of the sum of ST-segment elevation in all leads (van't Hof et a., 1997; Schröder et al., 1994; de Lemos JA & Braunwald, 2001; Zeymer et al., 2003). To this purpose, ST sum should take into account not only the ST shift in all leads showing ST elevation, but also the reciprocal ST deviation in leads showing ST depression. However, measuring ST resolution from all leads is time consuming and may be influenced by patient's position and by changes in position of lead electrodes. In order to simplify ST resolution assessment, other authors have proposed an alternative method based on measurement of ST resolution in only the single lead showing the maximum deviation before reperfusion: "the single lead ST resolution" (Schröder et al., 2001). In the single lead method, ST resolution is measured by comparing one ECG lead with the most prominent ST-segment shift at baseline and at a given time-point after reperfusion therapy, irrespective of the ECG lead measure at baseline. This method resulted as simple as accurate when compared to conventional model of sum ST resolution model. The optimal cut-off for defining reperfusion effectiveness and then mortality risk groups were assessed by statistical methods. Applying 2 cut-offs provides the most powerful stratification of high and low mortality risk group. To this purpose sum ST resolution is conventionally categorized as complete (≥ 70%), partial (<70% to 30%), and no (≤ 30%) ST-segment elevation resolution (Schroder et al., 1994). Although different time points have been reported across the studies evaluating the relationship between ST resolution and outcome, such as 30, 60, or even 90 minutes after reperfusion therapy, no significant differences between various time points were found, and the ideal time of measuring ST resolution remains unclear. However, these studies were mostly conducted in patients receiving fibrinolytic therapy, and may not directly applicable when assessing success of primary angioplasty. In fact, after fibrinolysis for STEMI the ECG for measuring ST resolution is usually taken 60 to 90 minutes after the onset of therapy, in order to detect by means of non-invasive tool the patency of epicardial vessel, rather than the reperfusion at microvascular level. In studies assessing the ST resolution on ECG, the timing of ECG after primary angioplasty was highly variable, ranging from 30 minutes after angioplasty to 60 minutes, or even several hours later. Strong evidences showed that ST resolution as evaluated 30 minutes after angioplasty correlated better with other markers of myocardial perfusion than ST resolution at 60 to 90 minutes. Indeed, recent evidences have shown that early complete ST recovery, as assessed immediately after last contrast injection in the catheterization laboratory, have a better preserved left ventricular ejection fraction and smaller infarct at magnetic resonance than patients showing ST resolution at 30 minutes or later (Haeck et al., 2011). These findings are not only consistent with the hypothesis that ST resolution implies effective microvascular and tissue reperfusion, but also relate the recovery of electrocardiografic changes to salvage of viable myocardium. Indeed, early assessment of ST recovery may represents the appropriate time to identify patients at higher risk of adverse events potentially benefit from additional novel therapies, ideally starting already at the catheterization laboratory.

7. ECG in stabilized myocardial infarction

The ECG in the stabilized phase of STEMI, after reperfusion therapy, represents a simply and universally applicable diagnostic tool to understand the prognosis and to guide further interventions. One method for determining the presence of pathological Q-waves related to myocardial infarction has been the Minnesota Code (Blackburn et a., 1960). This method was developed for diagnosis of infarction rather than the quantification of its size and correlates poorly with anatomically measured infarct size (Pahlm et al., 1998). An improved correlation of changes in the QRS complex with infarct size was the development of a QRS scoring system by Selvester et al. The Selvester QRS scoring system included 54 criteria from the QRS complexes in 10 of the standard leads, which totaled 32 points, each equivalent to approximately 3% of the left ventricular wall (Startt-Selvester et al., 1989). Recently, studies using cardiac magnetic resonance have show that Q-wave predict the location and size of myocardial infarction (Wu E et al., 2001.). Historically the presence of Q-wave on ECG after myocardial infarction has been used in clinical practice to stratify patients in Q-wave and non-Q-wave myocardial infarction, according to larger necrosis and worse outcome discovered in Q-wave infarctions (Stone PH et al., 1988). On these basis, for many years after the original report by Prinzmetal in animal model (Prinzmetal et al., 1954), the presence of Q-wave has been related to transmural infarction, whereas its absence was categorize as non-transmural infarction. Recently, studies based on cardiac magnetic resonance have clarified that, even if this distinction still appears useful to stratify the risk after myocardial infarction, the presence of Q-wave on surface ECG is determined by the total size of necrosis rather than transmural extent of underlying myocardial infarction (Moon et al., 2004). A relative small number of patients after myocardial infarction still show persistence of ST-segment elevation even days and month after the acute event. Historically, this late persistence of ST-segment elevation has been ascribed to left ventricular aneurysm or impending rupture of free wall or ventricular septum, identifying patients at very high risk for heart failure and death (Chon et al., 1967). However, this association is among the most controversial in electrocardiography, since previous studies, including echocardiography and angiography, clearly showed a more severe systolic dysfunction and wall motion abnormalities in patients with persistent STE, but failed to demonstrate a definite relationship between this electrocardiographic pattern and left ventricular aneurysm. Moreover, the explanation of the underlying mechanism of persistent STE and its pathological correlates are still unclear (Bar et al., 1984 & Lidsay J et al., 1984 ; Bhatnagar, 1994). Recently, using cardiac magnetic resonance, correlations between this ECG pattern and type of myocardial damage have been reported. Particularly, the presence of persisting ST-elevation seems related to the presence of large microvascular damage in the context of transmural necrosis (Figure 3). These findings suggest that in this scenario late persistence of ST elevation indicates not only, as predictable, a greater extent of myocardial necrosis, but also, and more interestingly, the presence of severe microvascular damage as shown by cardiac magnetic resonance. Patients exhibiting persistent ST elevation showed more frequently left ventricular aneurysm, even though this difference did not achieve a statistical significance. Taking into account the findings of previous studies, these observations lead to the criticism about wall motion abnormalities as mechanism of electrocardiographic alterations. Recently, Li et al provided direct evidence in animals that opening of sarcolemmal KATP channels underlies ST elevation during ischemia (Li RA et al., 2000). It has also been demonstrated in a swine model that mechanical stimuli can induce marked ST elevation , by producing the stretching activation of KATP channel (Link et al., 1999). On these basis it has been hypothesized that outward bulging of myocardial necrotic wall, producing an abnormal stretch on the adjacent tissue, may alter cellular activity, generating injury currents at this level responsible for the ST elevation (Gussak et al., 2000). Thus patients exhibiting persistence of ST elevation had not only more severe myocardial

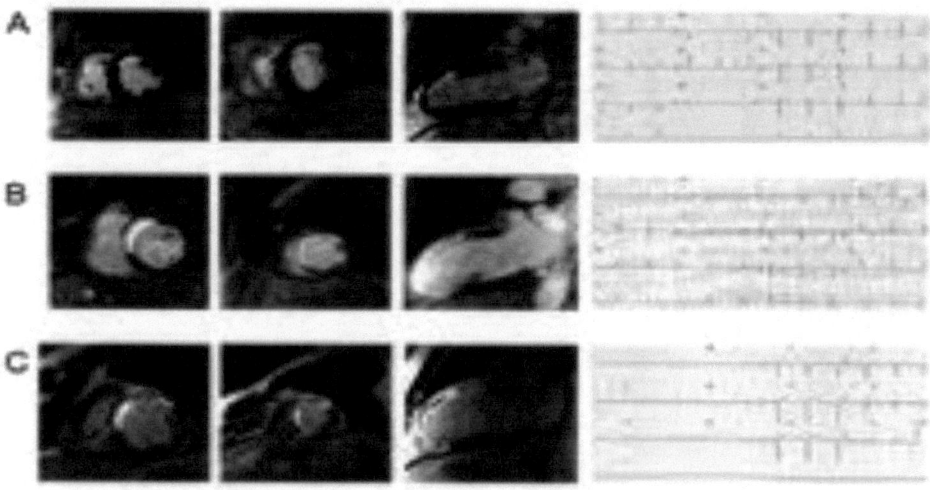

Panel A: ECG shows neither ST-segment elevation nor pathological Q-wave; the ce-MRI detects non-trasmural necrosis (middle and apical segments) of anterolateral wall, without either persistent microvascular obstruction or left ventricular aneurysm. **Panel B**: ECG shows pathological Q-wave in leads V4 to V6, with persistent ST elevation; the corresponding ce-MRI shows transmural necrosis of the septum, anterolateral wall (middle and apical segments), and apex, with evidence of persistent microvascular obstruction in the setting of necrotic core, without aneurysm. **Panel C :** ECG shows Q-wave in leads V1 through V6, DI, aVL, and STE in leads V1 through V6. The corresponding ce-MRI shows a large trasmural necrosis in the septum and anterolateral wall (middle and apical segments), and of the apical segments of inferior wall, with evidence of persistent microvascular obstruction in the necrotic core.

Fig. 3. Different patterns of myocardial structural abnormalities detected by contrast-enhanced magnetic resonance imaging (ce-MRI) and corresponding 12-leads electrocardiogram (ECG).

damage, but also more frequently coexistence of microvascular damage within it, that could account for diffuse alterations in myocardial skeletal favoring myocardial bulging and mechanical activation of KATP channels in the adjacent tissue. Finally, these findings may also explain the temporal discrepancy between developing of aneurysm and ECG alterations.

8. Conclusion

The ECG is the most important diagnostic tool in the diagnosis of evolving ST-segment elevation myocardial infarction, influencing therapeutic strategies and management. Moreover, ECG remains a simple but valuable method to estimate the risk of STEMI patients either before and after reperfusion therapy. Finally the value of ECG in the prognostic stratification after stabilized STEMI have still a role in current management of these patients.

9. References

Aldrich, H.R. (1988). Use of initial ST-segment deviation for prediction of final electrocardiographic size of acute myocardial infarcts. *Am J Cardiol*, Vol.61, pp. 749-753, 0002-9149

American College Cardiology (ACC)/American Heart Association (AHA) (2009). Guidelines for the management of patients with acute myocardial infarction. *J Am Coll Cardiol*, Vol. 34, pp 1890 –1911, 0735-1097

Antman, E.M. (2004). ACC/AHA guidelines for the management of patients with ST-elevation myocardial infarction--executive summary. *J Am Coll Cardiol,* Vol.44, pp. 671-719, 0735-1097

Antman, E.M. (2006). Enoxaparin versus unfractionated heparin with fibrinolysis for ST elevation MI (EXTRACT TIMI 25 trial). *N Eng J Med,* Vol.354, pp. 1477-1488, 1533-4406

Antman, E.M. (2008). Focused Update of the ACC/AHA 2004 Guidelines for the Management of Patients With ST-Elevation Myocardial Infarction. *JACC,* Vol.51, 2, pp. 210-247, 0735-1097

Antman, E.M. (2008). Focused update of the ACC/AHA 2004 guidelines for the management of patients with ST-elevation myocardial infarction: a report of the American College of Cardiology/American Heart Association Task Force on Practice Guidelines. *J Am Coll Cardiol,* Vol.51, pp. 210-47, 0735-1097

Antoniucci, D. (2004). Abciximab-supported infarct artery stent implantation for acute myocardial infarction and long-term survival: A prospective, multicenter, randomized trial comparing infarct artery stenting plus abciximab with stenting alone. *Circulation,* Vol.109, pp.1704–6, 0009-7322

Bairey, C.N. (1987). Electrocardiographic differentiation of occlusion of the left circumflex versus the right coronary artery as a cause of inferior acute myocardial infarction. *Am J Cardiol,* Vol.60, pp. 456-69, 0002-9149

Bär, F.W. (1996). Development of ST- segment elevation and Q-and R-wave changes in acute myocardial infarction and the influence of thrombolytic therapy. *Am J Cardiol,* Vol.77, pp.337-43, 0002-9149

Bar, FW. (1984). Prognostic value of Q waves, R/S ratio, loss of R wave voltage, ST-T segment abnormalities, electrical axis, low voltage and notching: correlation of electrocardiogram and left ventriculogram. *J Am Coll Cardiol,* Vol.4, pp. 17-27, 0735-1097

Barbagelata, A. (1997). Thrombolysis and Q wave versus non-Q wave first acute myocardial infarction: a GUSTO-I substudy. *J Am Coll Cardiol,* Vol 29, pp. 770-7, 0735-1097

Bayes de Luna, A. (2006a). Concordance of electrocardiographic patterns and healed myocardial infarction detected by cardiovascular magnetic resonance. *Am J Cardiol,* Vol.97, pp. 443-451, 0002-9149

Bayes de Luna, A. (2006b). A new terminology for the left ventricular walls and location of myocardial infarcts that present Q-wave on the standard of cardiac magnetic resonance imaging. *Circulation,* Vol114, pp. 1755-1760, 0009-7322

Betriu, A. (2005). Comparison of mortality rates in acute myocardial infarction treated by percutaneous coronary intervention versus fibrinolysis. *Am J Cardiol,* Vol.95, pp. 100–101, 0002-9149

Bhatnagar, SK. (1994). Observation of the relationship between left ventricular aneurysm and ST segment elevation in patients with a first acute anterior Q wave myocardial infarction. *Eur Heart,* Vol.15, pp. 1500-1504, 1522-9645

Birnbaum, Y. (1993). Prediction of the level of left descending coronary artery obstruction during anterior wall acute myocardial infarction by the admission electrocardiogram. *Am J Cardiol,* Vol.72, pp 823-826, 0002-9149

Blackburn, H. (1960). Electrocardiogram in population studies: a classification system. *Circulation,* Vol.21, pp. 1160-75, 0009-7322

Boersma, E. (2006). Does time matter? A pooled analysis of randomized clinical trials comparing primary percutaneous cor- onary intervention and in-hospital fibrinolysis in acute myocardial infarction patients. *Eur Heart J ,* Vol.27, pp. 779–788, 1522-9645

Brady, W.J. (2001). Electrocardiographic STsegment elevation: the diagnosis of acute myocardial infarction by morphologic analysis of the ST segment. *Acad Emerg Med,* Vol.8, pp. 961-967, 1069-6563

Brener, S.J. (1998). Randomized, placebo-controlled trial of platelet glycoprotein IIb/IIIa blockade with primary angioplasty for acute myocardial infarction. ReoPro and Primary PTCA Organization and Randomized Trial (RAPPORT) Investigators. *Circulation,* Vol. 98, pp. 734-41, 0009-7322.

Cannon, C.P. (2000). Relationship of symptom- onset-to-balloon time and door-to-balloon time with mortality in patients undergoing angioplasty for acute myocardial infarction. *JAMA,* Vol 283, pp. 2941–2947, 0098-7487

Cerqueira, M.D. (2002). Standardized myocardial segmentation and nomenclature for tomographic imaging of the heart. *Circulation,* Vol.105, pp. 539-542, 0009-7322

Chon, K. (1967). Use of electrocardiogram as an aid in screening for left ventricular aneurysm. J Electrocardiol. 1976;9:53-58. Herman MV, et al. Localized disorders in myocardial contraction. Asynergy and its role in congestive heart failure. *N Engl J Med,* Vol.277, pp. 222-232, 1533-4406

Chong, E. (2010). Two-year clinical registry follow-up of endothelial progenitor cell capture stent versus sirolimus-eluting bioabsorbable polymer-coated stent versus bare metal stents in patients undergoing primary percutaneous coronary intervention for ST elevation myocardial infarction. *J Inter Cardiol,* Vol 23, pp.101-8, 0167-5273

Claeys, M.J. (1999). Determinants and prognostic implications of persistent ST-segment elevation after primary angio- plasty for acute myocardial infarction: Importance of microvascular reperfusion injury on clinical outcome. *Circulation,* Vol.99, pp.1972-7, 0009-7322

Co, M. (2008). Use of endothelial progenitor cell capture stent (Genous Bio-Engineered R Stent) during primary percutaneous coronary intervention in acute myocardial infarction. *American Heart Journal,* Vol.155, pp. 128-32, 0002-8703

Correale, E. (1999). Electrocardiographic patterns in acute inferior myocardial infarction with and without right ventricular involvement: classification, diagnostic and prognostic value, masking effect. *Clin Cardiol,* Vol.22, pp. 37-44,

Cropp, G.J. (1960). Manning GW. Electrocardiographic changes simulating myocardial ischemia and infarction associated with spontaneous intracranial hemorrhage. *Circulation,* Vol 22, pp. 25-38, 0009-7322

Daemen, J. (2007). Comparison of three-year clinical outcome of sirolimus- and paclitaxel-eluting stents versus bare metal stents in patients with ST-segment elevation myocardial infarction. *Am J Cardiol,* Vol.99, pp 1027–32, 0002-9149

De Lemos, J.A. (2001). ST segment resolution as a tool for assessing the efficacy of reperfusion therapy. *J Am Coll Cardiol,* Vol 38, pp. 1283-94, 0735-1097

De Lemos, JA. (2000) . ST-segment resolution and infarct-related artery patency and flow after thrombolytic therapy. TIMI-14 14 Investigators. *Am J Cardiol* , Vol.85, pp. 299-304, 0002-9149

De Lemos, JA. (2001). ST segment resolution as a tool for assessing the efficacy of reperfusion therapy. *J Am Coll Cardiol,* Vol.38, pp. 1283-1294, 0735-1097

De Lemos, JA. (2001). ST-segment resolution as a tool for assessing the efficacy of reperfusion therapy. *J Am Coll Cardiol,* Vol.38, pp. 1283-1294, 0735-1097

De Luca, G. (2003). Myocardial Infarction Study Group. Symptom onset to balloon time and mortality in patients with acute myocardial infarction treated by primary angioplasty. *J Am Coll Cardiol,* Vol.42, pp. 991–997, 0735-1097

Dressler, W. (1947). High T waves in the earliest stage of myocardial infarction. *Am Heart J,* Vol.34, pp. 627-645, 0002-8703

Edwards, J. (2005). The COMMIT trial investigators: Addition of clopidogrel to aspirin in 45,852 patients with AMI: a randomized placebo controlled trial. *Lancet,* Vol.366, pp. 1607-1621, 0140-6736

Engelen, D.J. (1999). Value of electrocardiogram in localizing the occlusion site in the left anterior descending coronary artery in acute myocardial infarction. *J Am Coll Cardiol,* Vol.34, pp 389-395, 0735-1097

Essen, R. (1979). Spontaneous course of ST-segment elevation in acute anterior myocardial infarction. *Circulation,* Vol.59, pp. 105-12, 0009-7322

Fuster, V. (2006). ACC/AHA/ESC 2006 Guidelines for the Management of Patients with Atrial Fibrillation. *Circulation,* Vol.114, pp. e257–e354, 0009-7322

Goldberger A.L. 4th ed. (1991). *Myocardial infarction: electrocardiographic differential diagnosis,*): Mosby; St. Louis

Goldschlager, N. (1989). Principles of clinical electrocardiography, In: *Appleton and Lange,* Norwalk Conn, pp. 110-2. 13th ed

Goldstein, JA. (2005). Patterns of coronary compromise leading to bradyarrhytmias and hypotension in inferior myocardial infarction. *Coron Artery Dis* 2005, Vol.16, pp. 265-274

Gurm, HS. (2008). The relative safety and efficacy of abciximab and eptifibatide in patients undergoing primary percutaneous coronary intervention: insights from a large regional registry of contemporary percutaneous coronary intervention. *J Am Coll Cardiol* , Vol 51, pp. 529–35, 0735-1097

Gussak, I. (2000). Exercise induced ST segment elevation in Q wave leads in postinfarction patients: defining its meaning and utility in today's practice. *Cardiology,* Vol.93, pp. 205-209

Haeck, JDE. (2011). Impact of early, late, and no ST-segment resolution measured by continuous ST Holter monitoring on left ventricular ejection fraction and infarct size as determined by cardiovascular magnetic resonance imaging. *J Electrocardiol,* Vol.44, pp. 36-41

Haines, D.E. (1983). Anatomic and prognostic significance of new T-wave inversion in unstable angina. *Am J Cardiol,* Vol.52, pp.14-8, 0002-9149

Hamby, R.I. (1983). Left bundle branch block: a predictor of poor left ventricular function in coronary heart disease. *Am Heart J,* Vol.106, pp. 471-477, 0002-8703

Henkel, DM. (2006). Ventricular arrhytmias after acute myocardial infarction: a 20 year community study. *Am Heart J,* Vol.151, pp. 806-812, 0002-8703

Herz, M. (1997). New electrocardiographic criteria for predicting either the right or left circumflex artery as the culprit coronary artery in inferior wall acute myocardial infarction. *Am J Cardiol,* Vol.80, pp. 1343-1345, 0002-9149

Huikuri, H. (2001). Sudden death due to cardiac arrhytmias. *N Engl J Med,* Vol.345, pp. 1473-1482, 1533-4406

Keeley, E.C. (2003). Primary angioplasty versus intravenous throm- bolytic therapy for acute myocardial infarction a quantitative review of 23 ran- domized trials. *Lancet,* Vol.361, pp 13–20, 0140-6736

Krucoff, M.W. (1993). Continuous 12-lead ST- segment recovery analysis in the TAMI 7 study. Performance of a non invasive method for real-time detection of failed myocardial reperfusion. *Circulation,* Vol.88, pp. 437-46, 0009-7322.

Lee, K.L. (1995). Predictors of 30-day mortality in the era of reperfusion for acute myocardial infarction. *Circulation,* Vol. 91, pp. 1659-1568, 0009-7322

Lee, Y.P. (2010). Endothelial progenitor cell capture stent implantation in patients with ST-segment elevation acute myocardial infarction: one year follow-up. *Eurointervention,* Vol.5, pp. 698-702, 1969-6213

Lemos, P.A. (2004). Unrestricted utilization of sirolimus-eluting stents compared with conventional bare stent implantation in the "real world": the Rapamycin- Eluting Stent Evaluated at Rotterdam Cardiology Hospital (RESEARCH) registry. *Circulation,* Vol.109, pp. 190-5, 0009-7322

Li, RA. (2000). Molecular basis of electrocardiographic ST-segment elevation. *Circ Res,* Vol.87, pp. 837-39

Lidsay, J Jr. (1984). Relation of ST-segment elevation after healing of acute myocardial infarction to the presence of left ventricular aneurysm. *Am J Cardiol,* Vol.54, pp. 84-6, 0002-9149.

Link, MS. (1999). Selective activation of the KATP channel is mechanism by which sudden death is produced by low energy chest wall impact. *Circulation,* Vol 100, pp. 413-418, 0009-7322.

Mandel, W.J.(1968). Analysis of T-wave abnormalities associated with myocardial infarction using a theoretic model. *Circulation,* Vol.38, pp. 178-88, 0009-7322

Meine, TJ. (2005). Incidence, predictors, and outcomes ESC Guidelines of high-degree atrioventricular block complicating acute myocardial infarction treated with thrombolytic therapy. *Am Heart J* , Vol.149, pp. 670–674, 0002-8703

Menown, I.B. (2000). Optimizing the initial 12-lead electrocardiographic diagnosis of acute myocardial infarction. *EurHeart J,* Vol.21, pp. 275-283, 1522-9645

Mills, R.M. (1975). Natural history of S-T segment elevation after acute myocardial infarction. *Am J Cardiol,* Vol 35, pp. 609-14, 0002-9149

Montalescot, G. (2001). Platelet glycoprotein IIb/IIIa inhibition with coronary stenting for acute myocardial infarction. *N Engl J Med,* Vol.344, pp. 1895–903, 1533-4406

Moon, JCC. (2004). The Pathologic basis of Q-wave and non-Q wave myocardial infarction. *JAm Coll Cardiol,* Vol 44, pp. 554-60, 0735-1097

Nallamothu, B.K. (2003). Percutaneous coronary intervention versus fibrinolytic therapy in acute myocardial infarction is timing (almost) everything? *Am J Cardiol,* Vol.92:, pp. 824–826, 0002-9149

Newby, KH. (1996). Incidence and clinical relevance of the occurrence of bundle-branch block in patients treated with thrombolytic therapy. *Circulation,* Vol.94, pp. 2424–2428, 0009-7322.

Oliva, P.B. (1993). Electrocardiographic diagnosis of postinfarction regional pericarditis. Ancillary observations regard- ing the effect of reperfusion on the rapidity and amplitude of T wave inversion after acute myocardial infarction. *Circulation,* Vol 88, pp. 896-904, 0009-7322

Opolski, G. The effect of infarct size on atrioventricular and intraventricular conduction disturbances in acute myocardial infarction. *Int J Cardiol,* Vol.10, pp. 141-147

Pahlm, US. (1998). Comparison of various electrocardiografic scoring codes for estimating anatomically documented size and single and multiple infarcts of the left ventricle. *Am J Cardiol,* Vol.81, pp. 809-15, 0002-9149

Parikh, A. 2nd ed. (1997). New insights into the electrocardiogram of acute myocardial infarction, In: *Acute myocardial infarction,* Gersh BJ Rahimtoola SH editors, Chapman and Hall, New York

Perera, D. (2004). Dynamics of ST segment in ischaemic heart disease, In: *Dynamic electrocardiography,* Malik M, Camm AJ, editors.. 1st ed. Elmsford (NY)

Pinto, D.S. (2006). Hospital delays in reperfusion for ST-elevation myocardial infarction. Implications when selecting a reperfusion strategy. *Circulation,* Vol.114, pp. 2019–2025, 0009-7322.

Pinto, D.S. (2007). Hospital delays in reperfusion for ST-elevation myocardial infarction: implications when selecting a reperfusion strategy. *Circulation,* Vol.114, pp. 2019-2025, 0009-7322

Poli, A. (2002). Integrated analysis of myocardial blush and ST-segment elevation recovery after successful primary angioplasty: real-time grading of microvascular reperfusion and prediction of early and late recovery of left ventricular function. *Circulation,* Vol 106, pp. 313-8, 0009-7322

Prinzmetal, M. (1954).Studies on the mechanism of ventricular activity. The depolarization complex in pure subendocardial infarction: role of subendocardial region in the normal electrocardiogram. *Am J Med,* Vol.16, pp. 469-88

Raitt, M.H. (1995). Appearance of abnormal Q waves early in the course of acute myocardial infarction: implications for efficacy of thrombolytic therapy. *J Am Coll Cardiol,* Vol 25, pp.1084-8, 0735-1097

Richardson, S.G. (1988). Relation of coronary arterial patency and left ventricular function to electrocardiographic changes after streptokinase treatment during acute myocardial infarction. *Am J Cardiol,* Vol.61, 0002-9149

Sabatine, M.S. (2005). Addition of clopidogrel to aspirin and fibrinolytic therapy for STEMI. *N Engl J Med,* Vol.352, pp. 1179-1189. 1533-4406

Schröder R. (2004). Prognostic Impact of early ST-segment resolution in acute ST-elevation myocardial infarction. *Circulation,* Vol 110, pp. e506-e510, 0009-7322

Schröder, K. (1994). Extent of early ST segment elevation resolution: a simple but strong predictor of outcome in patients with acute myocardial infarction. *J Am Coll Cardiol,* Vol.24, pp. 384-391, 0735-1097

Schröder, K. (2001). Extent of ST deviation in the single ECG lead of maximum deviation present 90 or 180 minutes after start of thrombolytic therapy best predicts outcome in acute myocardial infarction. *Z Kardiol 2001,* Vol.90, pp. 557-567

Sgarbossa, E.B. (1996). Early electrocardiographic diagnosis of acute myocardial infarction in the presence of ventricular paced rhythm. *Am J Cardiol,* Vol.77, pp. 423–424, 0002-9149

Sgarbossa, E.B. (1998). Electrocardiographic diagnosis of evolving acute myocardial infarction in the presence of left bundle-brach block. *N Engl J Med,* Vol.334, pp. 81–87, 1533-4406

Smith, S.W. (2005). Acute coronary syndromes: acute myocardial infarction and ischemia. In: *ECG in emergency medicine and acute care,* Chan TC, Brady WJ, Harrigan RA, editors, 1st edition, pp. (151-63). Mosby, Philadelphia

Smith, S.W. (2006). Acute coronary syndromes. *Emerg Med Clin North,* Vol 24, pp. 53-89.

Somers, M.P. (2002). The prominant T wave: electrocardiographic differential diagnosis. *Am J Emerg Med,* Vol 20, pp. 243-251, 0735-6757

Startt-Selvester, RH. (1989). Myocardial infarction. In: *Comprehensive Electrocardiology: theory and practice in health disease,* Macfarlane PW Lawrie TDV editors, pp. 565-629, Pergamon Press, New York

Stenestrand, U. (2006). RIKS-HIA Registry. Long-term outcome of primary percutaneous coronary intervention vs prehospital and in-hospital thrombolysis for patients with ST-elevation myocardial infarction. *JAMA,* Vol.296, pp. 1749–1756, 0098-7484

Stone, G.W. (2008). Bivalirudin during primary PCI in acute myocardial infarction. *N Engl J Med,* Vol.358, pp. 2218-30. 1533-4406

Stone, PH (1988). Prognostic significance of location and type of myocardial infarction. *J Am Coll Cardiol,* Vol 11, pp. 453-63, 1735-1097

Tamura, A. (1999). Significance of spontaneous normalization of negative T waves in infarct-related leads during healing of anterior wall acute myocardial infarction. *Am J Cardiol,* Vol.84, pp.1341-4, 0002-9149

Tanimoto, S. (2006). Drug-eluting stent implantation in acute myocardial infarction. Do we need another randomized trial? (TYPHOON, PASSION and HORIZONS trials). *EuroIntervention,* Vol.2, pp. 23-7, 1969-6213

Tarantini, G. (2005). Expla-nation for the survival benefit of primary angioplasty over thrombolytic therapy in patients with ST-elevation acute myocardial infarction. *Am J Cardiol,* Vol.96, pp. 1503–1505, 0002-9149

Tarantini, G. (2010). Acceptable reperfusion delay to prefer primary angioplasty over fibrin-specific thrombolytic therapy is affected (mainly) by the patient's mortality risk: 1 h does not fit all. *Eur Heart J,* Vol 31, pp. 676–683, 1522-9645.

Tcheng, J.E. (2003). Benefits and risks of abciximab use in primary angioplasty for acute myocardial infarction: the Controlled Abciximab and Device Investigation to Lower Late Angioplasty Complications (CADILLAC) trial. *Circulation,* Vol.108, pp. 1316–23, 0009- 7322

Thune, J.J. (2005). DANAMI-2 Investigators. Simple risk stratification at the admission to identify patients with reduced mortality from primary angioplasty. *Circulation,* Vol.112, pp. 2017–2021, 0009-7322.

Valgimigli, M. (2008). Comparison of angioplasty with infusion of tirofiban or abciximab and with implantation of sirolimus-eluting or uncoated stents for acute myocardial infarction, the MULTISTRATEGY randomized trial. *JAMA,* Vol.299, pp. 1788–99, 0098-7484

Van't Hof, AW. (1997). Clinical value of 12-lead electrocardiogram after successful reperfusion therapy for acute myocardial infarction. *Lancet,* Vol.350, pp. 615-619, 0140- 6736

Verouden, N.J. (2209). Distinguishing the right coronary artery from the left circumflex coronary artery as the infarct-related artery in patients undergoing primary percutaneous coronary intervention for acute inferior myocardial infarction. *Europace,* Vol.11, pp 1517-1521,

Wagner, G.S. (2009). Electrocardiography and Arrhythmias Committee. AHA/ACCF/HRS Recommendations for the standardization and interpretation of the electrocardiogram. *J Am Coll Cardiol,* Vol.53, pp. 1003-1011, 0735-1097

Wu, E. (2001). Visualization of presence, location, and transmural extent of healed Q-wave and non-Q-wave myocardial infarction. *Lancet,* Vol.357, pp 21-8, 0140-6736

Yusuf, S. (2006). Effects of fondaparinux on mortality and reinarction in patients with acute ST-segment elevation myocardial infarction. The OASIS-6 randomized trial. *JAMA,* Vol.295, pp.1519-30, 0098-7484

Zeymer, U. (2001).Non-invasive detection of early infarct vessel patency by resolution of ST-segment elevation in patients with thrombolysis for acute myocardial infarction. *Eur Heart J,* Vol .2, pp. 769-775, 1522-9645.

Zeymer, U. (2003). Primary percutaneous transluminal coronary angioplasty accelerates early myocardial reperfusion compared to thrombolytic therapy in patients with AMI. *Am Heart J,* Vol.146, pp. 686-691, 0002-8703

Zipes, DP. (2006). ACC/AHA/ESC 2006 guidelines for management of patients with ventricular arrhythmias and the prevention of sudden cardiac death—executive summary. *Eur Heart J,* Vol.27, pp. 2099–2140, 1522-9645

9

Mechanisms of Postinfarction Electrophysiological Abnormality: Sympathetic Neural Remodeling, Electrical Remodeling and Gap Junction Remodeling

Guoqiang Zhong, Jinyi Li, Honghong Ke,
Yan He, Weiyan Xu and Yanmei Zhao
Department of Cardiology, The First Affiliated Hospital of Guangxi Medical University, Nanning, China

1. Introduction

Of various functional impairments of electrical events in the heart, ventricular arrhythmias underlie the majority of deaths in patients with left ventricular dysfunction and heart failure after myocardial ischemia and infarction. As heart failure develops, pathophysiological remodeling of cardiac function occurs at multiple levels, spanning the spectrum from molecular and subcellular changes to those occurring at the organ system levels (Jin et al., 2008).

Although advances in anti-arrhythmic agents and implantation of direct-current defibrillator have resulted in improved prevention of death due to arrhythmia in myocardial infarction, morbidity and mortality due to arrhythmias are still high in all over the world. In addition, in patients with severe congestive heart failure, ventricular arrhythmia is also a critical determinant of prognosis, because conservative anti-arrhythmia therapies are not very effective. Therapeutic strategies for arrhythmias have been focused mainly on electrophysiological aspects with little consideration of structural or cellular bases for arrhythmogenesis. Thus, the exact cellular mechanism underlying lethal arrhythmias is undetermined. Identification of arrhythmogenic substrates from viewpoints other than electrophysiological ones is essential (Takamatsu, 2008).

Despite decades of investigation, the precise mechanisms that underlie the electrophysiological abnormality remain elusive. In this chapter we therefore focus on three main issues with an emphasis on the mechanisms responsible for these adaptations: sympathetic neural remodeling, electrical remodeling and gap junction remodeling.

2. Cardiac sympathetic neural remodeling

2.1 The sympathetic nervous system in the heart

Cardiac innervation comes from both extrinsic and intrinsic sources. The extrinsic sympathetic innervation arises from the stellate ganglia and paravertebral sympathetic ganglia. The vagal nerves are sources of extrinsic parasympathetic nerves that innervate the heart. In addition to the extrinsic cardiac nervous system, there is also an extensive intrinsic cardiac nervous system that includes collections of ganglionated plexuses (Armour, 2010). The major neurotransmitter mediating sympathetic response is norepinephrine; of note, epinephrine release during activation is negligible (Fig 1) (Esler et al., 1990).

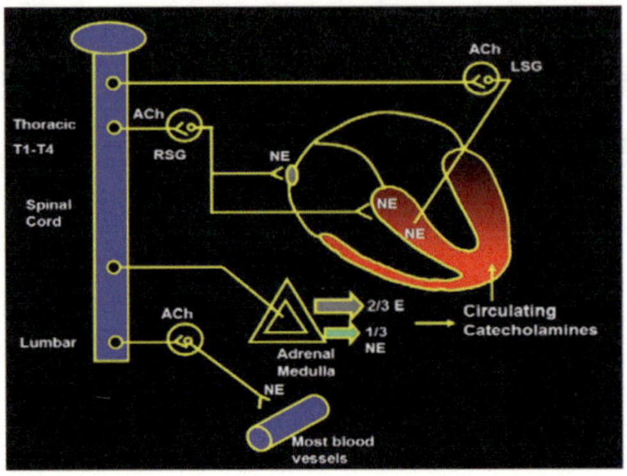

Fig. 1. Cardiac sympathetic control. NE, norepinephrine; Ach, acetylcholine; E, epinephrine (Esler et al., 1990).

Each ganglionated plexuses contains both sympathetic and parasympathetic neurons that are associated with complex synaptology. The sympathetic innervation to the ventricles follows a course along the common pulmonary artery into the plexus supplying the main left coronary artery. The sympathetic nerves are distributed to the myocardium in superficial epicardial layers. They penetrate the myocardium along with the coronary arteries (Figure 2) (Zipes, 1990). Immunocytochemical techniques have allowed investigators to stain many nerve cells and nerve tissues including the Schwann cells and autonomic nerves using different antibodies with different stains (Oki et al., 1995; Gulbenkian et al., 1993; Chow et al., 1998).

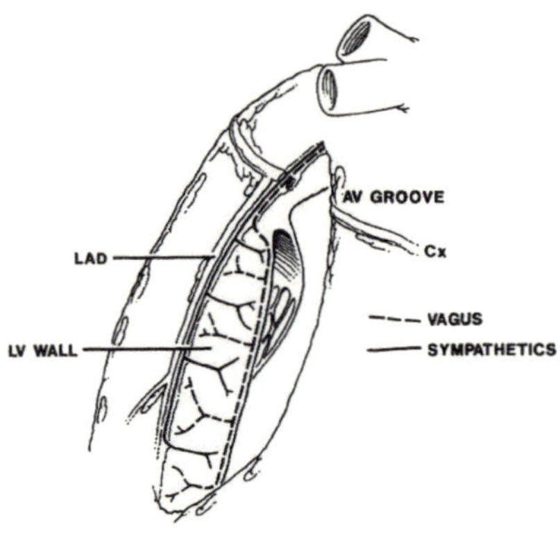

Fig. 2. Schematic of sagittal view of left ventricular wall showing pathways of vagal and sympathetic afferent and efferent nerves. Postganglionic sympathetic axons are located superficially in periadventia of coronary arteries; postganglionic vagal axons cross the atrioventricular groove in subepicardium but are located in subendocardium. Cx, circumflex coronary artery; LAD, left ventricular descending coronary artery (Zipes, 1990).

2.2 Sympathetic neural remodeling after myocardial infarction

In ischemic hearts, regional heterogeneity of sympathetic innervation usually occurs as a result of ischemia- or infarction-induced neural axons necrosis and nerve sprouting (Zipes, 1990). Sympathetic neural remodeling characterized by heterogeneous cardiac nerve sprouting and sympathetic hyperinnervation was also observed; see Figure 3 (Cao et al., 2000).

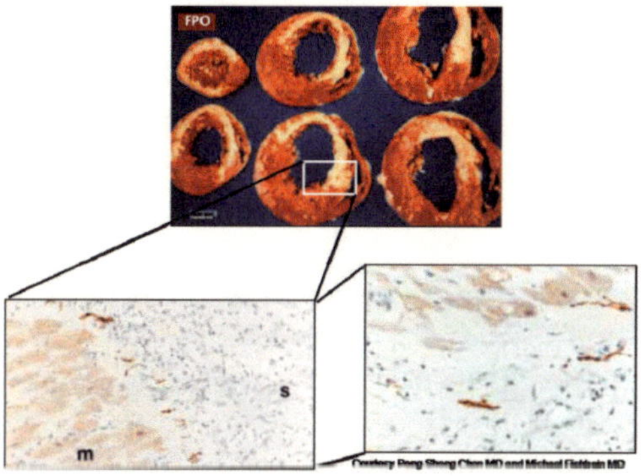

Fig. 3. Neural remodeling and nerve sprouting (Cao et al., 2000).

The density of nerve fibers immunopositive for Growth-associated protein-43 upregulated after myocardial infarction at different periods, indicating nerve fibers undergoing sprouting activity shortly after myocardial infarction (Oh et al., 2006; Zhou et al., 2004). However, sprouting nerve fibers may regress unless nerve terminals can form synaptic contacts with target cells. Therefore, the density of growth-associated protein-43 positive nerve fibers is a measurement for nerve sprouting activity instead of a measurement for stable innervation.

Myocardial infarction induced nerve sprouting activity in both peri-infarct and remote areas. Nerve sprouting, which resulted in sympathetic (but not parasympathetic) hyperinnervation, was greater in the outer loop of the heart. The difference in the outer and inner loops started within 3 hours and persisted for 2 months after myocardial infarction (Figure 4) (Oh et al., 2006).

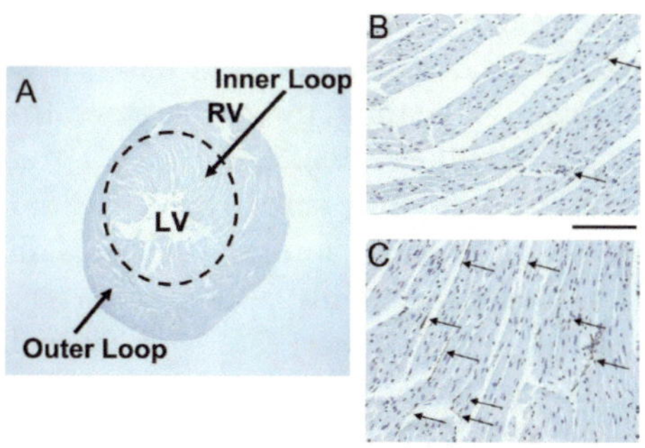

Fig. 4. Nerve fiber densities in the outer versus the inner loop of normal mouse heart. A, Cross-section of a normal mouse ventricle. The fiber orientation in the inner loop is roughly perpendicular, whereas the outer loop fibers are parallel to the circumference of the ventricles. B, C: Growth-associated protein-43 immunopositive nerves in the inner and outer loops, respectively. More nerve fibers are present in the outer loop than the inner loop. Arrows point to brown nerve twigs (20×objective) (Oh et al., 2006).

Necrotic injury to the rat myocardium results in denervation followed by proliferative regeneration of schwann cells and axons (Nori et al., 1995). Abnormal patterns of neurilemma proliferation have been documented in infarsitescted human and rat hearts (Vracko, 1990, 1991). Rencently, Huazhi et al (Huazhi et al., 2010) showed that sympathetic nerve sprouting at the peri-infarct zone in infarcted hearts at 8 weeks post myocardial infarction was more excessive and heterogeneous than that in the corresponding zone in normal hearts. Excessive nerve sprouting may result in abnormal patterns of myocardial innervation and may potentially increase cardiac arrhythmia. Wei et al (Wei et al., 2004) identified a number of changes, including substantial denervation of the left ventricular and areas of apparent hyperinnervation at the border of innervated and denervated myocardium after myocardial infarction.

2.3 Mechanisms of sympathetic neural remodeling after myocardial infarction

The sympathetic innervation of the heart regulates cardiac function by stimulating heart rate, contractility, and conduction velocity through the release of norepinephrine and the activation of cardiac β1-adrenergic receptors. Sympathetic innervation of the heart is sculpted during development by chemoattractive and chemorepulsive factors (Ieda et al., 2007). For example, nerve growth factor supports sympathetic neuron survival and promotes cardiac axon outgrowth during development (Crowley et al., 1994), whereas the chemorepulsive factorsemaphorin 3a (Sema3a) attenuates sympathetic axon extension in the heart (Ieda et al., 2007) and in the peripheral vasculature (Long et al., 2009).

The nerve fiber regeneration process is triggered by up-regulation of nerve growth factor or other neurotrophic factor genes in the non-neuronal cells around the site of injury. Up-regulation of nerve growth factor was more prominent in the area near the infarct than in the area remote to the infarct (Oh et al., 2006). Nerve growth factor mRNA was significantly up-regulated within 3 hours after myocardial infarction and persisted for 1 month in both the infarcted myocardium and the noninfarcted left ventricular free wall (Oh et al., 2006; Zhou et al., 2004).

Neurotrophins such as nerve growth factor act through two distinct types of receptors: tropomyosin-related tyrosine kinase (Trk) receptors and the lower-affinity p75 neurotrophin receptor ($p75^{NTR}$) (Kuruvilla et al., 2004; Kaplan & Miller, 2003). Nerve growth factor acts through TrkA to promote the extension of sympathetic axons into the heart (Kuruvilla et al., 2004), whereas $p75^{NTR}$ modulates signaling by coreceptors that can either stimulate or inhibit axon outgrowth (Kaplan & Miller, 2003). $p75^{NTR}$ has a great functional impact on the cardiovascular system and cardiac rhythm stability (Christina et al., 2010), which were particularly relevant to myocardial infarction and heart failure where heterogeneous sympathetic innervation was correlated with altered neurotrophin expression and the development of ventricular arrhythmias (Rubart & Zipes, 2005).

In addition to nerve growth factor, other neurotrophic factors are also up-regulated after myocardial infarction. For example, Leukemia inhibitory factor protein was increased by 40% at 48 hours after myocardial infarction in mice (Fuchs et al., 2003). IL-1α was increased after myocardial infarction, primarily at peri-infarct sites. And IL-1, IL-1β, and IL-6 were increased at only one time point after myocardial infarction (Oh et al., 2006; Nian et al., 2004). IL-6 mRNA was induced in myocytes at the viable border zone in dogs subjected to ischemia-reperfusion (Gwechenberger et al., 1999). Table 1 describes detailly neurotrophic factors gene expression in the myocardium after myocardial infarction.

	Peri-infarct					Remote				
	3 hours	3 days	1 week	1 month	2 months	3 hours	3 days	1 week	1 month	2 months
NGF-α	1.97	2.00	0.70	0.80	1.35	9.64	2.57	3.42	1.18	11.03
NGF-β	**5.63 (2.14)**	**8.02 (2.40)**	0.69 **(1.79)**	0.81 **(1.39)**	**4.15 (1.40)**	1.98	2.26	0.95	0.28	0.39
NGF-γ	5.31	1.91	1.42	1.59	0.57	1.09	1.74	0.92	**3.48**	**4.47**
BDNF	1.54	1.93	1.89	1.22	1.22	1.34	0.67	0.72	0.30	0.67
NT-3	1.10	0.38	0.27	0.24	0.46	0.78	0.38	0.36	0.78	0.14
FGF	0.37	0.09	0.07	0.23	0.14	0.15	0.28	0.10	0.15	2.46
EGF	2.12	0.48	0.39	3.33	0.62	0.64	0.08	0.09	0.09	0.24
IGF 1-1	1.53	1.20	0.94	0.96	0.95	0.98	0.54	0.55	0.42	0.67
IGF 1-2	**3.72**	**8.55**	**8.18 (5.80)**	**3.78**	**3.47 (4.04)**	2.15	**7.54**	**4.68**	1.50	2.31
IGF 2-1	16.86	0.71	0.43	0.71	0.48	0.98	1.09	2.82	1.28	4.65
IGF 2-2	1.40	1.12	1.18	0.76	0.75	0.85	0.65	0.42	0.34	0.51
GDNF	1.15	0.79	0.92	0.69	1.64	1.01	0.27	0.86	0.53	0.85
LIF	**4.70 (1.01)**	**6.43 (4.23)**	**3.75 (2.06)**	2.93 **(1.15)**	**6.28 (2.93)**	1.17	3.36	0.98	0.89	32.1
TGF-α	0.63	1.75	0.65	0.82	2.64	1.05	0.56	1.30	0.51	3.77
TGF-β_1	1.48	1.05	0.77	0.91	0.88	0.50	0.91	0.79	0.26	0.59
TGF-β_2	2.67	3.35	1.15	2.27	0.24	1.61	0.40	1.74	0.22	7.01
TGF-β_3	**3.25**	**4.26**	**14.46 (13.27)**	**7.23**	**3.34 (2.71)**	**3.85**	**4.07**	2.69	1.98	5.84
IL-1α	**3.50**	**4.03**	**3.33 (2.54)**	2.55	**3.60 (5.11)**	0.85	1.48	1.09	0.63	1.41
IL-1β	1.20	1.51	3.45	2.03	1.45	0.91	1.23	0.93	0.43	0.51
IL-6	4.92	0.42	1.03	0.38	0.14	65.34	2.01	3.13	0.36	1.15
TNF-α	2.35	1.02	1.07	1.33	0.84	1.45	1.78	1.39	0.97	2.02
TNF-β	0.73	1.27	1.47	0.36	2.89	1.41	1.09	0.43	0.75	2.11

Table 1. Neurotrophic factors gene expression in the myocardium after myocardial infarction Numbers indicate ratio to normal control. Bold numbers indicate those $>3\times$ of control in at least two consecutive time points. Bold numbers in parentheses are obtained with quantitative reverse-transcriptase polymerase chain reaction. Other numbers are obtained using DNA microarray. BDNF = brain-derived neurotrophic factor; EGF = epidermal growth factor; FGF = fibroblast growth factor; GDNF = glial cell-derived neurotrophic factor; IGF = insulin-like growth factor; IL = interleukin; LIF = leukemia inhibitory factor; NT-3 = neutrophin-3; NGF, nerve growth factor; TGF = transforming growth factor; TNF = tumor necrosis factor (Oh et al., 2006).

Increase of neurotrophic factors sometimes can be injurious. Thus, both exogenous and endogenous nerve growth factor can induce cardiac nerve sprouting, but they also can increase the incidence of ventricular arrhythmias and sudden death in canine models (Cao et al., 2000a). Increased neurotrophic factor expression and heterogeneous innervation also could induce side effects that contribute to the increased risk for sudden death after myocardial infarction (Luisi et al., 2002; Canty et al., 2004).

2.4 The interaction between sympathetic neural remodeling and electrical remodeling

Regional heterogeneity of sympathetic innervation is also closely related to electrical inhomogeneity. Previous study revealed that electrical heterogeneity is exacerbated after initial nerve injury by sympathetic nerve sprouting and subsequent regional myocardial hyperinnervation (Figure 6) (Rubart & Zipes, 2005). The enhanced spatial inhomogeneity in cardiac sympathetic innervation could amplify the spatial inhomogeneity of these electrophysiological properties and therefore facilitate the initiation of ventricular arrhythmias (Cao et al., 2000b).

Nerve growth factor overexpression and nerve sprouting affected the expressions and functions of certain potassium channels and thus increases the susceptibility to ventricular tachyarrhythmia. Nerve sprouting suppressed the expressions and functions of myocardial transient outward current (I_{to}) and inward rectifier current (I_{K1}) channels. Myocardial necrotic injury plus intensified sympathetic nerve sprouting further decreased Kir2.1 expression and I_{K1} current density. All of these changes affected the repolarization of myocardial cells and hence increased the vulnerability to ventricular arrhythmia (Ren et al., 2008).

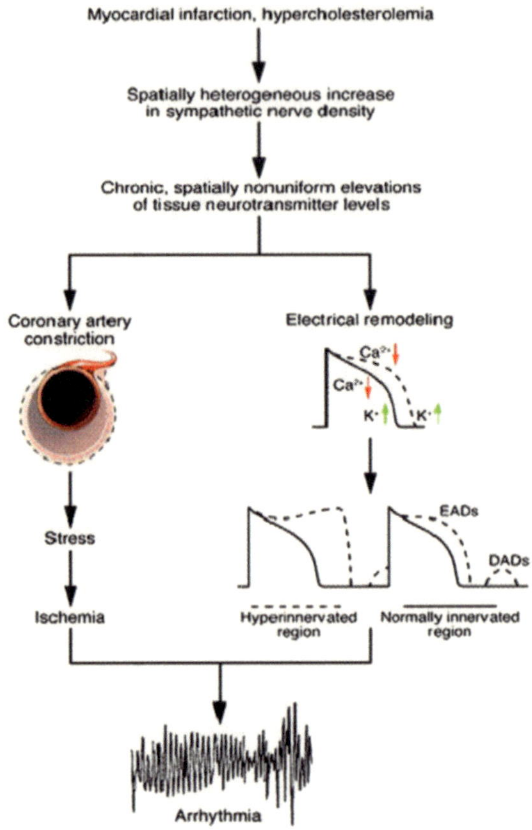

Fig. 6. Factors contributing to arrhythmogenesis in hearts with heterogeneous sympathetic innervation (Rubart & Zipes, 2005).

Besides, the coexistence of sympathetic denervation zones (infarct zones), sympathetic reinnervation zones (ischemic zones) and sympathetic normal zones in the ischemic heart could increase the heterogeneity of electrical communication which is facilitative to the abnormality of cardiac autorhythmicity and triggered activity. Sympathetic neural remodeling can raises the norepinephrine concentration, which encourage the early afterdepolarization (EAD) and delayed afterdepolarization (DAD) by affect the calcium influx and repolarization potassium current, and then trigger arrhythmia. Neurotransmitters such as norepinephrine can cause focal vasoconstriction and myocardial ischemia which is facilitative to the arrhythmogenesis.

2.5 Relationship between sympathetic neural remodeling and ventricular arrhythmia

The initiation of lethal arrhythmias needs a substrate and a trigger. Myocardial remodeling (structural and/or functional) is considered the substrate. In recent years, the concept "cardiac nerve remodeling" and its potentiality as a trigger for lethal arrhythmia have entered the scope of arrhythmia research (Ren et al., 2008). Abnormally increased post-injury sympathetic nerve density may be in part responsible for the occurrence of ventricular arrhythmia and sudden cardiac death in patients with severe heart failure (Cao et al., 2000b). Cardiac nerve sprouts detering occured after myocardial infarction even without exogenous nerve growth factor.

Infusion of nerve growth factor accelerated and intensified the magnitude of nerve sprouting, resulting in a high incidence of sudden cardiac death (Cao et al., 2000a).

The left stellate ganglion is known to be important in cardiac arrhythmogenesis (Schwartz & Stone, 1980). Left cardiac sympathetic denervation, including left stellate ganglion resection, decreases the incidence of ventricular arrhythmia in patients with myocardial infarction (Schwartz et al., 1992). Increased sympathetic tone is important in the generation of ventricular arrhythmia and sudden cardiac death (Rubart & Zipes, 2005). In dogs with both complete atrioventricular block and myocardial infarction, high-amplitude spiky discharges frequently cause premature ventricular contractions or even ventricular tachycardia (Figure 7). These findings suggest that high-amplitude spiky discharges is highly arrhythmogenic in diseased hearts. However, because high-amplitude spiky discharges is also present in normal hearts, the presence of these types of discharge by itself is not pathological (Zhou S, et al., 2008).

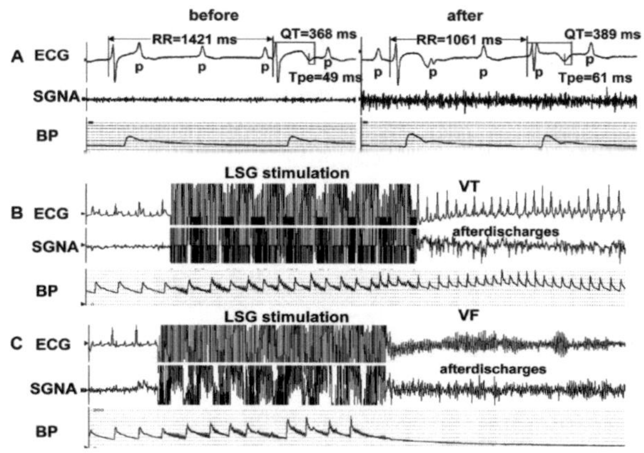

Fig. 7. A, Electrical stimulation of left stellate ganglion lengthened the corrected QT (QTc) from 325 to 402 ms and the corrected Tpe (Tpec) from 45 to 82 ms (at 10 mA). B, Left stellate ganglion stimulation induced ventricular tachycardia (VT); C, ventricular fibrillation (VF) in the experimental group. Afterdischarges were present in left stellate ganglion recordings after electrical stimulation. BP = blood pressure; SGNA = stellate ganglion nerve activity (Zhou S, et al., 2008).

2.6 Therapeutic implications of sympathetic neural remodeling after myocardial infarction

As sympathetic tone was known to be increased in cardiomyopathy patients, interventions that aim to reduce sympathetic tone could reduce the risk of sudden cardiac death and ventricular tachyarrhythmias (Fig 8， Marmar & Kalyanam, 2008).

Selective sympathetic blockade was an effective theraty， which was applied in animal models and human during myocardial ischemia (Issa et al., 2005; Nademanee et al., 2000). In a canine model, intrathecal clonidine, when delivered via a catheter at T2–T4 spinal segments, significantly reduced the occurrence of ventricular tachycardia and fibrillation during transient myocardial ischemia (Issa et al., 2005). Electrical storm, defined as recurrent multiple ventricular fibrillation (VF) episodes, often occurs in patients with recent myocardial infarction. Sympathetic blockade was proved to be superior to the antiarrhythmic therapy in treating electrical storm patients, and sympathetic blockade - not class 1 antiarrhythmic drugs - should be the treatment of choice for electrical storm

(Nademanee et al., 2000). Successful treatment of recurrent ventricular tachycardia, refractory to antiarrhythmic therapy, can be achieved by neuraxial modulation at the level of the spinal cord. The benefit of thoracic epicardial anesthesia was reported in a patient with ischemic cardiomyopathy and recurrent ventricular arrhythmia refractory to intubation and sedation, with the use of 0.25% Bupicavaine at T1–T2 interspace, reducing the number of ICD shocks from 86 in 48 hours to zero (Mahajan et al., 2005).

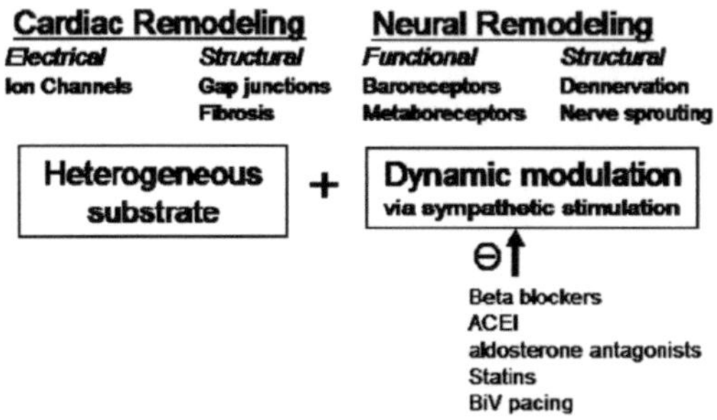

Fig. 8. Structural and functional basis of ventricular tachycardia and fibrillation (Marmar & Kalyanam, 2008).

β-blockers, angiotensin-converting enzyme inhibitors, angiotensin receptor blockers, aldosterone antagonists (Cittadini et al., 2003), statins (Gao et al., 2005), and fish oil have been shown to decrease risk of sudden cardiac death in ischemic cardiomyopathy and significantly improve mortality through modulating the autonomic nervous system to decrease sympathetic tone (Marmar & Kalyanam,2008). In a recent study, carvedilol ameliorated electrical remodeling at peri-infarct zones after myocardial infarction by improving the spatial distribution of the sympathetic nerve reinnervation (Huazhi et al., 2010). Moreover, attenuation of oxidative stress and inflammatory response after resveratrol treatment, a naturally occurring compound, significantly inhibited nerve growth factor expression, and protected against sympathetic neural remodeling (Ping et al., 2010). Ghrelin, a novel growth hormone-releasing peptide, which was showed to inhibite neural remodeling in rats with myocardial infarction, likely mediated through nerve growth factor suppression, might be used as a new potential way to treat and prevent sudden cardiac death after myocardial infarction (Ming-Jie et al., 2009).

3. Myocardial electrical remodelling

3.1 The cardiac action potential

The normal sequence and synchronous contraction of the atria and ventricles require the rapid activation of groups of cardiac cells. An activation mechanism must enable rapid changes in heart rate and also respond to the changes in autonomic tone. The propagating cardiac action potential fulfils these roles. The action potential is a key determinant of cardiac electrical activity and is shaped by underlying ionic currents and transporters (Nerbonne & Kass 2005). A schematic representation of a cardiac action potential and the principal currents involved in its various phases are shown in Figure 9A (Nattel & Carlsson 2006). The action potentials of pacemaker cells in the sinoatrial (SA) and atrioventricular (AV) nodes are significantly different from those in working myocardium. Figure 9B depicts action potential characteristics in different regions of the heart (Michael et al., 2009).

The average duration of the ventricular action potential duration is reflected in the QT interval in the ECG. Factors that prolong the action potential duration (eg, a decrease in outward K^+ currents or an increase in inward late Na^+ current) prolong the action potential duration and the QT interval in the ECG. The QT interval of males and females is equal during early childhood. However, at puberty the interval of males shortens (Rautaharju et al., 1992).

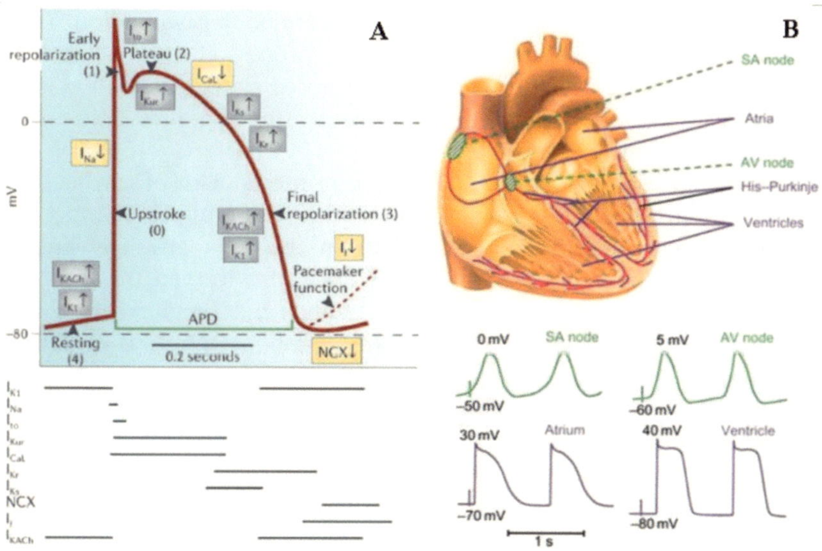

Fig. 9. A, Membrane currents that generate the normal action potential duration. Resting (4), upstroke (0), early repolarization (1), plateau (2), and final repolarization are the 5 phases of the action potential. A decline of potential at the end of phase 3 in pacemaker cells, such as the sinus node, is shown as a broken line. The inward currents, I_{Na}, I_{Ca}, and I_f, are shown in yellow boxes; the sodium-calcium exchanger (NCX) is also shown in yellow. It is electrogenic and may generate inward or outward current. I_{KACh}, I_{K1}, I_{to}, I_{Kur}, I_{Kr}, and I_{Ks} are shown in gray boxes. The action potential duration is approximately 200ms. B, Various specialized tissues in the heart and typical corresponding action potentials. The short vertical lines indicate the time of onset of activity in the sinus atrial node for one beat. Green, slow-channel tissue (nodes); violet, fast-channel tissues (Nattel & Carlsson 2006).

3.2 General properties of ion channels

Ion channels have two fundamental properties, ion permeation and gating (Hille, 1978). Ion permeation describes the movement through the open channel. The selective permeability of ion channels to specific ions is a basis of classification of ion channels (eg, Na^+, K^+, and Ca^{2+} channels). Size, valency, and hydration energy are important determinants of selectivity (Augustus, 2009). Ion channels provide multiple binding sites for ions as they traverse the membrane. Like an enzyme-substrate interaction, the binding of the permeating ion is saturable. Most ion channels are singly occupied during permeation; certain K^+ channels may be multiply occupied (Augustus, 2009).

Gating is the mechanism of opening and closing of ion channels and is their second major property. Ion channels are also subclassified by their mechanism of gating: voltagedependent, ligand-dependent, and mechano-sensitive gating. Voltage-gated ion channels change their conductance in response to variations in membrane potential. Voltage-dependent gating is the commonest mechanism of gating observed in ion channels. A majority of ion channels open in response to depolarization. The pacemaker current channel (I_f channel) opens in response to membrane hyperpolarization. The steepness of the voltage dependence of opening or activation varies between channels (Hille, 1978).

Ion channels have two mechanisms of closure. Certain channels like the Na^+ and Ca^{2+} channels enters a closed inactivated state during maintained depolarization. To regain their ability to open, the channel must undergo a recovery process at hyperpolarized potentials. The inactivated state may also be accessed from the closed state. Inactivation is the basis for refractoriness in cardiac muscle and is fundamental for the prevention of premature reexcitation (Hille, 1978; Leblanc & Hume, 1990).

Ligand-dependent gating is the second major gating mechanism of cardiac ion channels. The acetylcholine (Ach)-activated K^+ channel, an inward-rectifying K^+ channel (I_{KAch}), is one of this class. I_{KAch} channels are most abundant in the atria and the sinus atrial and atrioventricular nodes. The ATP-sensitive K^+ channel, also termed the ADP-activated K^+ channel, is a ligand-gated channel distributed abundantly in all regions of the heart. Energy depletion during ischemia increases the [ADP]/ [ATP] ratio, activates I_{KATP}, and abbreviates the action potential. The abbreviated action potential results in less force generation and may be cardioprotective. This channel also plays a central role in ischemic preconditioning (Hille, 1978).

3.3 Significance and arrhythmic consequences of Ionic currents remodeling associated with myocardial infarction

Myocardial infarction refers to the death of cardiac tissue, most often caused by critical decreases in coronary artery blood flow induced by obstructive coronary artery disease. Several mechanisms, including reentry and triggered activity due to early and delayed afterdepolarizations, contribute to ventricular tachyarrhythmia (Janse & Wit, 1989; Qin et al., 1996). Remodeling of ion-channel and transport processes cause important changes in cellular electrical activity and impulse propagation over days and weeks following acute infarction (Friedman et al., 1975; Spear et al., 1977).

Generally, by 24–48h after total coronary artery occlusion the action potentials and maximal action potential upstroke velocity (Vmax) decreased, as well as an increase in total time of repolarization. On the other hand, the cells of the epicardial border zone of the canine infarction model show a reduction in Vmax, and a shortening and triangularization of the action potential by 5 days after total artery occlusion. By 14 days post occlusion further shortening of the action potential occurs. Then by the time of the healed infarct (2 months), action potential voltage profiles have returned to nearly normal suggesting the presence of a process that might be termed 'reverse remodeling' (Figure 10) (Ursell et al., 1985). We found that the PR, QRS, QT and QTc intervals in myocardial infarction mice were significantly longer than normal mice after 4, 8, and 12 weeks (LI et al., 2009c).

These abnormalities cause severe conduction disturbances that strongly promote reentry. A particularly important arrhythmia mechanism is anisotropic reentry in the peri-infarction border zone (Dillon et al., 1988; Restivo et al., 1990). Acute myocardial infarction causes longer term (remodeling) changes over days to weeks, as well as important very early (within minutes to hours) functionally based ion-channel abnormalities. Figure 11 illustrates how different forms of ionchannel remodeling contribute to anisotropic reentry in the presence of a healed myocardial infarction (Nattel S et al., 2007).

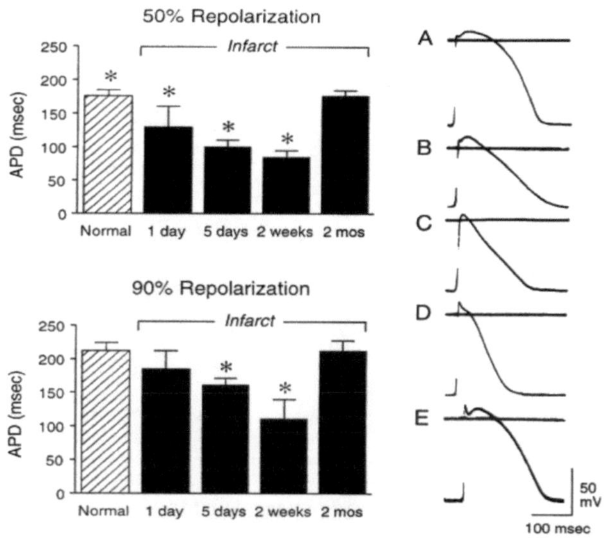

Fig. 10. Changes in action potential duration measured to 50% (above left) and 90% repolarization (below left) of epicardial muscle fibers with increasing time after coronary artery occlusion. Asterisks denote values significantly different from control. At the right are shown representative transmembrane potential recordings; A, normal; B, 1 day; C, 5 days; D, 2 weeks; E, 2 months. Note that action potentials in the 1- and 5-day-old infarcts show loss of the plateau phase during repolarization. Action potential duration is decreased more in 5-day-old than in 1-day-old infarcts (Ursell et al., 1985).

3.4 Alterations in K^+ currents

Cardiac K^+ channels fall into three broad categories: Voltagegated (I_{to}, I_{Kur}, I_{Kr}, and I_{Ks}), inward rectifier channels (I_{K1}, I_{KAch}, and I_{KATP}), and the background K^+ currents (TASK-1, TWIK-1/2). Voltage-gated K^+ channels consist of principal α-subunits and multiple β-subunits. The channel functional units also include the complementary proteins K_V-channel associated protein, KChAP, and the K_V channel interacting protein, KChIP. The major subfamilies of α-subunits include K_VN.x (n=1 to 4), the HERG channel (gene KCNH2), and K_vLQT1 (gene KCNQ1). They are important in generating outward current in the heart (Augustus, 2009). Myocardial infarction causes substantial changes in K^+ current expression, density, and function (Janse & Wit, 1989).

3.4.1 Changed K^+ current function in surviving border-zone cells

A variety of K^+ currents are downregulated in border-zone cells. Background K^+ conductance is reduced in surviving canine subendocardial Purkinje fibers (Boyden et al., 1989), due to reduced I_{K1} and altered delayed-rectifier currents (Pinto & Boyden, 1998). Border-zone left ventricular cardiomyocytes show reduced I_{to} (Lue & Boyden, 1992). I_{to} decreases are most prominent within days of acute infarction and tend to resolve over the subsequent 2 months (Dun et al., 2004). The expression of subunits encoding I_{Kr} (ERG) and I_{Ks} (KvLQT1 and minK) is downregulated in 2-day postinfarction border-zone cells (Dun & Boyden, 2005; Jiang et al., 2000). Overall, the multiple forms of K^+-channel dysfunction postinfarction impair repolarization and lead to early afterdepolarizations.

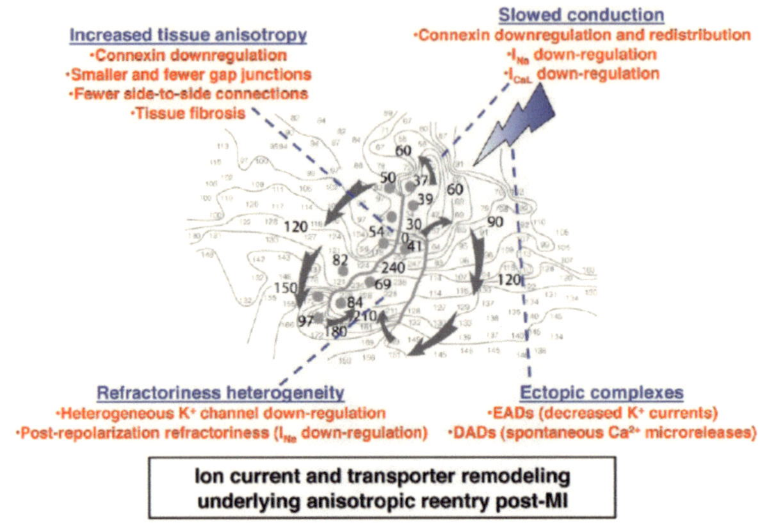

Fig. 11. Contributors to anisotropic reentry in myocardial infarction. A principal mechanism underlying potentially lethal ventricular tachyarrhythmias post-myocardial infarction is anisotropic reentry, represented schematically by the black activation map in the central part of the figure (Peters et al., 1997). The numbers indicated on the map are times of electrical activation, and the curved lines (isochrones) indicate zones of tissue activated within 10 ms of each other. Crowded isochrones denote very slow conduction. Thicker black lines show lines of functional conduction block parallel to fiber orientation, due to the impaired transverse conduction (increased anisotropy) post-myocardial infarction. The impulse travels slowly in two parallel streams (thick arrows) around the lines of block, which come together to conduct through the central corridor (thinner arrows) of the reentrant pathway. The ways in which ion-channel remodeling post-myocardial infarction lead to this arrhythmia mechanism are indicated by the red points, organized into groups of dysfunction categories (blue underlined headings). Increased tissue anisotropy, which causes the unidirectional block needed for reentry initiation, arises because of connexin downregulation, reduced gap junction number and size, fewer side-to-side connections, and tissue fibrosis around muscle bundles. Unidirectional block is also favored by refractoriness heterogeneity due to spatially heterogeneous K^+ channel downregulation coupled with postrepolarization refractoriness. Slowed conduction, which allows enough time for the proximal part of the central corridor to recover excitability when the reentering impulse returns, is caused by connexin downregulation, I_{Na} decreases, and reduced I_{CaL} (I_{CaL} is particularly important for conduction in conditions of impaired coupling). Finally, the ectopic complexes needed to engage spatially variable refractoriness and initiate reentry are provided by early afterdepolarizations promoted by K^+ current downregulation and delayed afterdepolarizations caused by spontaneous diastolic Ca^{2+} releases (Nattel S et al., 2007).

3.4.2 Changes in K^+ currents in normal zones of hearts with prior myocardial infarction

Action potential duration increases and ventricular arrhythmias are features of normal-zone tissues from postinfarction rat (Perrier et al., 2004) and rabbit (Liu et al., 2004) hearts. Both reentries associated with spatial refractoriness heterogeneity and triggered activity is involved (Liu et al., 2004). Decreases in I_{to}, I_{K1}, and total delayed-rectifier current (I_K) occur in rabbit hearts (Liu et al., 2004). In rats, I_{to} decreases correlate most closely with downregulation of Kv4.2 subunits (Perrier et al., 2004). There may be compensatory upregulation of Kv1.4 subunits (Kaprielian et al., 2002), although downregulation of Kv1.4 has also been reported (Gidh-Jain et al., 1996). Decreases in rat I_K correlate with downregulation of the putative α-subunit Kv2.1 (Huang et al., 2001b). The effects of postinfarction remodeling on spatial dispersion of electrophysiological properties in noninfarcted tissues are controversial, with one study showing increases in dispersion (Huang et al., 2001b) and another decreased spatial heterogeneity (Kaprielian et al., 2002).

3.5 Alterations in Ca^{2+} currents and cellular Ca^{2+} handling

Calcium ions are the principal intracellular signaling ions. They regulate excitation-contraction coupling, secretion, and the activity of many enzymes and ion channels. $[Ca^{2+}]_i$ is highly regulated despite its marked fluctuation between systole and diastole. Calcium channels are the principal portal of entry of calcium into the cells; a system of intracellular storage sites, and transporters such as the sodium-calcium exchanger, also play important roles in $[Ca^{2+}]_i$ regulation. In cardiac muscle, two types of Ca^{2+} channels, the L- (low threshold type) and T-type (transient-type), transport Ca^{2+} into the cells. The L-type channel is found in all cardiac cell types. The T-type channel is found principally in pacemaker, atrial, and Purkinje cells. The unqualified descriptor Ca^{2+} channel refers to the L-type channel. Table 2 contrasts the properties of the two types of channels (Augustus, 2009). Changes in Ca^{2+} handling contribute importantly to arrhythmogenesis postinfarction.

	L-Type	T-Type
Activation		
Range	Low Em (≈ −30 mV)	High Em (≈ −60 mV)
Inactivation		
Range	Low Em (≈ −40 mV)	Hyperpolarized
Voltage dependence	Slow	Fast
$[Ca^{2+}]_i$ dependent	Yes	No
Pharmacologic sensitivity		
Dihydropyridnes	Yes	No
Cd	High	Low
N_i	Low	High
Isoproternol	Yes	No

Table 2. A comparisons of the L-type and T-type Ca2+ channels (Augustus, 2009).

3.5.1 Changes in Ca^{2+} current

I_{CaL} is diminished in border-zone cells of dogs (Dun et al., 2004), sheep (Kim et al., 2002), cats (Pinto et al., 1997), and rabbits (Litwin et al., 2000). I_{CaL} kinetic properties also change, with slowed recovery (Dun et al., 2004) and hyperpolarizing shifts in inactivation voltage dependence (Pinto et al., 1997). The I_{CaL} response to dihydropyridine agonists (Pu et al., 1999) and tyrosine kinase inhibitors (Yagi & Boyden, 2002) is preserved in the border zone. T-type Ca^{2+} current (I_{CaT}) varies over time, being unchanged 5 days postinfarction (Aggarwal & Boyden, 1995) and increasing thereafter (Dun et al., 2004). In surviving subendocardial Purkinje cells, both I_{CaL} and I_{CaT} are reduced (Boyden & Pinto, 1994).

3.5.2 Changes in cellular Ca^{2+} handling

Ca^{2+} transients in border-zone cells are decreased in amplitude and show slowed recovery and decay (Kim et al., 2002). SERCA2A, the sarcoplasmic reticulum Ca^{2+} ATPase, is downregulated (Kim et al., 2002). The diminished and slowed Ca^{2+} transients are due to impaired spatial coordination of quantal Ca^{2+} releases, or sparks (Litwin et al., 2000). Na^{+}-Ca^{2+} exchange function is unaltered, and action potential abnormalities are not responsible for Ca^{2+} handling abnormalities (Pu et al., 2000). Surviving subendocardial Purkinje cells show marked abnormalities in subcellular Ca^{2+} release events, with spontaneous and spatiotemporally nonuniform microreleases that can trigger arrhythmic episodes (Boyden et al., 2003). Drugs that suppress Ca^{2+} microreleases by either inhibiting sarcoplasmic reticulum Ca^{2+} release channels or inositol trisphosphate receptors may constitute a novel antiarrhythmic approach postinfarction (Boyden et al., 2004).

3.6 Alterations in Na^{+} current

The human cardiac sodium channel hNa$_V$1.5 is a member of the family of voltage-gated sodium channels (hNa$_V$1 to 9). The channel consists of a primary α-and multiple secondary β-subunits. The sodium channel consists of 4 homologous domains, DI through DIV (Noda et al., 1984) arranged in a 4-fold circular symmetry to form the channel (Figure 12) (Herbert & Chahine, 2006).

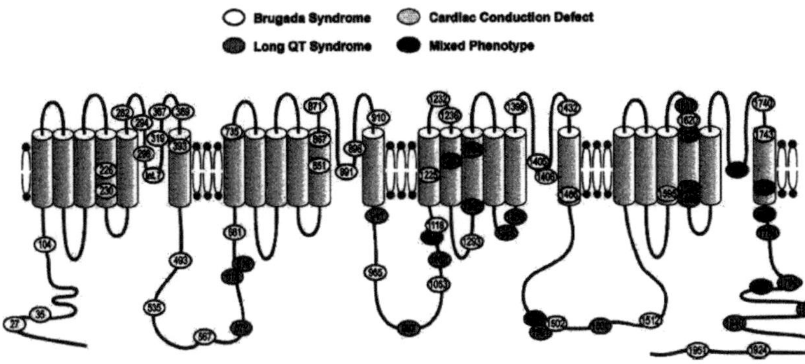

Fig. 12. Putative transmembrane organization of the sodium channel. The channel consists of 4 homologous domains, DI through DIV. The amino and carboxyl termini are intracellular. (Herbert & Chahine, 2006).

Each sodium channel opens very briefly (<1ms) during more than 99% of depolarizations (Patlak & Ortiz, 1985). The channel occasionally shows alternative gating modes consisting of isolated brief openings occurring after variable and prolonged latencies and bursts of openings during which the channel opens repetitively for hundreds of milliseconds. The isolated brief openings are the result of the occasional return from the inactivated state. The bursts of openings are the result of occasional failure of inactivation (Patlak & Ortiz, 1985). The cardiac sodium channel has consensus sites for phosphorylation by protein kinase, protein kinase C, and Ca-calmodulin kinase (Frohnwieser et al., 1997).

3.6.1 Na^{+} current changes

Surviving border-zone tissue is characterized by reduced phase 0 amplitude and upstroke velocity (dV/dtmax), suggestive of reduced I_{Na} (Spear et al., 1979). These abnormalities in excitability favor unidirectional block and reentry (Janse & Wit, 1989). Isolated border-zone cardiomyocytes also have reduced dV/dtmax (Lue & Boyden, 1992) and marked abnormalities in I_{Na}, including reduced current density, accelerated inactivation, and slowed reactivation (Pu & Boyden, 1997). Computer simulations suggest that both I_{Na} and I_{CaL} abnormalities contribute to conduction abnormalities in the reentry circuit (Baba et al., 2005), in keeping with the key role of I_{CaL} in the context of reduced coupling (Shaw & Rudy, 1997). Protein kinase A activators partially improve I_{Na} in peri-infarct zone cells, and the response to phosphatase inhibitors suggests that I_{Na} is hyperphosphorylated (Baba et al., 2004). In late postinfarction rat cardiomyocytes, changes in I_{Na} properties and in ion-channel subunit expression suggest the appearance of atypical I_{Na} isoforms (Huang et al., 2001a); these changes may be due to generalized cardiac hypertrophy/dysfunction rather than infarction per se.

3.6.2 Functional consequences

Oxidative stress in postinfarction tissues produces reactive intermediates that alter I_{Na} in a fashion similar to arrhythmogenic $Na_v1.5$ subunit mutations and potentiate the effects of Na^+ channel-blocking drugs (Fukuda et al., 2005). The I_{Na} blocker lidocaine differentially affects peri-infarct zone cardiomyocytes (Pu et al., 1998). These differential effects may contribute to the tendency of I_{Na} blockers to cause malignant ventricular tachyarrhythmias postinfarction (Ranger & Nattel, 1995). These paradoxical "proarrhythmic" effects of I_{Na}-blocking antiarrhythmic drugs on myocardial infarction tissues contribute to a mortality-enhancing potential (Cardiac Arrhythmia Suppression Trial (CAST) Investigators, 1989).

3.7 Therapeutic implications of ionic current and transporter remodeling

3.7.1 Remodeling-induced modification of the response to therapeutic interventions

Myocardial infarction greatly increases the risk of arrhythmic death, and associated remodeling sensitizes patients to the proarrhythmic effects of a variety of drugs. The risk of drug-induced Torsades de Pointes arrhythmias caused by early afterdepolarizations is approximately increased by myocardial infarction (Stanley et al., 2007). Drugs like β-adrenergic agonists and phosphodiesterase inhibitors, which increase cardiac contractility by increasing intracellular cAMP concentrations, Ca^{2+} loading and Ca^{2+}-induced Ca^{2+} release, have been used extensively to improve cardiac function in patients with severe cardiac dysfunction. Unfortunately, in the longer term they have arrhythmogenic actions and increase mortality (Gardner et al., 1985; Hagemeijer, 1993; Lubbe et al., 1992). Ionic remodeling likely contributes to these adverse responses.

Many of the changes responsible for adverse effects of antiarrhythmic drugs are caused by postinfarction myocardial remodeling: increased action potential duration, localized conduction slowing, downregulation of K^+ channels, abnormal diastolic Ca^{2+} handling, and impaired connexin function. Myocardial infarction predisposes to the proarrhythmic actions of Na^+ channel blocking drugs (Cardiac Arrhythmia Suppression Trial (CAST) Investigators, 1989; Ranger & Nattel, 1995) and I_{Kr} blocking agents (Waldo et al., 1996). Responses to I_{Kr} blocking drugs may be reduced in postinfarction cells, perhaps because of I_{Kr} downregulation (Yuan et al., 1999).

3.7.2 Ionic remodeling as a target for novel therapeutic approaches

Much less work has been done to study interventions targeting ion-handling processes postinfarction. An angiotensin-converting enzyme inhibitor attenuated increases in refractoriness heterogeneity and prevented afterdepolarization formation in normal zones of rats with prior infarctions (Li et al., 2004). The combined α- and β-adrenoceptor antagonist carvedilol suppresses downregulation of both Na^+ (Maltsev et al., 2002) and L-type Ca^{2+} (Li et al., 2005) currents following myocardial infarction. Protein kinase A activators can partially restore suppressed I_{Na} in the infarct border zone (Baba et al., 2004).

Advances in molecular cardiology have identified several potential targets for gene therapy. In a porcine model, focal gene transfer in the border zone of myocardial infarction to silence the KCNH2 potassium channel has been shown to abolish ventricular arrhythmias (Sasano et al., 2006). Furthermore, overexpression of the HERG potassium channel in isolated rabbit ventricular myocytes shortens action potential duration and reduces the frequency of early after-depolarizations (Nuss et al., 1999). Additional investigation is needed to confirm the safety and efficacy of targeted gene therapy in human. However, successful transition of gene therapy into clinical therapies will require the development of safe and efficient transgene vectors and delivery systems.

4. Cardiac gap junction remodeling

4.1 Gap junction structure, permeability and regulation

The gap junction, a type of cell-to-cell junction, is composed of low-resistance intercellular pathways and mediates electrical and metabolic coupling between adjacent cells. Each gap junction channel is formed by two end-to-end connected hemichannels (also known as connexons) contributed by each of the two adjacent cells. In chordates, hemichannels are hexameric structures formed by six connexins (Cx). Connexins have four transmembrane domains with two extracellular loops and with the N-terminal and C-terminal domains in the cytoplasm (Harris, 2001; Sosinsky, 2000). Twenty different connexin types have been identified in mouse and 21 in man (Sohl & Willecke, 2004). Cells can usually express a variety of connexins, and the six connexins forming a hemichannel may not be identical (for example Cx43 and Cx40), thus forming a heteromeric hemichannel. Although not all combinations are possible (Harris, 2001), hemichannels formed by a particular connexins can dock to hemichannels with a different composition (Harris, 2001). A principal ultrastructural feature of the intercalated disk and gap junction was illustrated in Figure 13

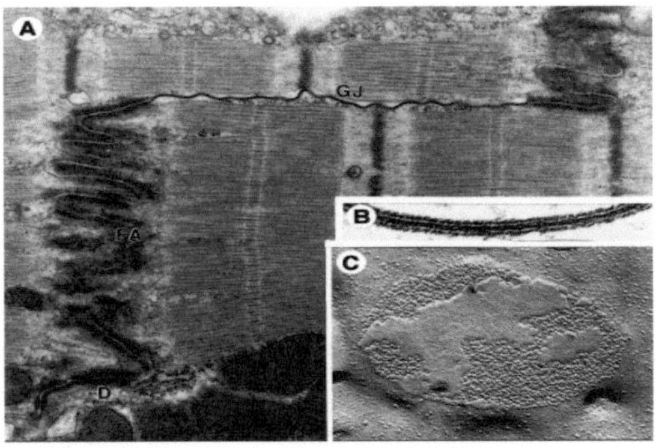

Fig. 13. Principal ultrastructural features of the intercalated disk and gap junction. A, Thin-section electron micrograph showing the appearance of the 3 types of cell-cell junction, the gap junction (GJ), fascia adherens (FA), and desmosome (D). B, Higher magnification thin-section of a gap junction. C, Structure of gap junction as revealed by freeze-fracture electron microscopy. The gap junction is seen as a cluster of particles. Each particle represents a connexon hemichannel. (a) ×36,250; (b) ×350,000; (c) ×98,000 (Severs et al., 1993).

(Severs et al., 1993). Gap junction are permeable to relatively large molecules (Harris, 2001). Depending on the connexins type, pore diameter ranges between approximately 6.5 and 15A °(Harris, 2001), which is wide enough to allow the passage of water, all relevant cations and anions, including Na^+, K^+, and Ca^{2+} and most second messengers as IP_3, cAMP, and cGMP (Figure 14) (Harris, 2001; Wong et al., 2008).

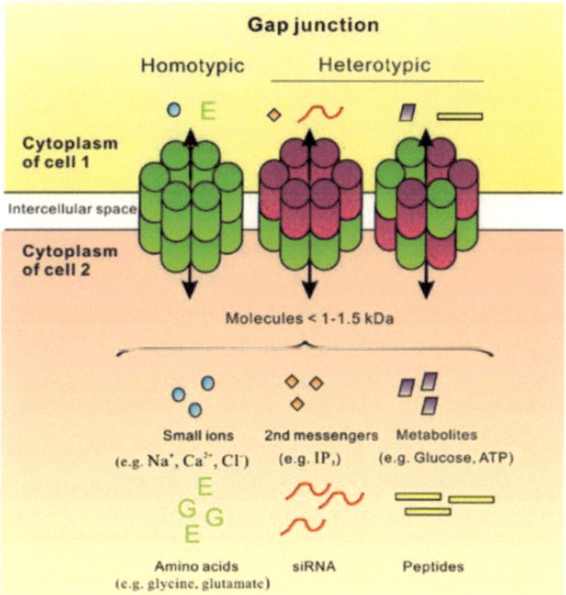

Fig. 14. Organisation of connexins into gap junctions and molecules capable of diffusing through gap junctions (Wong et al., 2008).

The mechanisms by which gap junction channel close or open are not fully elucidated. Gating can take place in at least two independent ways: a rapid, voltage-driven mechanism that can change the channel conformation between a fully open and a nearly completely closed state within a few ms (voltage gating), and a slower (up to 30 ms) mechanism (Harris, 2001; Moreno et al., 2002a). Phosphorylation alters the probability of the different conductance states as well as intracellular trafficking and assembly of connexins depending on the connexins type, the phosphorylation site and, possibly, the biochemical environment (Van et al., 2001). The half-life of connexins is relatively short (less than 2h for Cx43) (Laing & Beyer, 2000) so that changes in the rates of synthesis or degradation are rapidly translated into changes in the number of operative gap junction channel.

4.2 Diversity of connexin expression in the normal heart

Three principal connexins are expressed in cardiac myocytes, Cx43, Cx40, and Cx45. Although Cx43 predominates in the heart as a whole, it is typically co-expressed in characteristic combinations and relative quantities with Cx40 and/or Cx45 in a chamber-related and myocyte-type-specific manner (Vozzi et al., 1999). Although a few other connexins have been reported in cardiac tissue, these are minor components, species variants, or not been confirmed. Figure 15 gives an overview of the typical connexin expression patterns of the normal adult mammalian heart (Severs et al., 2008).

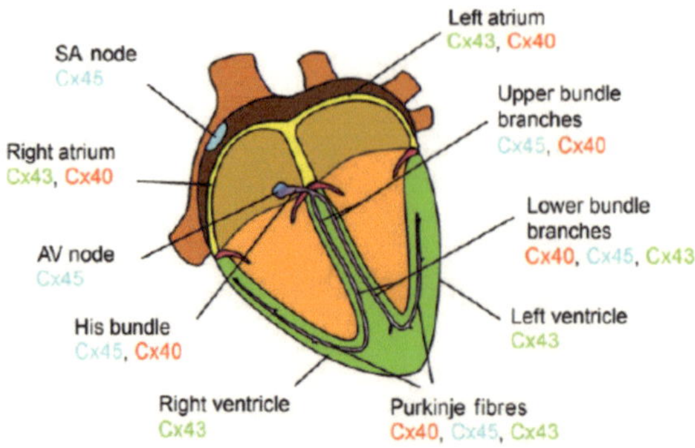

Fig. 15. Summary of the typical connexin expression patterns of the mammalian heart (Severs et al., 2008).

The working cardiomyocytes of the ventricle are extensively interconnected by clusters of connexin43-containing gap junctions located at the intercalated disks (Figure 16) (Severs et al., 2004). The intercalated disks of working ventricular myocardium have a step-like configuration, with the gap junctions situated predominantly in the membrane segments that lie parallel with the long axis of the cell (Severs, 1990), with larger gap junctions typically circumscribing the disk periphery (Gourdie et al., 1991). This and other features of gap junction organization and aspects of tissue architecture such as the size and shape of the cells combine to ensure preferential propagation of the impulse in the longitudinal axis and hence the normal pattern of anisotropic spread of the impulse of healthy ventricular myocardium.

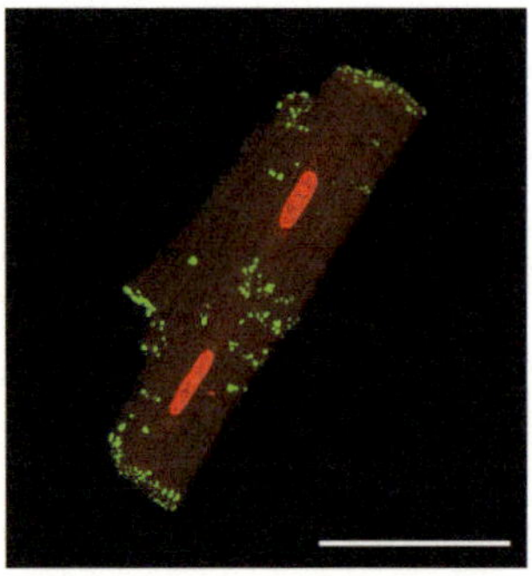

Fig. 16. An isolated ventricular myocyte labelled for Cx43 (green) illustrating localization of the gap junctions in clusters at the intercalated disks (Severs et al., 2004).

The gap junctions of atrial myocytes contain abundant Cx40 (Vozzi et al., 1999; Dupont et al., 2001), co-localized with Cx43 within the same individual gap-junctional plaques (Severs et al., 2001). Working ventricular myocytes, by contrast, normally lack detectable Cx40. In both ventricular and atrial working myocardium, Cx45 is present in very low quantities (Vozzi et al., 1999; Dupont et al., 2001). The specialized cardiomyocytes of the impulse generation and conduction system are distinct from the working ventricular and atrial cells both in terms of general morphology (Severs, 1989) and connexin expression profiles (Figure 17) (Coppen et al., 1999).

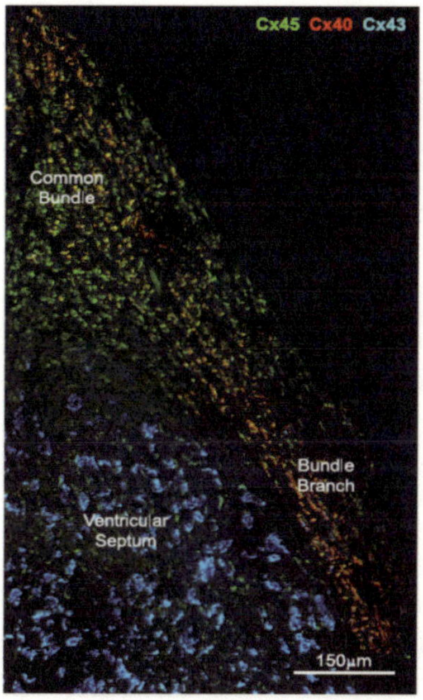

Fig. 17. Expression patterns of Cx43, Cx40 and Cx45 in different cardiomyocyte sub-types. This triple-labelled confocal montage shows part of the conduction system (common bundle and right bundle branch) which expresses Cx40 and Cx45). These two connexins are not detected in the adjacent working ventricular myocytes of the septum, which instead express Cx43. This example comes from rat heart (Coppen et al., 1999).

4.3 Gap junction remodeling in myocardial infarction

4.3.1 Connexin 43 remodeling in myocardial infarction

Two principal gap junction-related alterations have been reported in the diseased ventricle: disturbances in the distribution of gap junctions and reduced levels of their major component, Cx43. "Lateralization"of Cx43 gap junction label is a prominent feature of the border zone of surviving myocytes around infarct scar tissue in the human ventricle (Smith et al., 1991). Electron microscopy reveals that both laterally disposed gap junctions connecting adjacent cells, and internalized (non-functional) gap junctional membrane, contribute to this abnormal pattern (Smith et al., 1991).

By 6–12h after ligation, the normal distribution was lost for Cx43, desmoplakin, and cadherin at the intercalated disks in the infarct zone. By 24–48 h after ligation, the expression of Cx43 markedly decreased, to 5% of the levels of shamoperated hearts (Figure 18) (Takamatsu, 2008). At 4 days post-infarction in a dog model, lateral gap junction label in the extended infarct border zone has been correlated spatially with electrophysiologically identified figure-of-eight re-entrant circuits (Peters et al., 1997).

Gap junctional changes distant from the infarct scar tissue, in particular reduction in the size and the number of gap junctions per unit length of intercalated disc, and fewer side-to-side connections between myocytes, have been described as longer term remodelling events in dog myocardium (Kostin et al., 2003). Our study showed that Cx43 mRNA and Cx43 protein reduced significantly at ischemic zone at 4, 8 and 12 weeks of myocardial infarction mice (Figure 19) (LI et al., 2010; Zhao et al., 2009).

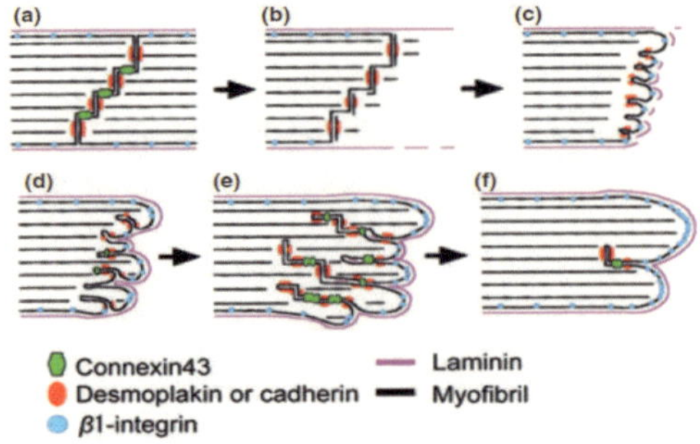

Fig. 18. Remodeling process of cell-cell and cell–extracellular matrix (cell–ECM) interactions at the stump of myocardial infarction. (a) Normal; (b) 24–48 h. At early phase after ligation (to 48 h), borderline cardiomyocytes facing the infarct lose neighboring cells and form blunt-ended stumps while maintaining some desmoplakin, and cadherin loses Cx43. (c) 48 h–day 3. By day 3, integrins such as b1-integrin cluster at stumps where basement membranes are partially formed. The formation of intracellular junctions composed of desmoplakin and cadherin is initiated between cell processes. (d) Days 3–4; (e) days 8–15, After day 3, stumps change into fine cytoplasmic processes toward the infarct. Cx43 expression between cell processes forms intracellular junctional complexes with desmoplakin and cadherin, similar to those of typical intercalated disks. Cx43 expression is also observed at transverse cell boundaries of borderline and vicinity cardiomyocytes. (f) In the chronic phase (days 60–90), integrin–ECM couplings at the tips of cell processes and collagen accumulation around the processes increase as wound healing proceeds. Cell processes fuse together, and the intercalated disk-like structures diminish (Takamatsu, 2008).

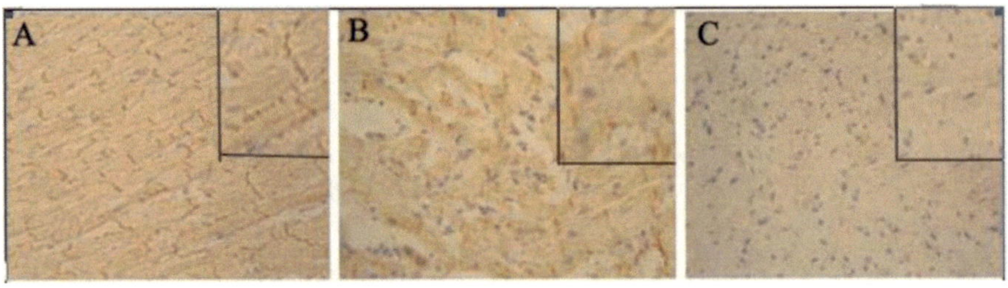

Fig. 19. A, Cx43 expression at normal zones in myocardial infarction mice after 4 weeks; B, Cx43 expression at ischemic zones in myocardial infarction mice after 4 weeks; C, Cx43 expression at infarcted zones in myocardial infarction mice after 4 weeks (×400) (LI et al., 2010).

Apart from alterations in connexin43 level, rapid dephosphorylation of Cx43 and translocation of Cx43 from gap junctions into the cytosol has been reported when electrical uncoupling is induced by acute ischaemia in the Langendorff-perfused rat heart (Beardslee et al., 2000). These processes are reversible upon reperfusion and substantially reduced with ischemic preconditioning (LI et al., 2009a). Dephosphorylated Cx43 is associated with the laterally distributed gap junction label, while those gap junctions that remain in the classic, polar intercalated disc orientation contain phosphorylated Cx43 (Lampe et al., 2006).

A rather different form of gap junction remodelling is associated with 'hibernating myocardium' in patients with ischemic heart disease (Kaprielian et al., 1998). The term 'hibernating myocardium' refers to regions of ventricular myocardium that do not contract properly but which recover after normal blood flow is restored following coronary artery by-pass surgery. In hibernating myocardium, the large Cx43 gap junctions typically found at the periphery of the intercalated disc are smaller in size, and the overall amount of immunodetectable Cx43 per intercalated disc is reduced, compared with normally perfused myocardial regions of the same heart (Kaprielian et al., 1998). These findings were the first indication that Cx43 gap junction remodelling contributes to impaired ventricular contraction, in addition to arrhythmia, in human ischemic heart disease (Kaprielian et al., 1998).

4.3.2 Connexin 45 remodeling in myocardial infarction

Because Cx45 is not expressed widely in working ventricular myocytes in the normal adult heart, there is no report on the alternation of distribution and expression of Cx45 after myocardial infarction. However, previous study showed that expression of Cx45 in the failing human ventricle was up-regulated, alongside the reduction in Cx43, thus significantly altering the Cx43: Cx45 ratio (Yamada et al., 2003). Our datas showed that Cx45 mRNA and Cx45 protein increased significantly at ischemic zone at 4, 8 and 12 weeks in myocardial infarction mice (Figure 20) (Zhao et al., 2009). Up-regulation of Cx45 in myocardial infarction hearts inplicates a novel mechanism whereby connexin remodeling may promote arrhythmogenesis.

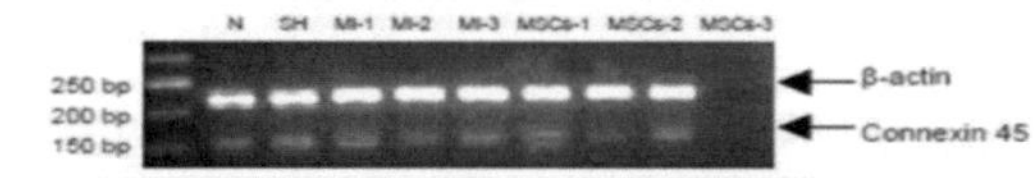

Group	4 wk		
	Normal area	Ischemic zone	Infarcted zone
Normal control	0.314±0.016	-	-
Sham operation	0.309±0.021	-	-
Myocardial infarction	0.314±0.018	0.648±0.015[a]	0.020±0.016[b]
MSCs	0.306±0.018	0.441±0.021[ac]	0.019±0.015[b]

Fig. 20. Ratio change of connexin 45/β-actin for myocardial infarction mice after 4, 8 and 12 weeks MSCs, bone marrow mesenchymal stem cells; [a]P < 0.01, vs. the normal area in the same group; [b]P < 0.01, vs. the ischemic zone in the same group; [c]P < 0.01, vs. myocardial infarction group (Zhao et al., 2009).

4.3.3 Possibility of formation of heteromeric gap junction channels in myocardial infarction

Expression of multiple connexin isoforms induces the formation of hetero-multimeric gap junction channels with distinct gating and permeability properties than their homo-multimeric counterparts. Cx43 and Cx45 can form heterotypic channels that have unitary conductances lower than those of homotypic Cx43 channels and that fail to pass the fluorescent dye Lucifer yellow (Zhong et al., 2002; Moreno et al., 2002b; Moreno et al., 1995). When Cx43-expressing ROS cells are transfected to coexpress Cx45, electrical coupling is reduced even though Cx43 abundance, phosphorylation, and localization do not change (Koval et al., 1995). Coexpression of Cx45 with Cx43 in HeLa cells reduced the number of neighboring cells that were chemically coupled. Thus, increased Cx45 expression may

reduce coupling and slow conduction or create microheterogeneities in coupling without slowing macroscopic conduction (Yamada et al., 2003).
Previos studies showed that heterotypic combination of Cx45 and Cx43 in mammalian cell lines impairs voltage gating of Cx43 and alters residual conductances, suggesting that connexon interactions may play a distinct role in modulation of intercellular communication (Elenes et al., 2001; Thomas et al., 2004). Cx43 and Cx45 formed heteromeric channels that exhibit reduced single channel conductance compared with Cx43 homomeric channels (Martinez et al., 2002). Our datas demonstrated colocalization of Cx45 and Cx43 in both control and ischemic ventricular myocardium (Figure 21).
Not only do Cx45 and Cx43 form hybrid channels in vitro, colocalization of these connexins in ventricular myocyte gap junctions provides and opportunity for hybrid channel formation in vivo, where interaction between Cx45 and Cx43 in hybrid channels could alter conductance states and gating responsiveness relative to the biophysical properties of homotypic channels (Yamada et al., 2003; Moreno et al., 2004). Our dates further suggested that enhanced expression of Cx45 in the ischemic heart occurs in junctions containing reduced levels of Cx43, raising the intriguing possibility that the relative stoichiometries of Cx45 and Cx43 within gap junctional plaques may be dramatically altered in the ischemic heart (Zhao et al., 2009). The limitation for our study is that the colocalization data are qualitative. In the absence of technological support of electrophysiologic confirmation of hybrid gap junction channels connecting ventricular myocytes in vivo, we can only speculate on the functional effects of increased Cx45 in the myocardial infarction heart.

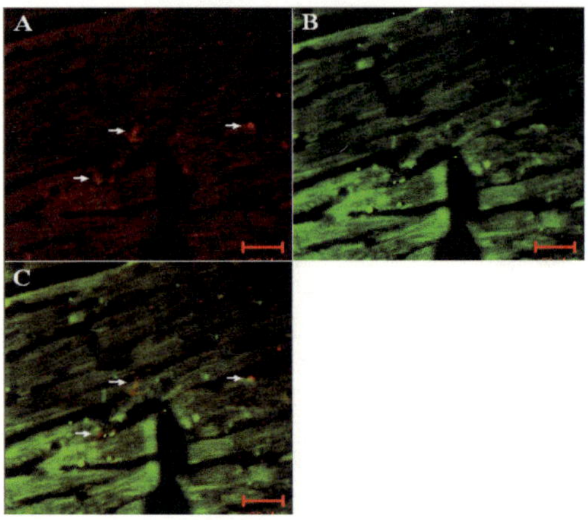

Fig. 21. Colocalizations (white arrows) of Cx45 and Cx43 in ischemic ventricular myocardium after 12 weeks in myocardial infarction mice by confocal microscopy examination (Scale bar = 20µm).

4.3.4 Mitochondrial Cx43 in myocardial infarction

Although it is generally assumed that Cx43 is exclusively localized at the sarcolemma, Cx43 has been found recently at cardiomyocyte mitochondria linner and outer membrane (Boengler et al., 2005; Rodriguez-Sinovas et al., 2006; Goubaeva et al., 2007). Boengler et al (Boengler et al., 2005) presented evidence at first for the presence of Cx43 in mitochondria from mouse, rat, pig and human left ventricular myocardium obtained from fluorescence-activated cell sorting and western blot analyses, as well as confocal and immunoelectron microscopy (Figure 22).

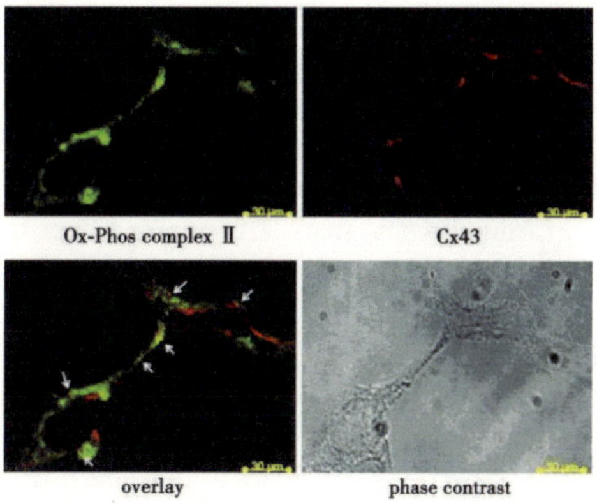

Fig. 22. Cultured mice atrial HL-1 cardiomyocytes were stained with antibodies against Cx43 (red) and mitochondria (Ox-Phos Com plex II, green) and analyzed by confocal laser scan microscopy. Merged image demonstrates colocalization as yellow po ints (arrows). Additional ly, the phase contrast image was shown (Boengler et al., 2005).

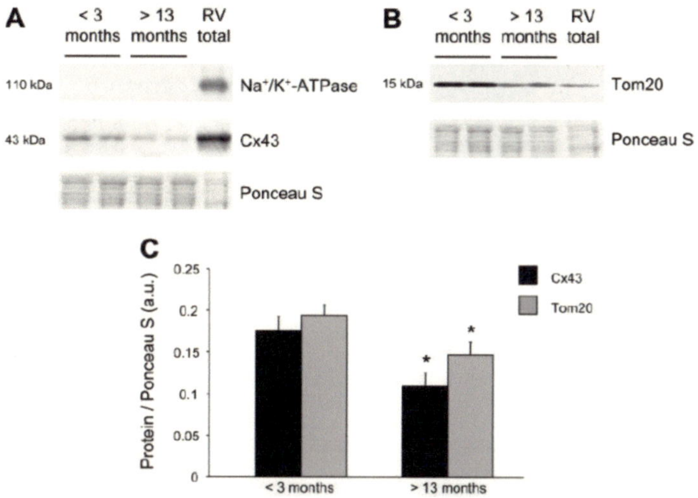

Fig. 23. Cx43 and translocase of the outer membrane 20 (Tom20) protein level in mitochondria isolated from left ventricular mycardium from young and aged mice. A: Western blot analysis was performed on mitochondrial protein extracts from young (< 3 mo) and aged (> 13mo) mice and on total right ventricular proteins (< 3 mo) for Na-K-ATPase and Cx43. Ponceau S staining demonstrates equal protein loading. B: Western blot analysis was performed for Tom20 on mitochondrial protein extracts from young and aged mice and on total right ventricular proteins. Ponceau S staining demonstrates equal protein loading. C: quantification of the Cx43 and Tom20 immunoreactivity in mitochondria of young (<3 mo, n = 14) and aged (> 13 mo, n = 10) mice normalized to Ponceau S staining. *P<0.05 vs. <3 mo (Boengler et al., 2007).

In Antonio et al (Rodriguez-Sinovas et al., 2006) study, treatment of isolated mitochondria with digitonin resulted in a marked reduction of voltage dependent anion channel immunoreactivity (VDA), whereas an adenine nucleotide transporter (ANT) specific signal was detected by confocal laser scan microscopy. An observations, by using western blotting and immunofluorescence with anti-VDAC as a marker for the outer mitochondrial membrane and with anti-ANT as a marker for the inner mitochondrial membrane, confirmed that Cx43 was not only present in the inner and outer mitochondrial membrane, but the mitochondrial Cx43 is phosphorylated (Goubaeva et al., 2007). Furthermore, with progressing age, GJ and mitochondrial levels of Cx43 in ventricular and atrial tissue homogenates are reduced. In mice hearts, sarcolemmal Cx43 content was reduced in aged (> 13 month) com pared with young (< 3 month). Also in mitochondria isolated from aged mice left ventricular myocardium, western blot analysis indicated a 40% decrease in Cx43 content compared with mitochondria isolated from young mice hearts. The reduced levels of Cx43 may contribute to the age-related loss of cardioprotection (Figure 23) (Boengler et al., 2007).

There is very little research on the relationship between mitochondria connexin and myocardial infarction until now, and Cx43 is the only connexin that has been found at cardiomyocyte mitochondria. Recentlly, our data showed that Heptanol (a GJ blocker) preconditioning protects myocardium from ischemia-reperfusion injury. The mechanism may be related to increasing in mitochondrial membrane potential and attenuating the decrease in mitochondria Cx43 expression induced by isehemia-reperfusion (Figure 24) (HE, 2009, 2010).

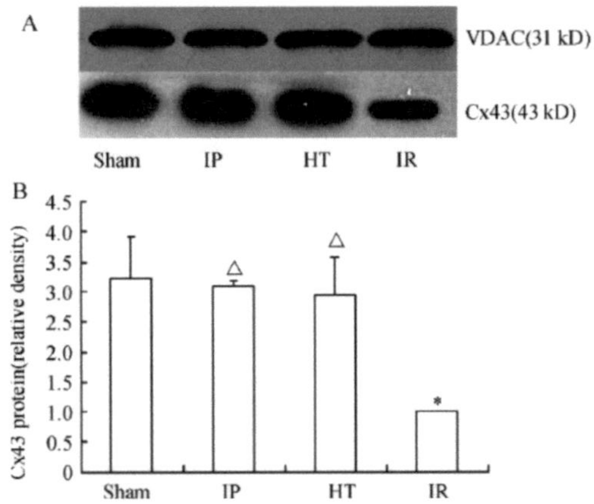

Fig. 24. Western blotting (30 μg total protein / lane) shows the increase of Cx43 protein in myoca rdial mitochondria in heptanol preconditioning on myocardial isehemia/reperfusion injury of rabbits. A: expression of Cx43 protein detected by Western blotting; B: results of the relative density of Cx43 protein; n = 3. △P<0.05 vs IR; *P< 0.05 vs sham (HE, 2009, 2010).

4.4 Electrophysiological consequences of gap junction remodeling

Reductions in intercellular coupling lead to slowing of impulse propagation and amplification of the normal electrical heterogeneity within the ventricular myocardium. Individually, each of these electrophysiological effects of uncoupling are predicted to favor reentry, and together they may very well synergistically enhance arrhythmic risk (Kleber & Rudy, 2004).

Anatomic evidence of GJ remodeling, typically documented by immunohistochemical means, has been correlated with functional measures of aberrant cell-cell coupling such as slowing of impulse propagation and changes in anisotropy, as well as arrhythmogenicity

(Fishman, 2005). In the healing canine infarct model, areas of GJ remodeling characterized by redistribution of Cx43 to lateral cell borders, correlates with the location of the central common pathway of figure-of-eight reentrant circuits (Peters et al., 1997). Additionally, junctional conductance of side-to-side coupled cells from the epicardial border zone is markedly diminished (Yao et al., 2003).

What needs to be noted is that dysregulated connexin expression occurs as but one element of a widespread remodeling process - one that in volves many of the ion-handling proteins that regulate cardiac excitability (Fishman, 2005). Cardiac-specific Cx43 gene-targeted mutant mice showed significant slowing of impulse propagation and despite the relatively small mass of the murine ventricle, they all succumb to spontaneous or easily inducible sustained ventricular tachyarrhythmias (Fishman, 2005). Moreover, optical mapping studies suggest that most, if not all of these arrhythmias are due to reentry (Gutstein et al., 2001).

On the other hand, studies of several additional genetic models in which Cx43 expression is modified are instructive, including the heteryzygous ($Cx43^{+/-}$) germline knockout mice, chimeric ($Cx43^{-/-}/Cx43^{+/+}$) mice, as well as the recently described Cx43 O-CKO mice (Guerrero et al., 1997). Taken together, data from these murine models suggest that in the absence of additional pathologic stimuli, less widespread or more modest reductions in cell-cell coupling are insufficient to support sustained ventricular arrhythmias (Fishman, 2005).

For example, Cx43 germline heterozygous mice subjected to myocardial infarction reportedly have no increase in the frequency of spontaneous or inducible arrhythmias compared to wildtype mice with infarcts (Betsuyaku, 2004). Moreover, the imposition of ischemia in isolated-perfused hearts from $Cx43^{+/-}$ mice provokes only non-sustained ventricular tachycardia (Lerner et al., 2000). Cx43 chimeric mice, which have relatively large foci of uncoupled myocytes within the ventricle, display a substantial increase in spontaneous PVCs and short runs of VT (Gutstein et al., 2005). The O-CKO mice only develop inducible or spontaneous sustained VT when the anatomic extent of knockout is marked, encompassing more than 60% of the myocardium (Danik et al., 2004). Thus, the spatial extent and magnitude of uncoupling of Cx43 is likely to be insufficient to support the development of sustained ventricular tachyarrhythmias in the absence of additional pathologic pro-arrhythmic"hits" (Fishman, 2005).

4.5 Therapeutic Implications of gap junction remodeling after myocardial infarction

4.5.1 Pharmacological therapeutic implications

Pharmacology of GJ intercellular communication is still at its beginnings. Figure 26 shows a schematic view of a gap junction channel as a target of pharmacology (Salameh & Dhein, 2005). Potential mechanisms controlling the level of intercellular communication in the heart include regulation of connexin turnover (synthesis and degradation), cellular distribution and phosphorylation. There are numerous data showing that some compounds can up-regulate Cx43 via modulation either synthesis or degradation and enhance gap junctional communication (Salameh & Dhein, 2005). Although many substances have effects on Gap junction-mediated intercellular communication (GJMIC), there is a lack of powerful and specific GJ blockers (Dhein, 1998, 2005).

Substances, such as AAP10 (Weng et al., 2002) or its derivative ZP123 (Xing et al., 2003), that increase intercellular coupling have presented themselves as valuable new tools to investigate the role of intercellular coupling in physiology and pathophysiology. It has been shown that uncoupling correlates with the development of some types of arrhythmias, and in several cases application of drugs that increase coupling has confirmed this role (Axelsen

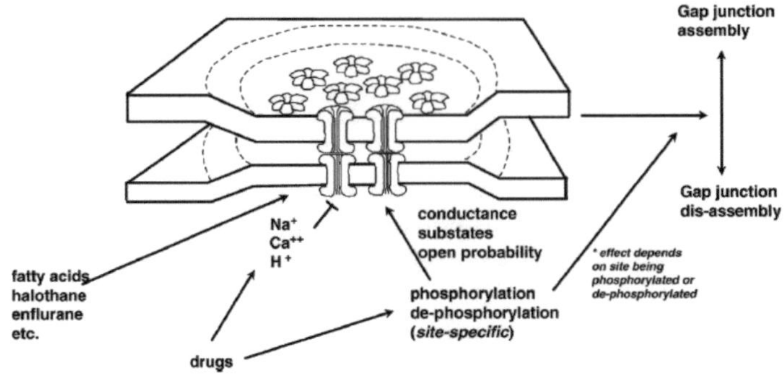

Fig. 26. Schematic view of a gap junction channel and its constituent component, the connexin, as a target of pharmacology (Salameh & Dhein, 2005).

et al., 2007). Two recent studies showed (Haugan et al. 2005, Axelsen et al. 2007 (Haugan et al., 2005; Axelsen et al., 2007) that an increase of gap junctional conductance by specific peptide, rotigaptide, can prevent atrial conduction slowing or re-entrant ventricular tachycardia in ischemic heart. Suppression of ischemia-induced dephosphorylation of connexin seems to be one of the mechanisms involved. This mechanism was thought to be involved in the antiarrhythmic effects of ischemic preconditioning (Schulz et al., 2007). On the other hand, the reduction in gap junction communication that takes place during ischemia has been regarded as a beneficial and protective measure (Garcia-Dorado et al., 2004). Several investigators have examined the role of uncoupling GJ communication on myocardial infarct size. Thus, pharmacological uncoupling of GJ communication with nonselective uncouplers of GJ communication has been reported to reduce infarct size in animal experiments. Addition of the GJ blocker heptanol at concentration has a marked protective effect when applied at the time of reperfusion (Garcia-Dorado et al., 1997). Recent studies analyzing the effect of GJ uncouplers when administered during reoxygenation or reperfusion have consistently documented a reduction of necrosis (enzyme release or infarct size) (Saltman et al., 2002; Sebbag et al., 2003). Besides, electrical uncoupling by heptanol significantly lowers defibrillation threshold and dispersion of ventricular fibrillation cycle length without altering refractoriness (Qi et al., 2003). Although the beneficial and protective effort of GJ uncouplers delighted our researches, an important limitation is the lack of specific, rapid, reversible, and safe inhibitors of GJ intercellular communication.

Modulation of GJ intercellular coupling may open interesting new therapeutic approaches for a large number of diseases including myocardial infarction. However, in many respects, we have not completely understood the complex networking and its long-term regulation. This again underlines the need for in vivo and organbased models to evaluate the possibilities of pharmacological approaches towards an acute or chronic modulation of gap junctions. Moreover, the development of connexin- or organ specific gap junction modulator drugs is a challenging task for pharmacologists.

4.5.2 Stem cell therapy

Stem cell transplantation has emerged as a potential treatment strategy for heart failure secondary to acute or chronic ischaemic heart disease (Laflamme & Murry, 2005). But currently two autologous cell types, namely bone marrow (BM) cells and skeletal myoblasts (SMs), which were used in clinical trials in patients after myocardial infarction (Murry et al.,

2005), seem to provide only modest improvement of contractile heart function (Janssens et al., 2006) because neither BM cells (Murry et al., 2004) nor SMs (Reinecke et al., 2002) adopt a cardiac cell fate or couple electrically with the host myocardium (Leobon et al., 2003; Murry et al., 2004). Moreover, VT has been reported in several of the patients transplanted with SMs (Hagege et al., 2006), raising concerns as to whether engraftment of cells enhances the risk of VT, the most frequent cause of sudden death after myocardial infarction (Solomon et al., 2005; Henkel et al., 2006). So it is very important to fully answer these two questions before cell or stem cell therapy was proposed widely in clinic: whether cell or stem cell can differenciate into cardiomyocytes? Whether cell or stem cell can form functional coupling with the host, which is important for the physiological communication between cardiac myocytes?

A study (Virginijus et al., 2004) showed that human mesenchymal stem cells (hMSCs) can express connexins and couple to one another via Cx43 and Cx40. In addition, they formed functional gap junction channels with cells tranfected with Cx43, Cx40 or Cx45 as well as canine ventricular cardiomyocytes. Those are the foundermantal conditions for mesenchymal stem cells therapy for heart disease including myocardial infarction (see Figure 27).

Besides, another study (Wilhelm et al., 2007) showed that cardiomyocyte transplantation has the potential to impart electrical stability to the injured heart, thereby markedly reducing the major factor leading to sudden death. This protective effect was independent of the documented modest augmentation of left ventricular function and was associated with improved electrical coupling within the infarct by the engraftment of Cx43-expressing embryonic cardiomyocytes (eCMs). This enhanced coupling reduced vulnerability to VT by decreasing the incidence of conduction block within the infarct and/or by a modulatory effect on border-zone cardiomyocytes. This study also found that expression of the cardiac gap-junction protein Cx43 is the critical factor underlying augmented intercellular electrical conduction and protection from arrhythmia, because engraftment of Cx43-expressing SMs

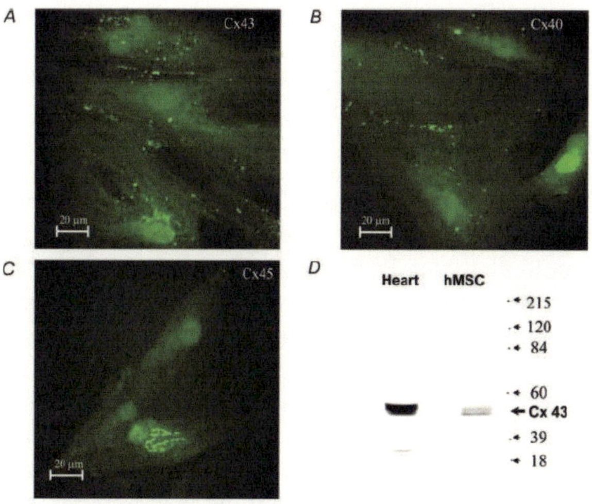

Fig. 27. Identification of connexins in gap junctions of hMSCs Immunostaining of Cx43 (A), Cx40 (B) and Cx45 (C). D, immunoblot analysis of Cx43 in canine ventricular myocytes and hMSCs. Whole cell lysates (120µg) from ventricular cells or hMSCs were resolved by SDS, transferred to membrans, and blotted with Cx43 antibodies. Migration of molecular weight markers is indicated to the right of the blot (Virginijus et al., 2004).

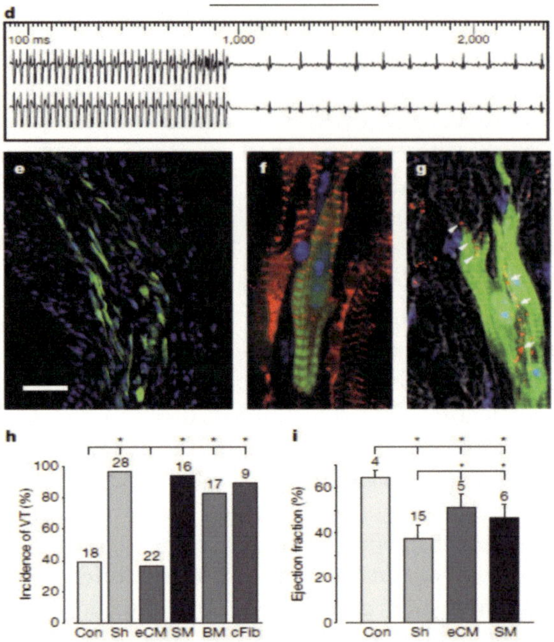

Fig. 28. d, Ventricular burst stimulation does not induce VT. Upper trace, surface ECG; lower trace, His-level electrogram. e, EGFP-positive eCMs integrate into the infarct. f, EGFP positive eCMs are striated (α-actinin staining, red) and are in direct contact with EGFP-negative host cardiomyocytes. g, Cx43 staining (red) illustrates gap-junction formation between engrafted EGFP-positive eCMs (arrows) and with native cardiomyocytes (arrowheads). h, Summary of VT inducibility. Note strongly elevated susceptibility to VT induction in shaminjected group (Sh) compared with control group; eCM engraftment reduces VT inducibility compared with sham injection. Conversely, VT remains frequent after transplantation of SMs, BM and cardiac myofibroblasts (cFib). i, Improvement of left ventricular ejection fraction after eCM or SM transplantation. Numbers above bars indicate n; error bars show s.d. Scale bar, 60 mm (e), 5 mm (f), and 11mm (g).

protected against VT induction (see Figure 28). Thus, cell therapy including stem cell therapy in combination with Cx43 gene transfer represents a promising therapeutic strategy to decrease the risk of potentially fatal arrhythmias in injured heart.

In our recently study on mice, Laser Scanning Confocal Microscope examination found that DAPI-labeled MSCs distributed widely at the host ischemic zone and expressed Cx43. Fluorescence PCR, Immunohistochemistry, Immunofluorescence and immuno-electron microscope studies showed that Cx43 mRNA and Cx43 protein exprssions were statistically higher in MSCs group compared to MI group; Cx45 mRNA and Cx45 protein expressions were statistically lower in MSCs group compared to MI group (see Figure 29). We concluded that MSCs transplantation, which could survive at the host ischemic zone and express Cx43, can modulate the electrophysiological abnormality of myocardial infarction by up-regulating Cx43 and down-regulating Cx45 both at Protein and mRNA levels. In a word, MSCs have the plasticity of differentiating into cardiac muscle cell-like cells, which can modulate the electrophysiological abnormality via regulation of Cx43 and Cx45 remodeling following with myocardial infarction (Li et al., 2009b, 2010; Zhao et al., 2009, 2010).

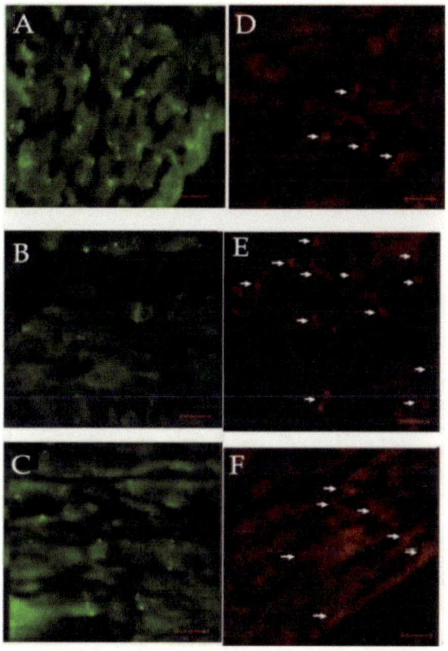

Fig. 29. A, Cx43 staining by FITC (green) at normal zones of ventricular myocardium. B, Cx43 staining by FITC at ischemic zones of ventricular myocardium. C, Cx43 staining by FITC at ischemic zones of ventricular myocardium after MSCs transplantation. D, Cx45 staining by TR (red) at normal zones of ventricular myocardium. E, Cx45 staining by TR at ischemic zones of ventricular myocardium. F, Cx45 staining by TR at ischemic zones of ventricular myocardium after MSCs transplantation.

5. Conclusions and perspective

In this chapter, we have presented mechanisms of sympathetic neural remodeling, electrical remodeling and gap Junction remodeling, which closely relate to the electrophysiological abnormality after myocardial infarction. Pathophysiological remodeling in myocardial infarction is multifactorial and complex, which involves changes in the structure and function of the myocardium. Although we anthropogenically divided the arrhythogenic mechamism of myocardial infarction into three parts, we have emphasized the importance of interrelationship among them which occurs at the cellular and molecular levels. Elucidating the role of myocardial remodeling and its molecular underpinnings present opportunities for the development of novel gene- and cell-based strategies as well as more pharmacotherapies. Besides, the localization of Cx43 at mitochondria opens a new door for us to reveal the cardioprotection against myocardial infarction. Stem cells, especially MSCs, give us a new hope on the potential treatment strategy for reducing life-threatening post-infarct arrhythmias and for heart failure secondary to acute or chronic ischaemic heart disease.

6. Acknowledgment

This work was supported by grants from the National Natural Science Foundation of China (No. 30560051); the Science Foundation for Returnees of Guangxi Zhuang Autonomous

Region of China (No.0448014) and the Key Scientific Research Subject of Medical Treatment and Public Health of Guangxi Zhuang Autonomous Region of China (No.200301).

7. References

Aggarwal R & Boyden PA. (1995). Diminished Ca^{2+} and Ba^{2+} currents in myocytes surviving in the epicardial border zone of the 5-day infarcted canine heart. *Circ Res,* Vol.77, No.6, pp. 1180–1191. ISSN 0009-7330

Armour, JA. (2010). Functional anatomy of intrathoracic neurons innervating the atria and ventricles. *Heart Rhythm,* Vol.7, No.7, pp. 994-996. ISSN 1547-5271

Augustus O. Grant. (2009). Cardiac Ion Channels. *Circ Arrhythm Electrophysiol.* 2, 185-194. ISSN 1941-3149

Axelsen LN, Haugan K, Stahlhut M, Kjølbye AL, Hennan JK, Holstein-Rathlou NH, Petersen JS & Nielsen MS. (2007). Increasing Gap Junctional Coupling: A Tool for Dissecting the Role of Gap Junctions. *J Membrane Biol,* Vol.216, No.1, pp. 23-35. ISSN 0022-2631

Baba S, Dun W & Boyden PA. (2004). Can PKA activators rescue Na^{+} channel function in epicardial border zone cells that survive in the infarcted canine heart? *Cardiovasc Res,* Vol.64, No.2, pp. 260–267. ISSN 0008-6363

Baba S, Dun W, Cabo C & Boyden PA. (2005). Remodeling in cells from different regions of the reentrant circuit during ventricular tachycardia. *Circulation,* Vol.112, No.16, pp. 2386–2396. ISSN 0009-7322

Beardslee MA, Lerner DL, Tadros PN, Laing JG, Beyer EC, Yamada KA, Kléber AG, Schuessler RB & Saffitz JE. (2000). Dephosphorylation and intracellular redistribution of ventricular connexin43 during electrical uncoupling induced by ischemia. *Circ Res,* Vol.87, No.8, pp. 656-62. ISSN 0009-7330

Betsuyaku T, Kanno S, Lerner DL, Schuessler RB, Saffitz JE & Yamada KA. (2004). Spontaneous and inducible ventricular arrhythmias after myocardial infarction in mice. *Cardiovasc Pathol,* Vol.13, No.3, pp. 156-164. ISSN 1054-8807

Boengler K, Dodoni G, Rodriguez-Sinovas A, Cabestrero A, Ruiz-Meana M, Gres P, Konietzka I, Lopez-Iglesias C, Garcia-Dorado D, Di Lisa F, Heusch G & Schulz R. (2005). Connexin 43 in cardiomyocyte mitochondria and its increase by ischemic preconditioning. *Cardiovasc Res,* Vol.67, No.2, pp. 234-244. ISSN 0008-6363

Boengler K, Konietzka I, Buechert A, Heinen Y, Garcia-Dorado D, Heusch G & Schulz R. (2007). Loss of ischemic preconditionings cardioprotection in aged mouse hearts is associated with reduced gap junctional and mitochondrial levels of connexin 43. *Am J Physiol Heart Circ Physiol,* Vol.292, No.4, pp. H1764-H1769. ISSN 0363-6135

Boyden PA, Albala A & Dresdner KP Jr. (1989). Electrophysiology and ultrastructure of canine subendocardial Purkinje cells isolated from control and 24-hour infarcted hearts. *Circ Res,* Vol.65, No.4, pp. 955–970. ISSN 0009-7330

Boyden PA & Pinto JM. (1994). Reduced calcium currents in subendocardial Purkinje myocytes that survive in the 24- and 48-hour infarcted heart. *Circulation,* Vol.89, No.6, pp. 2747–2759. ISSN 0009-7322

Boyden PA, Barbhaiya C, Lee T & ter Keurs HE. (2003). Nonuniform Ca^{2+} transients in arrhythmogenic Purkinje cells that survive in the infarcted canine heart. *Cardiovasc Res,* Vol.57, No.3, pp. 681–693. ISSN 0008-6363

Boyden PA, Dun W, Barbhaiya C & ter Keurs HE. (2004). 2APB- and JTV519(K201)-sensitive micro Ca^{2+} waves in arrhythmogenic Purkinje cells that survive in infarcted canine heart. *Heart Rhythm,* Vol.1, No.2, pp. 218–226. ISSN 1547-5271

Canty JM Jr, Suzuki G, Banas MD, Verheyen F, Borgers M & Fallavollita JA. (2004). Hibernating myocardium: chronically adapted to ischemia but vulnerable to sudden death. *Circ Res,* Vol.94, No.8, pp. 1142-1149. ISSN 0009-7330

Cao JM, Chen LS, KenKnight BH, Ohara T, Lee MH, Tsai J, Lai WW, Karagueuzian HS, Wolf PL, Fishbein MC & Chen PS. (2000a). Nerve sprouting and sudden cardiac death. *Circ Res,* Vol.86, No.7, pp. 816–821. ISSN 0009-7330

Cao JM, Fishbein MC, Han JB, Lai WW, Lai AC, Wu TJ, Czer L, Wolf PL, Denton TA, Shintaku IP, Chen PS & Chen LS. (2000b). Relationship between regional cardiac hyperinnervation and ventricular arrhythmia. *Circulation,* Vol.101, No.16, pp. 1960–1969. ISSN 0009-7322

Cardiac Arrhythmia Suppression Trial (CAST) Investigators. (1989). Preliminary report: effect of encainide and flecainide on mortality in a randomized trial of arrhythmia suppression after myocardial infarction. *N Engl J Med,* Vol.321, No.6, pp. 406–412. ISSN 0028-4793

Chow LT, Chow WH, Lee JC, Chow SS, Anderson RH & Gosling JA. (1998). Postmortem changes in the immunohistochemical demonstration of nerves in human ventricular myocardium. *J Anat,* Vol.192, No.1, pp. 73-80. ISSN 0021-8782

Cittadini A, Monti MG, Isgaard J, Casaburi C, Strömer H, Di Gianni A, Serpico R, Saldamarco L, Vanasia M & Saccà L. (2003). Aldosterone receptor blockade improves left ventricular remodeling and increases ventricular fibrillation threshold in experimental heart failure. *Cardiovasc Res,* Vol.58, No.3, pp. 555–564. ISSN 0008-6363

Coppen SR, Severs NJ & Gourdie RG. (1999). Connexin45 (a6) expression delineates an extended conduction system in the embryonic and mature rodent heart. *Dev Genet,* Vol.24, No.1-2, pp. 82-90. ISSN 0192-253X

Crowley C, Spencer SD, Nishimura MC, Chen KS, Pitts-Meek S, Armanini MP, Ling LH, McMahon SB, Shelton DL & Levinson AD. (1994). Mice lacking nerve growth factor display perinatal loss of sensory and sympathetic neurons yet develop basal forebrain cholinergic neurons. *Cell,* Vol.76, No.6, pp. 1001–1011. ISSN 0092-8674

Danik SB, Liu F, Zhang J, Suk HJ, Morley GE, Fishman GI & Gutstein DE. (2004). Modulation of cardiac gap junction expression and arrhythmic susceptibility. *Circ Res,* Vol.95, No.10, pp. 1035-1041. ISSN 0009-7330

Desplantez T, Halliday D, Dupont E & Weingart R. (2004). Cardiac connexins Cx43 and Cx45: formation of diverse gap junction channels with diverse electrical properties. *Pfluqers Arch,* Vol.448, No.4, pp. 363–375. ISSN 0031-6768

Dhein S. (1998). Gap junction channels in the cardiovascular system: pharmacological and physiological modulation. *Trends Pharmacol Sci,* Vol.19, No.6, pp. 229-41. ISSN 0165-6147

Dhein S, Polontchouk L, Salameh A & Haefliger J.-A. (2002). Pharmacological modulation and differential regulation of the cardiac gap junction proteins connexin 43 and connexin 40. *Biol Cell,* Vol.94, No.7-8, pp. 409-22. ISSN 0248-4900

Dillon SM, Allessie MA, Ursell PC & Wit AL. (1988). Influences of anisotropic tissue structure on reentrant circuits in the epicardial border zone of subacute canine infarcts. *Circ Res,* Vol.63, No.1, pp. 182–206. ISSN 0009-7330

Dun W, Baba S, Yagi T & Boyden PA. (2004). Dynamic remodeling of K^+ and Ca^{2+} currents in cells that survived in the epicardial border zone of canine healed infarcted heart. *Am J Physiol Heart Circ Physiol,* Vol.287, No.3, pp. H1046–H1054. ISSN 0363-6135

Dun W & Boyden PA. (2005). Diverse phenotypes of outward currents in cells that have survived in the 5-day-infarcted heart. *Am J Physiol Heart Circ Physiol,* Vol.289, No.2, pp. H667–H673. ISSN 0363-6135

Dupont E, Ko Y, Rothery S, Coppen SR, Baghai M, Haw M & Severs NJ (2001). The gap-junctional protein, connexin40, is elevated in patients susceptible to post-operative atrial fibrillation. *Circulation,* Vol.103, No.6, pp. 842-9. ISSN 0009-7322

Elenes S, Martinez AD, Delmar M, Beyer EC & Moreno AP (2001). Heterotypic docking of Cx43 and Cx45 connexons blocks fast voltage gating of Cx43. *Biophys J,* Vol.81, No.3, pp. 1406-1418. ISSN 0006-3495

Esler M, Jennings G, Lambert G, Meredith I, Horne M & Eisenhofer G (1990). Overflow of catecholamine neurotransmitters to the circulation: source, fate, and functions. *Physiol Rev,* Vol.70, No.4, pp. 963–985. ISSN 0031-9333

Fishman GI. (2005). Gap junction remodeling and ventricular arrhythmias. *Heart Rhythm,* Vol.2, No.8, pp. 887-9. ISSN 1547-5271

Friedman PL, Fenoglio JJ & Wit AL. (1975). Time course for reversal of electrophysiological and ultrastructural abnormalities in subendocardial Purkinje fibers surviving extensive myocardial infarction in dogs. *Circ Res,* Vol.36, No.1, pp. 127–144. ISSN 0009-7330

Frohnwieser B, Chen, L-Q, Schreibmayer W & Kallen RG. (1997). Modulation of the human cardiac sodium channel a-subunit by cAMP-dependent protein kinase and the responsible sequence domain. *J Physiol,* Vol.498, No.2, pp. 309-318. ISSN 0022-3751

Fuchs M, Hilfiker A, Kaminski K, Hilfiker-Kleiner D, Guener Z, Klein G, Podewski E, Schieffer B, Rose-John S & Drexler H. (2003). Role of interleukin-6 for LV remodeling and survival after experimental myocardial infarction. *FASEB J,* Vol.17, No.4, pp. 2118-2120. ISSN 0892-6638

Fukuda K, Davies SS, Nakajima T, Ong BH, Kupershmidt S, Fessel J, Amarnath V, Anderson ME, Boyden PA, Viswanathan PC, Roberts LJ 2nd & Balser JR. (2005). Oxidative mediated lipid peroxidation recapitulates proarrhythmic effects on cardiac sodium channels. *Circ Res,* Vol.97, No.12, pp. 1262–1269. ISSN 0009-7330

Gao L, Wang W, Li YL, Schultz HD, Liu D, Cornish KG & Zucker IH. (2005). Simvastatin therapy normalizes sympathetic neural control in experimental heart failure: roles of angiotensin II type 1 receptors and NAD(P)H oxidase. *Circulation,* Vol.112, No.12, pp. 1763–1770. ISSN 0009-7322

Garcia-Dorado D, Inserte J, Ruiz-Meana M, González MA, Solares J, Juliá M, Barrabés JA & Soler-Soler J. (1997). Gap junction uncoupler heptanol prevents cell-to-cell progression of hypercontracture and limits necrosis during myocardial reperfusion. *Circulation,* Vol.96, No.10, pp. 3579-3586. ISSN 0009-7322

Garcia-Dorado D, Rogriguez-Sinovas A & Ruiz-Meana M. (2004). Gap junction-mediated spread of cell injury and death during myocardial ischemia-reperfusion. *Cardiovas Res,* Vol.61, No.3 pp. 386-410. ISSN 0008-6363

Gardner PI, Ursell PC, Fenoglio JJ Jr & Wit AL. (1985). Electrophysiologic and anatomic basis for fractionated electrograms recorded from healed myocardial infarcts. *Circulation,* Vol.72, No.3, pp. 596–611. ISSN 0009-7322

Gidh-Jain M, Huang B, Jain P & el-Sherif N. (1996). Differential expression of voltage-gated K^+ channel genes in left ventricular remodeled myocardium after experimental myocardial infarction. *Circ Res,* Vol.79, No.4, pp. 669–675. ISSN 0009-7330

Goubaeva F, Mikami M, Giardina S, Ding B, Abe J & Yang J. (2007). Cardiac mitochondrial connexin 43 regulates apoptosis. *Biochem Biophys Res Commun,* Vol.352, No.1, pp. 97-103. ISSN 0006-291X

Gourdie RG, Green CR & Severs NJ. (1991). Gap junction distribution in adult mammalian myocardium revealed by an antipeptide antibody and laser scanning confocal microscopy. *J Cell Sci,* Vol.99, No.1, pp. 41–55. ISSN 0021-9533

Guerrero PA, Schuessler RB, Davis LM, Beyer EC, Johnson CM, Yamada KA & Saffitz JE. (1997). Slow ventricular conduction in mice heterozygous for a connexin43 null mutation. *J Clin Invest,* Vol.99, No.8, pp. 1991-1998. ISSN 0021-9738

Gulbenkian S, Saetrum Opgaard O, Ekman R, Costa Andrade N, Wharton J, Polak JM, Queiroz e Melo J & Edvinsson L. (1993). Peptidergic innervation of human epicardial coronary arteries. *Circ Res,* Vol.73, No.3, pp. 579–588. ISSN 0009-7330

Gutstein DE, Morley GE, Tamaddon H, Vaidya D, Schneider MD, Chen J, Chien KR, Stuhlmann H & Fishman GI. (2001). Conduction slowing and sudden arrhythmic death in mice with cardiac-restricted inactivation of connexin43. *Circ Res,* Vol.88, No.3, pp. 333-339. ISSN 0009-7330

Gutstein DE, Danik SB, Lewitton S, France D, Liu F, Chen FL, Zhang J, Ghodsi N, Morley GE & Fishman GI. (2005). Focal gap junction uncoupling and spontaneous ventricular ectopy. *Am J Physiol Heart Circ Physiol,* Vol.289, No.3, pp. H1091-8. ISSN 0363-6135

Gwechenberger M, Mendoza LH, Youker KA, Frangogiannis NG, Smith CW, Michael LH & Entman ML. (1999). Cardiac myocytes produce interleukin-6 in culture and in viable border zone of reperfused infarctions. *Circulation,* Vol.99, No.4, pp. 546-551. ISSN 0009-7322

Hagège AA, Marolleau JP, Vilquin JT, Alhéritière A, Peyrard S, Duboc D, Abergel E, Messas E, Mousseaux E, Schwartz K, Desnos M & Menasché P (2006). Skeletal myoblast transplantation in ischemic heart failure: long-term follow-up of the first phase I cohort of patients. *Circulation,* Vol.114, No. (1 Suppl), pp. 1108–13. ISSN 0009-7322

Hagemeijer F. (1993). Calcium sensitization with pimobendan: pharmacology, haemodynamic improvement, sudden death in patients with chronic congestive heart failure. *Eur Heart J,* Vol.14, No.4, pp. 551–566. ISSN 0195-668X

Harris AL. (2001). Emerging issues of connexin channels: biophysics fills the gap. *Q Rev Biophys,* Vol.34, No.3, pp. 325-472. ISSN 0033-5835

Haugan K, Olsen KB, Hartvig L, Petersen JS, Holstein-Rathlou NH, Hennan JK & NlelsenI MS. (2005). The antiarrhythmic peptide analog ZP123 prevents atrial conduction slowing during metabolic stress. *J Cardiovasc Electrophysiol,* Vol.16, No.5, pp. 537-545. ISSN 1045-3873

HE Yan, ZENG Zhi-yu, ZHONG Guo-qiang, LI Jin-yi, LI Wei-ke & LI Wei. (2009). Cx43 in mitochondria participates in the protection for heptanol preconditioning on myocardial ischemia/reperfusion injury of rabbits. *Chinese Pharmacological Bulletin,* Vol.25, No.12, pp. 1660-1665. ISSN 1001-1978

HE Yan, ZHONG Guo-qiang, ZENG Zhi-yu, LI Wei-ke, LI Wei & LI Jin-yi. (2010). Effects of heptanol preconditioning on structure,function and Cx43 content of mitochondria in rabbit model of myocardial ischemia/reperfusion injury. *Chinese Journal of Pathophysiology,* Vol.26, No.3, pp. 461-465. ISSN 1000-4718

Henkel DM, Witt BJ, Gersh BJ, Jacobsen SJ, Weston SA, Meverden RA & Roger VL. (2006). Ventricular arrhythmias after acute myocardial infarction: a 20-year community study. *Am. Heart J,* Vol.151, No.4, pp. 806–812. ISSN 0002-8703

Herbert E & Chahine M. (2006). Clinical aspects and physiopathology of Brugada syndrome: review of current concepts. *Can J Physiol Pharmacol,* Vol.84, No.8-9, pp. 795-802. ISSN 0008-4212

Hille B. (1978). Ionic channels in excitable membranes. Current problems and biophysical approaches. *Biophys J.* Vol.22, No.2, pp. 283-94. ISSN 0006-3495

Huang B, El-Sherif T, Gidh-Jain M, Qin D & El-Sherif N. (2001a). Alterations of sodium channel kinetics and gene expression in the postinfarction remodeled myocardium. *J Cardiovasc Electrophysiol,* Vol.12, No.2, pp. 218–225. ISSN 1045-3873

Huang B, Qin D & El-Sherif N. (2001b). Spatial alterations of Kv channels expression and K(+) currents in post-myocardial infarction remodeled rat heart. *Cardiovasc Res,* Vol.52, No.2, pp. 246–254. ISSN 0008-6363

Ieda M, Kanazawa H, Kimura K, Hattori F, Ieda Y, Taniguchi M, Lee JK, Matsumura K, Tomita Y, Miyoshi S, Shimoda K, Makino S, Sano M, Kodama I, Ogawa S & Fukuda K. (2007). Sema3a maintains normal heart rhythm through sympathetic innervation patterning. *Nat Med,* Vol.13, No.5, pp. 604–612. ISSN 1078-8956

Issa ZF, Ujhelyi MR, Hildebrand KR, Zhou X, Rosenberger J, Groh WJ, Miller JM & Zipes DP. (2005). Intrathecal clonidine reduces the incidence of ischemiaprovoked ventricular arrhythmias in a canine postinfarction heart failure model. *Heart Rhythm,* Vol.2, No.10, pp. 1122–1127. ISSN 1547-5271

Janse MJ & Wit AL. (1989). Electrophysiological mechanisms of ventricular arrhythmias resulting from myocardial ischemia and infarction. *Physiol Rev,* Vol.69, No.4, pp. 1049–1069. ISSN 0031-9333

Janssens S, Dubois C, Bogaert J, Theunissen K, Deroose C, Desmet W, Kalantzi M, Herbots L, Sinnaeve P, Dens J, Maertens J, Rademakers F, Dymarkowski S, Gheysens O, Van Cleemput J, Bormans G, Nuyts J, Belmans A, Mortelmans L, Boogaerts M & Van de Werf F. (2006). Autologous bone marrow-derived stem-cell transfer in patients with ST-segment elevation myocardial infarction: double-blind, randomised controlled trial. *Lancet,* Vol.367, No.9505, pp. 113–121. ISSN 0140-6736

Jiang M, Cabo C, Yao J, Boyden PA & Tseng G. (2000). Delayed rectifier K^+ currents have reduced amplitudes and altered kinetics in myocytes from infarcted canine ventricle. *Cardiovasc Res,* Vol.48, No.1, pp. 34–43. ISSN 0008-6363

Jin H, Lyon AR & Akar FG. (2008). Arrhythmia mechanisms in the failing heart. *Pacing Clin Electrophysiol,* Vol.31, No.8, pp. 1048-56. ISSN 0147-8389

Kaplan DR & Miller FD. (2003). Axon growth inhibition: signals from the p75 neurotrophin receptor. *Nat Neurosci,* Vol.6, No.5 pp. 435–436. ISSN 1097-6256

Kaprielian R, Sah R, Nguyen T, Wickenden AD & Backx PH. (2002). Myocardial infarction in rat eliminates regional heterogeneity of AP profiles, I_{to} K^+ currents, $[Ca^{2+}]_i$

transients. *Am J Physiol Heart Circ Physiol,* Vol.283, No.3, pp. H1157-H1168. ISSN 0363-6135

Kaprielian RR, Gunning M, Dupont E, Sheppard MN, Rothery SM, Underwood R, Pennell DJ, Fox K, Pepper J, Poole-Wilson PA & Severs NJ. (1998). Down-regulation of immunodetectable connexin43 and decreased gap junction size in the pathogenesis of chronic hibernation in the human left ventricle. *Circulation,* Vol.97, No.7, pp. 651-660. ISSN 0009-7322

Kim YK, Kim SJ, Kramer CM, Yatani A, Takagi G, Mankad S, Szigeti GP, Singh D, Bishop SP, Shannon RP, Vatner DE & Vatner SF. (2002). Altered excitation-contraction coupling in myocytes from remodeled myocardium after chronic myocardial infarction. *J Mol Cell Cardiol,* Vol.34, No.1, pp. 63–73. ISSN 0022-2828

Kleber AG & Rudy Y. (2004). Basic mechanisms of cardiac impulse propagation and associated arrhythmias. *Physiol Rev,* Vol.84, No.2, pp. 431-488. ISSN 0031-9333

Kostin S, Rieger M, Dammer S, Hein S, Richter M, Klövekorn WP, Bauer EP & Schaper J. (2003). Gap junction remodeling and altered connexin43 expression in the failing human heart. *Mol Cell Biochem,* Vol.242, No.1, pp. 135–144. ISSN 0300-8177

Koval M, Geist ST, Westphale EM, Kemendy EM, Civitelli R, Beyer EC & Steinberg TH (1995). Transfected connexin 45 alters gap junction permeability in cells expressing endogenous connexin 43. *J Cell Biol,* Vol.130, No.4, pp. 987-995. ISSN 0021-9525

Kuruvilla R, Zweifel LS, Glebova NO, Lonze BE, Valdez G, Ye H & Ginty DD. (2004). A neurotrophin signaling cascade coordinates sympathetic neuron development through differential control of TrkA trafficking and retrograde signaling. *Cell,* Vol.118, No.2, pp. 243–255. ISSN 0092-8674

Laflamme, M. A. & Murry, C. E. (2005). Regenerating the heart. *Nature Biotechnol,* Vol.23, No.7, pp. 845–856. ISSN 1087-0156

Laing JG, Beyer EC. (2000). Degradation of gap junctions and connexins. In: *Gap junctions. Molecular basis of cell communication in health and disease.* Peracchia C, pp. 23-41, Academic Press, ISBN 0-12-153349-2, San Diego

Lampe PD, Cooper CD, King TJ & Burt JM. (2006). Analysis of Connexin43 phosphorylated at S325, S328 and S330 in normoxic and ischemic heart. *J Cell Sci,* Vol.119, No16, pp. 3435–3442. ISSN 0021-9533

Leblanc N & Hume JR. (1990). Sodium current-induced release of calcium from cardiac sarcoplasmic reticulum. *Science,* Vol.248, No.4953, pp. 372-376. ISSN 0036-8075

Leobon B, Garcin I, Menasche P, Vilquin JT, Audinat E & Charpak S. (2003). Myoblasts transplanted into rat infarcted myocardium are functionally isolated from their host. *Proc. Natl Acad. Sci,* Vol.100, No.13, pp. 7808–7811. ISSN 0027-8424

Lerner DL, Yamada KA, Schuessler RB & Saffitz JE. (2000). Accelerated onset and increased incidence of ventricular arrhythmias induced by ischemia in Cx43-deficient mice. *Circulation,* Vol.101, No.5, pp. 547-552. ISSN 0009-7322

LI Jinyi, ZHONG Guoqiang, HE Yan & LING Yun. (2009a). Cardiac Connexin 43 and Ischemic Cardioprotection. *South China Journal of Cardiovascular Diseases,* Vol.10, No.2, pp. 97-105. ISSN 1007-9688

Li Jin-yi, Zhong Guo-qiang, He Yan, Wen Li-na, Ke Hong-hong, Wei Zhuo, Deng Yan & Wu Zhi-fu. (2009b). Effects of allogenic bone marrow mesenchymal stem cell transplantation on electrophysiological abnormality and left ventricular remodeling in rats with myocardial infarction. *Journal of Clinical Rehabilitative Tissue Engineering Research,* Vol.13, No.27, pp. 5211-5216. ISSN 1671-5926

LI Jin-yi, ZHONG Guo-qiang, WEI Zhuo, XU Wei-yan, KE Hong-hong, NING Zong & WU ZHI-fu. (2009c). Establishment of a rat model of myocardial infarction and the post-infarction changes in electrophysiology and lef ventricular function. *Acta laboratorium animalis scientia sinica,* Vol.17, No.6, pp. 419-423. ISSN 1005-4847

LI Jinyi, ZHONG Guoqiang, KE Honghong, HE Yan, WEN Lina, WEI Zhuo & ZHAO Yanmei. (2010). Transplantation of allogenic mesenchymal stem cells up-regulates connexin 43 expression in rats with myocardial infarction. *Basic & Clinical Medicine,* Vol.30, No.4, pp. 337-342. ISSN 1001-6325

Li W, Knowlton D, Van Winkle DM & Habecker BA. (2004). Infarction alters both the distribution and noradrenergic properties of cardiac sympathetic neurons. *Am J Physiol Heart Circ Physiol,* Vol.286, No.6, pp. H2229-H2236. ISSN 0363-6135

Li X, Huang CX, Jiang H, Cao F & Wang T. (2005). The beta-adrenergic blocker carvedilol restores L-type calcium current in a myocardial infarction model of rabbit. *Chin Med J,* Vol.118, No.5, pp. 377–382. ISSN 0366-6999

Li Y, Xue Q, Ma J, Zhang CT, Qiu P, Wang L, Gao W, Cheng R, Lu ZY & Wang SW. (2004). Effects of imidapril on heterogeneity of action potential and calcium current of ventricular myocytes in infarcted rabbits. *Acta Pharmacol Sin,* Vol.25, No.11, pp. 1458–1463. ISSN 1671-4083

Litwin SE, Zhang D & Bridge JH. (2000). Dyssynchronous Ca($^{2+}$) sparks in myocytes from infarcted hearts. *Circ Res,* Vol.87, No.11, pp. 1040–1047. ISSN 0009-7330

Liu N, Niu H, Li Y, Zhang C, Zhou Q, Ruan Y, Pu J & Lu Z. (2004). The changes of potassium currents in rabbit ventricle with healed myocardial infarction. *J Huazhong Univ Sci Technolog Med Sci,* Vol.24, No.2, pp. 128–131. ISSN 1672-0733

Long JB, Jay SM, Segal SS & Madri JA. (2009). VEGF-A and semaphorin3A: modulators of vascular sympathetic innervation. *Dev Biol,* Vol.334, No.1, pp. 119–132. ISSN 0012-1606

Lorentz CU, Alston EN, Belcik T, Lindner JR, Giraud GD & Habecker BA. (2010). Heterogeneous ventricular sympathetic innervation, altered b-adrenergic receptor expression, and rhythm instability in mice lacking the p75 neurotrophin receptor. *Am J Physiol Heart Circ Physiol,* Vol.298, No.6, pp. H1652-H1660. ISSN 0363-6135

Lubbe WF, Podzuweit T & Opie LH. (1992). Potential arrhythmogenic role of cyclic adenosine monophosphate (AMP) and cytosolic calcium overload: implications for prophylactic effects of beta-blockers in myocardial infarction and proarrhythmic effects of phosphodiesterase inhibitors. *J Am Coll Cardiol,* Vol.19, No.7, pp. 1622–1633. ISSN 0735-1097

Lue WM & Boyden PA. (1992). Abnormal electrical properties of myocytes from chronically infarcted canine heart. Alterations in Vmax and the transient outward current. *Circulation,* Vol.85, No.3, pp. 1175–1188. ISSN 0009-7322

Luisi AJ Jr, Fallavollita JA, Suzuki G & Canty JM Jr. (2002). Spatial inhomogeneity of sympathetic nerve function in hibernating myocardium. *Circulation,* Vol.106, No.7, pp. 779–781. ISSN 0009-7322

Mahajan A, Moore J, Cesario DA & Shivkumar K. (2005). Use of thoracic epidural anesthesia for management of electrical storm: a case report. *Heart Rhythm,* Vol.2, No.12, pp. 1359–1362. ISSN 1547-5271

Maltsev VA, Sabbab HN & Undrovinas AI. (2002). Down-regulation of sodium current in chronic heart failure: effect of long-term therapy with carvedilol. *Cell Mol Life Sci,* Vol.59, No.9, pp. 1561–1568. ISSN 1420-682X

Marmar Vaseghi & Kalyanam Shivkumar. (2008). The Role of the Autonomic Nervous System in Sudden Cardiac Death. *Prog Cardiovasc Dis,* Vol.50, No.6, pp. 404–419. ISSN 0033-0620

Martinez AD, Hayrapetyan V, Moreno AP & Beyer EC: (2002). Connexin 43 and connexin 45 form heteromeric gap junction channels in which individual components determine permeability and regulation. *Circ Res,* Vol.90, No.10, pp. 1100-1107. ISSN 0009-7330

Michael G, Xiao L, Qi XY, Dobrev D & Nattel S. (2009). Remodelling of cardiac repolarization: how homeostatic responses can lead to arrhythmogenesis. *Cardiovasc Res,* Vol.81, No.3, pp. 491-9. ISSN 0008-6363

Moreno AP, Chanson M, Elenes S, Anumonwo J, Scerri I, Gu H, Taffet SM & Delmar M. (2002a). Role of the carboxyl terminal of connexin43 in transjunctional fast voltage gating. *Circ Res,* Vol.90, No.4, pp. 450-7. ISSN 0009-7330

Moreno AP, Zhong G, Hayrapetyan V. (2002b). Heteromultimeric gap junction channels: a connection with cardiac physiology and pathology. In: *Heart Cell Coupling and Impulse Propagation in Health and Disease-Basic Science for the Cardiologist,* WC. De Mello, M. Janse, pp. 89-108. Kluwer Academic Publishers. ISBN 1-4020-7182-5, Norwell.

Moreno AP, Hayrapetyan V, Zhong G. (2004). Homomeric and Heteromeric Gap Junctions. In: *Cardiac electrophysiololgy from cell to bedside.* Douglas P.Zipes and Jose Jalife. pp. 120-126, W.B Saunders Company, ISBN 0-7216-0323-8, Philadelphia

Murry CE, Soonpaa MH, Reinecke H, Nakajima H, Nakajima HO, Rubart M, Pasumarthi KB, Virag JI, Bartelmez SH, Poppa V, Bradford G, Dowell JD, Williams DA & Field LJ. (2004). Haematopoietic stem cells do not transdifferentiate into cardiac myocytes in myocardial infarcts. *Nature,* Vol.428, No.6983, pp. 664–668. ISSN 0028-0836

Murry CE, Field LJ & Menasche P. (2005). Cell-based cardiac repair: reflections at the 10-year point. *Circulation,* Vol.112, No.20, pp. 3174–3183. ISSN 0009-7322

Nademanee K, Taylor R, Bailey WE, Rieders DE & Kosar EM. (2000). Treating electrical storm: sympathetic blockade versus advanced cardiac life support-guided therapy. *Circulation,* Vol.102, No.7, pp. 742–747. ISSN 0009-7322

Nattel S & Carlsson L. (2006). Innovative approaches to anti-arrhythmic drug therapy. *Nat Rev Drug Discov,* Vol.5, No.12, pp. 1034-1049. ISSN 1474-1776

Nattel S, Maguy A, Le Bouter S, Yeh YH. (2007). Arrhythmogenic ion-channel remodeling in the heart: heart failure, myocardial infarction, and atrial fibrillation. *Physiol Rev.* Vol.87, No.2, pp. 425-56. ISSN 0031-9333

Nerbonne JM & Kass RS. (2005). Molecular physiology of cardiac repolarization. *Physiol Rev,* Vol.85, No.4, pp. 1205–1253. ISSN 0031-9333

Nian M, Lee P, Khaper N & Liu P. (2004). Inflammatory cytokines and postmyocardial infarction remodeling. *Circ Res,* Vol.94, No.12, pp. 1543–1553. ISSN 0009-7330

Noda M, Shimizu S, Tanabe T, Takai T, Kayano T, Ikeda T, Takahashi H, Nakayama H, Kanaoke Y, Minamino N, Kangawa R, Matsuo H, Raftery MA, Hirose T, Inayama S, Hayashida H, Miyata T & Numa S. (1984). Primary structure of electrophorus electricus sodium channel deduced from cDNA sequence. *Nature,* Vol.312, No.5990, pp. 121-127. ISSN 0028-0836

Nori SL, Gaudino M, Alessandrini F, Bronzetti E & Santarelli P. (1995). Immunohistochemical evidence for sympathetic denervation and reinnervation after necrotic injury in rat myocardium. *Cell Mol Biol,* Vol.41, No.6, pp. 799–807. ISSN 0145-5680

Nuss HB, Marbán E & Johns DC. (1999). Overexpression of a human potassium channel suppresses cardiac hyperexcitability in rabbit ventricular myocytes. *J Clin Invest,* Vol.103, No.6, pp. 889. ISSN 0021-9738

Oh YS, Jong AY, Kim DT, Li H, Wang C, Zemljic-Harpf A, Ross RS, Fishbein MC, Chen PS & Chen LS. (2006). Spatial distribution of nerve sprouting after myocardial infarction in mice. *Heart Rhythm,* Vol.3, No.6, pp. 728-736. ISSN 1547-5271

Oki T, Fukuda N, Kawano T, Iuchi A, Tabata T, Manabe K, Kageji Y, Sasaki M, Yamada H & Ito S. (1995). Histopathologic studies of innervation of normal and prolapsed human mitral valves. *J Heart Valve Dis,* Vol.4, No.5, pp. 496–502. ISSN 0966-8519

Patlak JB & Ortiz M. (1985). Slow currents through single sodium channels of adult rat heart. *J Gen Physiol,* Vol.86, No.1, pp. 89-104. ISSN 0022-1295

Perrier E, Kerfant BG, Lalevee N, Bideaux P, Rossier MF, Richard S, Gomez AM & Benitah JP. (2004). Mineralocorticoid receptor antagonism prevents the electrical remodeling that precedes cellular hypertrophy after myocardial infarction. *Circulation,* Vol.110, No.7, pp. 776–783. ISSN 0009-7322

Peters NS, Coromilas J, Severs NJ & Wit AL. (1997). Disturbed connexin43 gap junction distribution correlates with the location of reentrant circuits in the epicardial border zone of healing canine infarcts that cause ventricular tachycardia. *Circulation,* Vol.95, No.4, pp. 988–996. ISSN 0009-7322

Pinto JM, Yuan F, Wasserlauf BJ, Bassett AL & Myerburg RJ. (1997). Regional gradation of L-type calcium currents in the feline heart with a healed myocardial infarct. *J Cardiovasc Electrophysiol,* Vol.8, No.5, pp. 548–560. ISSN 1045-3873

Pinto JM & Boyden PA. (1998). Reduced inward rectifying and increased E-4031-sensitive K_ current density in arrhythmogenic subendocardial Purkinje myocytes from the infarcted heart. *J Cardiovasc Electrophysiol,* Vol.9, No.3, pp. 299–311. ISSN 1045-3873

Pu J & Boyden PA. (1997). Alterations of Na^+ currents in myocytes from epicardial border zone of the infarcted heart. A possible ionic mechanism for reduced excitability and postrepolarization refractoriness. *Circ Res,* Vol.81, No.1, pp. 110–119. ISSN 0009-7330

Pu J, Balser JR & Boyden PA. (1998). Lidocaine action on Na^+ currents in ventricular myocytes from the epicardial border zone of the infarcted heart. *Circ Res,* Vol. 83, No.4, pp. 431–440. ISSN 0009-7330

Pu J, Ruffy F & Boyden PA. (1999). Effects of Bay Y 5959 on Ca^{2+} currents and intracellular Ca^{2+} in cells that have survived in the epicardial border of the infarcted canine heart. *J Cardiovasc Pharmacol,* Vol.33, No.6, pp. 929–937. ISSN 0160-2446

Pu J, Robinson RB & Boyden PA. (2000). Abnormalities in Ca(i) handling in myocytes that survive in the infarcted heart are not just due to alterations in repolarization. *J Mol Cell Cardiol,* Vol.32, No.8, pp. 1509–1523. ISSN 0022-2828

Qi X, Varma P, Newman D & Dorian P. (2001). Gap junction blockers decrease defibrillation thresholds with out changes in ventricular refractoriness in isolated rabbit hearts. *Circulation,* Vol.104, No.13, pp. 1544-1549. ISSN 0009-7322

Qin D, Zhang ZH, Caref EB, Boutjdir M, Jain P & el-Sherif N. (1996). Cellular and ionic basis of arrhythmias in postinfarction remodeled ventricular myocardium. *Circ Res* , Vol.79, No.3, pp. 461–473. ISSN 0009-7330

Ranger S & Nattel S. (1995). Determinants and mechanisms of flecainideinduced promotion of ventricular tachycardia in anesthetized dogs. *Circulation,* Vol.92, No.5, pp. 1300–1311. ISSN 0009-7322

Rautaharju PM, Zhou SH, Wong S, Calhoun HP, Berenson GS, Prineas R & Davignon A. (1992). Sex differences in the evolution of the electrocardiographic QT interval with age. *Can J Cardiol,* Vol.8, No.7, pp. 690-695. ISSN 0828-282X

Reinecke H, Poppa V & Murry CE. (2002). Skeletal muscle stem cells do not transdifferentiate into cardiomyocytes after cardiac grafting. *J. Mol. Cell. Cardiol,* Vol.34, No.2, pp. 241–249. ISSN 0022-2828

Ren C, Wang F, Li G, Jiao Q, Bai J, Yu D, Hao W, Wang R & Cao JM. (2008). Nerve sprouting suppresses myocardial I(to) and I(K1) channels and increases severity to ventricular fibrillation in rat. *Auton Neurosci,* Vol.144, No.1-2, pp. 22–9. ISSN 1566-0702

Restivo M, Gough WB & el-Sherif N. (1990). Ventricular arrhythmias in the subacute myocardial infarction period. High-resolution activation and refractory patterns of reentrant rhythms. *Circ Res,* Vol.66, No.5, pp. 1310–1327. ISSN 0009-7330

Rodriguez-Sinovas A, Boengler K, Cabestrero A, Gres P, Morente M, Ruiz-Meana M, Konietzka I, Miró E, Totzeck A, Heusch G, Schulz R & Garcia-Dorado D. (2006). Translocation of Connexin 43 to the Inner Mitochondrial Membrane of Cardiomyocytes Through the Heat Shock Protein 90-Dependent TOM Pathway and Its Importance for Card ioprotection. *Circ Res,* Vol.99, No.1, pp. 93-101. ISSN 0009-7330

Roell W, Lewalter T, Sasse P, Tallini YN, Choi BR, Breitbach M, Doran R, Becher UM, Hwang SM, Bostani T, von Maltzahn J, Hofmann A, Reining S, Eiberger B, Gabris B, Pfeifer A, Welz A, Willecke K, Salama G, Schrickel JW, Kotlikoff MI & Fleischmann BK. (2007). Engraftment of connexin 43-expressing cells prevents post-infarct arrhythmia. *Nature,* Vol.450, No.7171, pp. 819-824. ISSN 0028-0836

Rubart M & Zipes DP. (2005). Mechanisms of sudden cardiac death. *J Clin Invest,* Vol.115, No.9, pp. 2305–2315. ISSN 0021-9738

Saltman AE, Aksehirli TO, Valiunas V, Gaudette GR, Matsuyama N, Brink P & Krukenkamp IB. (2002). Gap junction uncoupling protects the heart against ischemia. *J Thorac Cardiovasc Surg,* Vol.124, No.2, pp. 371-376. ISSN 0022-5223

Salameh A & Dhein S. (2005). Pharmacology of gap junctions. New pharmacological targets for treatment of arrhythmia, seizure and cancer? *Biochim Biophys Acta,* Vol.1719, No.1-2, pp. 36-58. ISSN 0005-2736

Sasano T, McDonald AD, Kikuchi K & Donahue JK. (2006). Molecular ablation of ventricular tachycardia after myocardial infarction. *Nat Med,* Vol.12, No.11, pp. 1256. ISSN 1078-8956

Schulz R, Boengler K, Totzeck A, Luo Y, Garcia-Dorado D & Heusch G. (2007). Connexin 43 in ischemic pre- and postconditioning. *Heart Fail Rev,* Vol.12, No.3-4, pp. 261-266. ISSN 1382-4147

Schwartz PJ & Stone HL. (1980). Left stellectomy in the prevention of ventricular fibrillation caused by acute myocardial ischemia in conscious dogs with anterior myocardial infarction. *Circulation,* Vol.62, No.6, pp. 1256-1265. ISSN 0009-7322

Schwartz PJ, Motolese M, Pollavini G, Lotto A, Ruberti U, Trazzi R, Bartorelli C & Zanchetti A. (1992). Italian Sudden Death Prevention Group. Prevention of sudden cardiac death after a first myocardial infarction by pharmacologic or surgical antiadrenergic interventions. *J Cardiovasc Electrophysiol,* Vol.3, No.1, pp. 2–16. ISSN 1045-3873

Sebbag L, Verbinski SG, Reimer KA & Jennings RB. (2003). Protection of ischemic myocardium in dogs using intracoronary 2, 3-butanedione monoxime (BDM). *J Mol Cell Cardiol,* Vol.35, No.2, pp. 165-176. ISSN 0022-2828

Severs NJ, (1989). Constituent cells of the heart and isolated cell models in cardiovascular research. In: *Isolated Adult Cardiomyocytes: Structure and metabolism,* Piper HM, Isenberg G, pp. 3-41, CRC Press, Boca Raton.

Severs NJ. (1990). The cardiac gap junction and intercalated disc. *Int J Cardiol,* Vol.26, No.2, pp. 137-73. ISSN 0167-5273

Severs NJ, Gourdie RG, Harfst E, Peters NS & Green CR. (1993). Intercellular junctions and the application of microscopical techniques: the cardiac gap junction as a case model. *J Microsc,* Vol.169, No.3, pp. 299–328. ISSN 0022-2720

Severs NJ, Rothery S, Dupont E, Coppen SR, Yeh HI, Ko YS, Matsushita T, Kaba R & Halliday D. (2001). Immunocytochemical analysis of connexin expression in the healthy and diseased cardiovascular system. *Microsc Res Tech,* Vol.52, No.3, pp. 301–22. ISSN 1059-910X

Severs NJ, Coppen SR, Dupont E, Yeh HI, Ko YS, Matsushita T. (2004). Gap junction alterations in human cardiac disease. *Cardiovasc Res.* Vol.62, No.2, pp. 368-77. ISSN 0008-6363

Severs NJ, Bruce AF, Dupont E & Rothery S. (2008). Remodelling of gap junctions and connexin expression in diseased myocardium. *Cardiovasc Res,* Vol.80, No.1, pp. 9-19. ISSN 0008-6363

Shaw RM & Rudy Y. (1997). Ionic mechanisms of propagation in cardiac tissue. Roles of the sodium and L-type calcium currents during reduced excitability and decreased gap junction coupling. *Circ Res,* Vol.81, No.5, pp. 727–741. ISSN 0009-7330

Smith JH, Green CR, Peters NS, Rothery S & Severs NJ. (1991). Altered patterns of gap junction distribution in ischemic heart disease. An immunohistochemical study of human myocardium using laser scanning confocal microscopy. *Am J Pathol,* Vol.139, No.4, pp. 801–821. ISSN 0002-9440

Sohl G & Willecke K. (2004). Gap junctions and the connexin protein family. *Cardiovasc Res,* Vol.62, No.2, pp. 228–232. ISSN 0008-6363

Solomon SD, Zelenkofske S, McMurray JJ, Finn PV, Velazquez E, Ertl G, Harsanyi A, Rouleau JL, Maggioni A, Kober L, White H, Van de Werf F, Pieper K, Califf RM & Pfeffer MA. (2005). Sudden death in patients with myocardial infarction and left ventricular dysfunction, heart failure, or both. *N Eng J Med,* Vol.352, No.25, pp. 2581–2588. ISSN 0028-4793

Sosinsky G. (2000). Gap junction structure: new structures and new insights. In: *Gap junctions. Molecular basis of cell communication in health and disease.* Peracchia C, pp. 1-22, Academic Press,: ISBN 0-12-153349-2, San Diego

Spear JF, Michelson EL, Spielman SR & Moore EN. (1977). The origin of ventricular arrhythmias 24 hours following experimental anterior septal coronary artery occlusion. *Circulation,* Vol.55, No.6, pp. 844–852. ISSN 0009-7322

Spear JF, Horowitz LN, Hodess AB, MacVaugh H 3rd & Moore EN. (1979). Cellular electrophysiology of human myocardial infarction. 1. Abnormalities of cellular activation. *Circulation,* Vol.59, No.2, pp. 247–256. ISSN 0009-7322

Takamatsu T. (2008). Arrhythmogenic substrates in myocardial infarct. *Pathol Int,* Vol.58, No.9, pp. 533-43. ISSN 1320-5463

Ursell PC, Gardner PI, Albala A, Fenoglio Jr. JJ & Wit AL. (1985). Structural and electrophysiological changes in the epicardial border zone of canine myocardial infarcts during infarct healing. *Circ Res,* Vol.56, No.3, pp. 436–451. ISSN 0009-7330

Valiunas V, Doronin S, Valiuniene L, Potapova I, Zuckerman J, Walcott B, Robinson RB, Rosen MR, Brink PR & Cohen IS. (2004). Human mesenchymal stem cells make cardiac connexins and form functional gap junctions.*J Physiol,* Vol.555, No.3, pp. 617–626. ISSN 0022-3751

Van Veen AA, van Rijen HV & Opthof T. (2001). Cardiac gap junction channels: modulation of expression and channel properties. *Cardiovasc Res,* Vol.51, No2, pp. 217–29. ISSN 0008-6363

Vozzi C, Dupont E, Coppen SR, Yeh HI & Severs NJ. (1999). Chamber-related differences in connexin expression in the human heart. *J Mol Cell Cardiol,* Vol.31, No5, pp. 991–1003. ISSN 0022-2828

Vracko R, Thorning D & Frederickson RG. (1990). Fate of nerve fibers in necrotic, healing, and healed rat myocardium. *Lab Invest,* Vol.63, No.4, pp. 490–501. ISSN 0023-6837

Vracko R, Thorning D & Frederickson RG. (1991). Nerve fibers in human myocardial scars. *Hum Pathol,* Vol.22, No.2, pp. 138–146. ISSN 0046-8177

Waldo AL, Camm AJ, deRuyter H, Friedman PL, MacNeil DJ, Pauls JF, Pitt B, Pratt CM, Schwartz PJ & Veltri EP. (1996). Effect of D-sotalol on mortality in patients with left ventricular dysfunction after recent and remote myocardial infarction. The SWORD Investigators survival with oral D-sotalol. *Lancet,* Vol.348, No.9019, pp. 7–12. ISSN 0140-6736

Wen H, Jiang H, Lu Z, Hu X, He B, Tang Q & Huang C. (2010). Carvedilol ameliorates sympathetic nerve sprouting and electrical remodelling after myocardial infarction in rats. *Biomedicine & Pharmacotherapy,* Vol.64, No.7, pp. 446–450. ISSN 0753-3322

Weng S, Lauven M, Schaefer T, Polontchouk L, Grover R & Dhein S. (2002). Pharmacological modification of gap junction coupling by an antiarrhythmic peptide via protein kinase C activation. *FASEB J,* Vol.16, No.9, pp. 1114–6. ISSN 0892-6638

Wong RC, Pera MF & Pébay A. (2008). Role of Gap Junctions in Embryonic and Somatic Stem Cells. *Stem Cell Rev,* Vol.4, No.4, pp. 283-292. ISSN 1550-8943

Xin P, Pan Y, Zhu W, Huang S, Wei M & Chen C. (2010). Favorable effects of resveratrol on sympathetic neural remodeling in rats following myocardial infarction. *European Journal of Pharmacology,* Vol.649, No.1-3, pp. 293-300. ISSN 0014-2999

Xing D, Kjølbye AL, Nielsen MS, Petersen JS, Harlow KW, Holstein-Rathlou NH & Martins JB. (2003). ZP123 increases gap junctional conductance and prevents reentrant ventricular tachycardia during myocardial ischemia in open chest dogs. *J Cardiovasc Electrophysiol*, Vol.14, No.5, pp. 510-20. ISSN 1045-3873

Yagi T & Boyden PA. (2002). Protein tyrosine kinases and L-type Ca^{2+} currents in cells that have survived in epicardial border zone of canine infarcted heart. *J Cardiovasc Pharmacol*, Vol.40, No.5, pp. 669–677. ISSN 0160-2446

Yamada KA, Rogers JG, Sundset R, Steinberg TH & Saffitz JE. (2003). Up-regulation of connexin45 in heart failure. *J Cardiovasc Electrophysiol*, Vol.14, No.11, pp. 1205–1212. ISSN 1045-3873

Yao JA, Hussain W, Patel P, Peters NS, Boyden PA & Wit AL. (2003). Remodeling of gap junctional channel function in epicardial border zone of healing canine infarcts. *Circ Res*, Vol.92, No.4, pp. 437-443. ISSN 0009-7330

Yuan F, Pinto JM, Li Q, Wasserlauf BJ, Yang X, Bassett AL & Myerburg RJ. (1999). Characteristics of I(K) and its response to quinidine in experimental healed myocardial infarction. *J Cardiovasc Electrophysiol*, Vol.10, No.6, pp. 844–854. ISSN 1045-3873

Yuan MJ, Huang CX, Tang YH, Wang X, Huang H, Chen YJ & Wang T. (2009). A novel peptide ghrelin inhibits neural remodeling after myocardial infarction in rats. *European Journal of Pharmacology*, Vol.618, No.1-3, pp. 52-57. ISSN 0014-2999

Zhao Yan-mei, Zhong Guo-qiang, Li Jin-yi, He Yan, Ke Hong-hong & Wang Dong-xu. (2009). mRNA expression of connectin 43 and connectin 45 following transplantation of allogenic bone marrow mesenchymal stem cells in rats with acute myocardial infarction. *Journal of Clinical Rehabilitative Tissue Engineering Research*, Vol.13, No.45, pp. 8895-8900. ISSN 1671-5926

Zhao Yan-mei, Zhong Guo-qiang, Ke Hong-hong & Li Jin-yi. (2010). Effects of different conditions on rat bone marrow mesenchymal stem cells differentiating into cardiomyocytes in vitro. *Basic & Clinical Medicine*, Vol.30, No.6, pp. 561-565. ISSN 1001-6325

Zhong G, Hayrapetyan V & Moreno AP. (2002). The Formation of mono-heteromeric Cx43-Cx45/43 gap junctions uncovers gating and selectivity properties of their channels. *Biophysical Journal*, Vol.82, No.1, pp. 633b. ISSN 0006-3495

Zhou S, Chen LS, Miyauchi Y, Miyauchi M, Kar S, Kangavari S, Fishbein MC, Sharifi B & Chen PS. (2004). Mechanisms of cardiac nerve sprouting after myocardial infarction in dogs. *Circ Res*, Vol.95, No.1, pp. 76–83. ISSN 0009-7330

Zhou S, Jung BC, Tan AY, Trang VQ, Gholmieh G, Han SW, Lin SF, Fishbein MC, Chen PS, Chen LS. (2008). Spontaneous stellate ganglion nerve activity and ventricular arrhythmia in a canine model of sudden death. *Heart Rhythm*. Vol.5, No.1, pp. 131-9. ISSN 1547-5271

Zipes DP. (1990). Influence of myocardial ischemia and infarction on autonomic innervation of heart. *Circulation*, Vol.82, No.4, pp. 95–105. ISSN 0009-7322.

10

Novel Porcine Models of Myocardial Ischemia/Infarction – Technical Progress, Modified Electrocardiograms Validating, and Future Application

Jianxun Liu and Xinzhi Li
Department of Pharmacology, Xiyuan Hospital,
China Academy of Chinese Medical Sciences, Beijing
China

1. Introduction

Cardiovascular diseases, the first killer for human being, constitute the global economic burden. The updated data from World Health Organization (WHO) addresses that the mortality rank of myocardial infarction will increase from No.5 in 2000 to Top One till 2020. And 30 percent of overall mortality is due to the cardiovascular diseases. Their prevalence has severely affected patients' healthy conditions. Therefore, it is the priority for us to enforce the research on the mechanisms of pathogenesis and treatment of cardiovascular diseases.

Heart attacks are most commonly caused by a fatty "plaque" dislodging from the blood vessel wall. Inflammation in vessels and heart also plays an important role in this process. This provokes tiny cells in the bloodstream known as platelets to clump together and block the blood circulation to important organs. To elucidate the exact mechanism of the mentioned process, researchers need to develop various pre-clinical approaches to simulate the clinical presentation in animal models, cell strains, or even in tube reactions. Among those methodologies, animal model are more acceptable than the others due to its easily "from bench to bed" translational property. The use of appropriate large-animal models is essential if some new therapeutic strategies are to be critically evaluated in a preclinical setting before their use in humans.

Over the past decade, swine have been increasingly used in studies of myocardial ischemia because of their numerous similarities to humans, including minimal preexisting coronary collaterals as well as similar coronary anatomy and physiology. In this chapter, the author will consequently review the most commonly used swine models of myocardial ischemia with special attention to regional myocardial blood flow and function and critically evaluates the strengths and weaknesses of each model in terms of utility for preclinical trials.

Also in this part, several porcine models of myocardial ischemia/infarction developed in our department will be summarized briefly regarding with the technical progress. We would also like to share our experiences about new adventures in the field of electrocardiogram mapping using multiple electrodes.

2. Animal models of myocardial ischemia/infarction

2.1 Myocardial ischemic or infarction models

High mortality and morbidity associated with myocardial ischemia or even the infarction necessitates modelling the process in animal. In a hospital setting, because the primary concern is resuscitation and maintaining of the patient's life, but not research in the underlying mechanism of the diseases. To study the pathophysiological changes associated with myocardial ischemic injury and how they lead to the establishment of cardiac cell death and regional infarction, animal models of clinical pathophysiology should gain our serious concern to overcome the limitations of clinical studies and to play an invaluable role in advancing mechanistic insight. Animal model studies will considerably provided new ideas and hypotheses that have been tested in clinical studies and have thus increased the level of knowledge regarding cardioprotection in the ischemic milieu.

Moreover, the use of experimental models of heart diseases in animals is an obligatory step for the understanding of mechanisms involved in pathologies consecutive to cardiac metabolic or functional disorders. As for any kind of therapeutic approach, to demonstrate its efficacy and safety there is also a need for animal models. Among factors of importance, there are animal species, coronary thrombosis induction method, thrombus composition and site of formation.

2.1.1 Acute ischemic and reperfusion animal models

Based on the clinical profiles of the sudden heart attach, people firstly sought for the mimic method to study myocardial ischemic condition by ligation of one of the three main arteries in heart. Back to 1975, myocardial ischemia was induced in swine by ligation of the anterior descending coronary artery for periods of 30 minutes to six hours. Electron microscopy was used to monitor normal and ischemic myocardium (Lichtig et al., 1975). Scientists from our institute did contribute quite a lot to this model, not in swine, but in dogs. The dog's heart was exposed by opening the chest. The acute ischemia models were prepared by ligating left anterior descending (LAD) artery. Meanwhile, timed monitoring hemodynamics and blood flow were determined by physiological polygraph and electromagnetic flow meter, respectively (Li, 1978). In another research group, the diagonal branches of the left anterior descending coronary artery in pigs were ligated for 5, 15, 30, 60 and 120 minutes. By using transmission electron microscopy, morphological observations indicated that initial leukocyte infiltration and inflammation during myocardial ischemia (Park et al., 1985).

These kinds of open-chest model were widely accepted during 1990s and were still prevalent in 2000s. With development of the diagnostic methods, more and more advanced technologies were employed in the research of heart diseases and animal modelling. In one of representative works, nine open-chest swine undergoing myocardial ischemia were instrumented for measurement of regional myocardial blood flow (microsphere method), contractile function (sonomicrometry), and hemodynamics. L-[1-^{14}C] Lactate or L-[U-^{13}C] lactate was infused intravenously using a primed continuous infusion technique to quantify regional myocardial lactate release. A close inverse relation between regional myocardial lactate release and regional subendocardial blood flow during graded ischemia was revealed (Guth et al., 1990). When researcher evaluated the utility of transplanting bone marrow stromal cells in a porcine myocardial infarction model, a myocardial infarction was created by occluding the distal left anterior descending artery in pigs with coils and Gelfoam sponge (Tomita et al., 2002). In this study, sestamibi technetium single-photon emission computed tomographic scans were performed to compare the stroke volume, regional perfusion, and wall motion in different treatment group.

Most of these myocardial infarction animal models using dogs or pigs is created by coronary artery ligation after surgical opening of the chest and exposure of the heart. Hereby, numerous disadvantages and experimental limitations may be associated with this technique: There is evidence suggesting that normal cardiac mechanics are disturbed in acute models after thoracotomy. Opening the chest and pericardium have both been suspected and reported to influence the pattern of left ventricular remodeling in chronic models (Kraitchman et al., 2000; Ludemann et al., 2007). Furthermore, the surgical trauma may cause a high rate of complications, resulting in high mortality. In addition, the trauma may render successful recovery from anesthesia in models of myocardial infarction more difficult, compared with closed chest procedures.

Besides, to date, there are various myocardial ischemic animal models, such as ligating the coronary artery (Takahashi et al., 2005), placing constrictors on the coronary artery (Laham et al., 2000), putting microembolus into the coronary artery (Huang et al., 2004), or injecting ferric chloride via the vein (Dogne et al., 2005). However, operations in these methods lead to much damage in animals, and channelization can not be restored in the obstructed coronary artery. More considerably, the mimic pathophysiological alterations deviate from clinical data, especially autopsy. Nowadays, cardiovascular medicine research requires the availability of appropriate experimental animal models that are as close to humans as feasible.

2.1.2 Mechanically chronic ischemic animal models

The most widely used porcine model of chronic ischemia has been the ameroid constrictor. Originally described by Litvak and colleagues in 1957, these constrictors are constructed of the hygroscopic material casein encased within a steel sleeve. When the device is implanted around an artery, the constrictor absorbs water and swells, compressing the artery and producing total coronary occlusion over a period of 14-30 or more days (Elzinga, 1969). The major advantage of the ameroid constrictor model is its simplicity. Inherent limitations to the use of these occluders include an inability to control the rate or degree (sometimes incomplete) of coronary occlusion (Inou et al., 1980).

Another large-animal model of chronic ischemia has involved placing an adjustable hydraulic occluder around an epicardial coronary artery to produce a fixed degree of coronary stenosis (Bolukoglu et al., 1992). This model is similar to the fixed stenosis model in that the coronary artery is reduced in diameter by an external device, although with this latter model the occluder is typically placed either proximal or distal to a myocardial flow probe. Another famous study using this animal is about the relationship between hibernating myocardium and cell autophage (Yan et al., 2005). Chronically instrumented pigs were studied with repetitive myocardial ischemia produced by coronary hydraulic stenosis. Autophagy, triggered by ischemia, could be a homeostatic mechanism, by which apoptosis is inhibited and the deleterious effects of chronic ischemia are limited (Yan et al., 2006).

2.1.3 Swine models with thrombosis formation in coronary artery

Coronary artery thrombosis is widely accepted as a major cause of myocardial infarction (MI). The abrupt transition from a stable, often clinically silent, disease to a symptomatic life-threatening condition results from endothelial injury or plaque disruption followed by thrombosis (Falk et al., 1995). Because of this acute intracoronary thrombotic occlusion, the primary goal of therapy is rapid, complete, and sustained restoration of infarct-related artery blood flow. In this case, the choice of the animal model of thrombosis to evaluate the efficiency of antiplatelet, antithrombotic or thrombolytic drugs in preclinical studies is crucial. Numerous animal models of thrombosis-induced MI have been proposed in the last decades (Leadley et al., 2000). Another example was from porcine model of myocardial infarction induced by topical application of ferric chloride to the LAD coronary artery, which was validated to quite close to clinical pathophysiological conditions, such as thrombus formation occurring after atherosclerotic plaque rupture (Dogne et al., 2005).

In dogs, left circumflex coronary artery (LCx) thrombosis was induced by vascular electrolytic injury (Hennan et al., 2001; Romson et al., 1980). After a flow probe and stenosis had been placed around the LCx, an intracoronary electrode was inserted through the LCx arterial wall, with the uninsulated portion positioned against the endothelial surface. An anodal current of 150 μA was applied to the endothelial surface to initiate the experiment. This operation is relatively difficult to master or needs much more practice, since the electrode is introduced into coronary artery. Another shortcoming is bleeding due to artery injury during procedure, especially the introduction of electrode.

In our department, to evaluate the thrombolytic effects of heparin-like drugs, swine's endoarterium was injuried and coronary thrombi were formed gradually through direct electrical stimulation on the coronary artery of animals (Liu et al., 2002). However, some limitations of this model should be pointed out. First, we are aware of the fact that the maintenance of pigs is expensive and difficult, and requires special facilities that are beyond the capabilities of most laboratories. Secondly, the pig presents a high myocardial sensitivity to hypoxia. Acute reduction of coronary blood flow can easily induce paroxystic ventricular fibrillation which may then requires the use of prophylactic antiarrythmic agents.

2.1.4 Making myocardial ischemic animal models via interventional techniques

Most models listed above in the pig, with or without subsequent reperfusion need thoracotomy. The majority of these employ surgical techniques of coronary occlusion following thoracotomy. During these complex operations, the subtle enviorment inside of the chest will be somewhat disturbed. The endovascular and minimal invasion techniques offer a series of advantages over the surgical technique such as a lower incidence of infections and of related complications which can compromise the survival of the animal and the validity of the results.

These disadvantages raise the demand for closed-chest models for myocardial infarction in large animals. To facilitate the surgical operation, we introduced the intervention technique and selective coronary angiography into our study. One ischemic model we used was developed in Chinese miniature swine, where myocardial ischemia was performed by injecting self-embolus into the middle segment of the left anterior descending (LAD) without thoracotomy (Liu et al., 2007b; Yu et al., 2007b). Embolization occurred in the LAD coronary artery of the Chinese miniature swine injected by self-embolus. There were significant myocardial ischemia and large cardiac muscle infarction in the Chinese miniature swine, which were accompanied with increased Body surface ECG (BS-ECG) (Liu et al., 2007b), decreased hemodynamic indexes of the cardiac output, cardiac index, left cardiac work and left cardiac work index, and increased systemic vascular resistance index.

Pathohistological analysis revealed myocardial degeneration, necrosis, fibrosis, inflammatory cell infiltration and granulation tissue hyperblastosis. Our data showed that myocardial ischemia induced by injecting self-embolus into the LAD coronary artery in Chinese miniature swine is quite close to clinical pathophysiological conditions. (Fig. 1.)

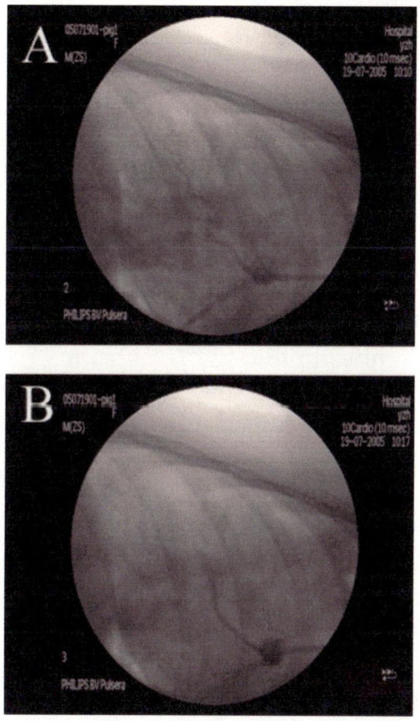

Fig. 1. Changes of coronary embolism were disclosed by the coronary angiography. (A) the LAD of the model group was normal at pre-operation; (B) the LAD of the model group was completely and instantly embolized, post-operation.

In other lab, injection of thrombogenic material, such as microcoils or thrombin fibrinogen mixtures, have also been proposed and explored (Koning et al., 1993; Naslund et al., 1992). In these studies, after injection into a coronary artery, the blood flow transports these materials downstream until their size matches the diameter of the coronary artery. Standardization of the infarction size is not possible because there is physiologic variation of the diameter of the coronary arteries between individual animals of similar body weight. Furthermore, with these approaches, either reperfusion is not possible or occurs after spontaneous lysis of the occluding material. This approach does not allow for controlling the duration of the occlusion.

On the other hand, X-ray-guided placement of a balloon catheter in the coronary artery and inflation of the balloon for coronary artery occlusion avoids extensive surgery and allows the control of both the location and the time of occlusion. This approach has been used in several studies. Balloon occlusion of the LAD can successfully be performed in pigs to create reperfused or occlusive myocardial infarction. The technique allows for a relatively short preparation time compared with open-chest surgery, control over the duration of ischemia, and standardization the location of the occlusion and infarcts size. The resulting changes of the myocardial function are solely due to the ischemic injury. This renders results obtained with this model more easily interpretable. Furhtermore, this model is advantageous for MRI studies because the heart is not exposed, so that susceptibility artifacts that arise from the myocardium-air border in open chest-models are avoided (Krombach et al., 2005).

2.1.5 Coronary atherosclerosis in swine

Recently, advanced coronary atherosclerosis in swine was produced by combination of balloon-catheter injury and cholesterol feeding (Li et al., 2009). In this study, twelve Chinese experimental miniature swine (CEMS) were randomly divided into Control and Model groups. In the model, fed with high fat diet for 2 weeks, the pigs underwent left coronary angiography and balloon over dilation in left anterior descending artery (LAD) followed by continuous feeding with high fat diet for 8 weeks. At the end of 10 weeks, an IVUS catheter was guided to the LAD artery. Intravascular ultrasound and virtual histology (IVUS-VH) data analysis was based on border contour calculation from gray scale. Coronary angiography with (IVUS) and virtual histology (VH) will help us to detect the process of coronary atherosclerosis during coronary heart disease (CHD). IVUS classified the plaque as concentric, with fibrous 62.8%, fibro-lipidic 12.7%, necrotic 15.5%, and calcific 8.9% tissue. In vitro histopathology correctly identified the different presence of fibrous tissue, and different extent of stenosis, which was consistently correlative to the result of IVUS-VH (Fig. 2.). These models provide essential help for researchers to better understand the pathophysiological implications of the heart diseases, from endothelium injury to plaque stability, from marker protein expressions to cell death pattern. All these findings will not only present one of the scientific answers to the pathogenesis of model animals with coronary atherosclerotic heart diseases (coronary heart disease, CHD), but also will facilitate to interpret the scientific insights of prevention and therapeutic strategy.

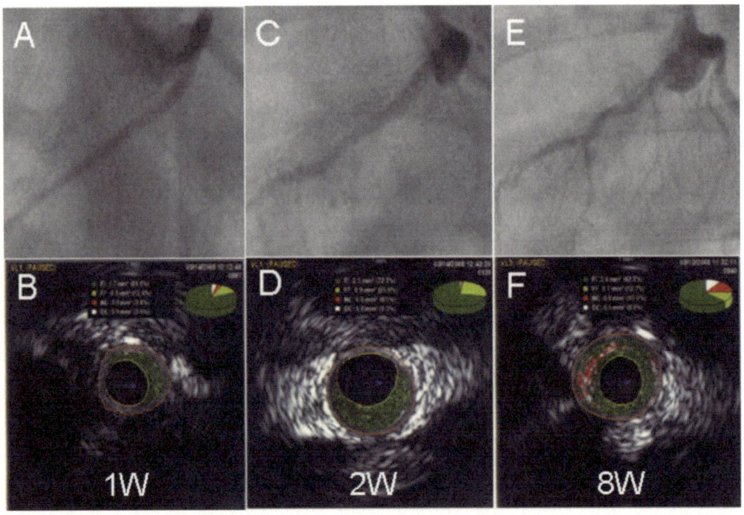

Fig. 2. LAD angiography and IVUS-VH after balloon injury in swine fed with high-fat diet for different time (1, 2, 8w). (A, C, E) LAD angiography; (B, D, F) IVUS-VH.

2.1.6 Transgenic animal models for cardiovascular diseases

For economic reasons and with the help of genetically targeted mouse manipulated in the laboratory, considerable basic and applied cardiovascular experimentation has been performed in mice and rats; on the assumption that the results can be translated to humans. Transgenic mice are widely accepted and used in many labs. To delve the roles of prostaglandin H synthase-1 and prostaglandin H-synthase-2, known colloquially as COX-1 (target of aspirin: first level heart disease prevention drug) and COX-2 (target of many anti-inflammatory drugs), in cardiovascular systems, Four different strains of mice were successfully generated and characterized including: (i) genetic knockdown of COX-1 (80-97% reduction) (Yu et al., 2005); (ii) genetic knockdown of COX-2 (80-95 % reduction) (Seta et al., 2009); (iii) knock-in of a point mutation at the COX-2 active site to abolish cyclooxygenase activity and leave peroxidase activity intact Ptgs2Y385F (Yu et al., 2006); and (iv) exchange of COX-1 into the COX-2 locus (Yu et al., 2007a). But before we head to set up more transgenic knock-in and/or knock-out mice, we should keep our own brain cool to think over the necessity and specific characters in each animal model.

Tiny mouse's heart muscle mass (<100 mg) as compared to about 500 g in the human heart presents problems of magnitude and architectural complexity. This may partially explain why so many effective investigational new drugs withdraw market after phase 3 clinical trials even they have show promising pharmacological effects in experimental animal models. Scientist resorted to another popular rodent animal: rat. But hampered by lacking specific techniques to manipulate the rat stem cells which have been working very well in mice, rats were kicked out of the transgenic game for a long time. Zinc-Finger Nucleases (ZFN) technology to generate knock-in rats in which foreign genes have been inserted, or 'knocked-in', into the rat genome in a precisely targeted manner (Geurts et al., 2009). This breakthrough achievement represents a major step forward in the creation of a transgenic animal, which may serve as more predictive models of human disease, especially in cardiovascular diseases. For example, first rat knockout in the renin-angiotensin system has demonstrated the efficacy of the ZFN technology for creating knockout rats for cardiovascular disease on any genetic background (Moreno et al., 2011).

2.1.7 Computer-based simulation of ischemia and reperfusion model

Experimental models, however, have their own set of limitations that hamper the comprehensive evaluation of heart functional mechanisms. At the end of the last century, some scientists pursued to develop a biochemically and biophysically detailed model that could provide a novel approach to studying myocardial ischaemia and reperfusion (Ch'en et al., 1998). Over the last decade, analysis of electrophysiological phenomena following coronary occlusion has been significantly augmented and advanced by the use of mathematical modeling and computer simulations, from the ionic channel to the whole organ. One of the major contributions of computational research in electrophysiology has been the ability of mathematical models to dissect various effects and to tease out important relations between electrophysiological parameters. This part has been well reviewed by others (Rodriguez et al., 2006).

2.2 Evaluation of myocardial ischemia and infarction

Conventional 12-lead electrocardiography (ECG) as well as analysis of serum markers still play a non-replaceable role clinically and even in the animal model research. In addition, a number of special techniques such as echocardiography, nuclear magnetic resonance imaging (MRI) (Wright et al., 2009), computed tomography (CT) (Baks et al., 2006; Buecker et al., 2005; Mahnken et al., 2005), single photon emission computed tomography (SPECT), and positron emission tomography (PET) have been devised to support diagnosis in the patients who show ambiguous symptoms and ECG findings. Major advantage of these latter methods is that infarct size can be non-invasively and repeatedly measured in vivo. Major limitation of the non-invasive imaging techniques in humans is the lack of quantification of the risk zone.

In preclinical small animal models, the use of above mentioned novel non-invasive imaging techniques is also limited due to several technical problems (e.g. lack of area at risk determination, insufficient temporal and spatial resolution, irradiation, etc.) and their high cost. Therefore, direct post-sacrifice techniques such as e.g. the triphenyltetrazolium (TTC) staining as well as nitroblue tetrazolium (NBT) staining, is still the most widely used, low-cost method to assess infarct size in animal models.

2.2.1 Modified ECG and multiple-electrode mapping

Identifying patients at risk of ST segment elevations (most frequently observed in heart attack) by use of body surface electrical measures is controversial. To probe the principal variations during myocardial ischemia, scientists have pursued to measure the electrophysiological changes of heart by modified ECG (s). In our lab, to circumvent some of these problems and to further our knowledge of the cardiovascular disorders we have undertook a series of investigations that consisted of designing novel modified ECG since 1970s. Two different modified ECGs were successfully developed and characterized including: epicardial electrograms (Li, 1978; Liu et al., 2002) and body surface ECG (BS-ECG) (Liu et al., 2007b). See the section "EECG and BS-ECG" below for the details.

Other lab worldwide besides our lab should also be reviewed here as to design very sensitive, multiple-electrode mapping technology. Mimicking the body 12-lead ECG, scientists from University of Oxford recorded ventricular epicardial electrograms from 5 anesthetized pigs with a 127-electrode sock and simultaneously investigated torso ECG using a specifically designed vest with 256 ECG electrodes. One of breakthroughs they have made in this study is that with chest reclosed, simultaneous arrays of epicardial electrograms and torso ECGs can be recorded during LAD occlusion and reperfusion (Nash et al., 2003).

The earlier identification of coronary occlusion with ST-segment elevation, the better outcomes patients undergoing heart attack may have due to timing of revascularization. Using an implantable, high-fidelity, intracardiac electrogram monitoring system with long-range telemetry in porcine subjected to acute coronary occlusion precipitated by stent thrombosis, researchers from Michigan State University real-timely detected acute ST-segment elevation and analyzed its correlations with thrombotic coronary occlusion. High sensitivity and specificity (100% and 100%, respectively) in such a system make it possible to advance the time frame of reperfusion therapy and potentially prevent, rather than interrupt, acute myocardial infarction in patients with coronary artery disease (Fischell et al., 2006).

In a porcine acute infarct and reperfusion model induced by balloon occlusion of the left anterior descending coronary artery for 45 minutes, endocardial electromechanical mapping (EMM) was performed to evaluat the extent of myocardial ischemia. Even though there was significant intersegmental threshold variability at baseline and after infarction, the electromechanical activity thresholds, for infarct detection, could be established. In this study, the capacity of separating myocardium with evolving necrosis from viable myocardium was so promising that would result in potential clinical uses (Odenstedt et al., 2003).

2.2.2 Advanced imaging systems

Conventional methods to quantify infarct size after myocardial infarction in mice are not ideal. Cardiologists therefore implemented a fast, high-resolution method to directly measure infarct size in vivo using three-dimensional (3D) late gadolinium enhancement MRI (3D-LGE). They had validated an improved 3D MRI method to noninvasively quantify infarct size in mice with unsurpassed spatial resolution and tissue contrast. This method is particularly suited to studies requiring early quantification of initial infarct size, for example, to measure damage before intervention with stem cells (Bohl et al., 2009). Another study group combined the small-animal PET and MRI data to acquire quantitative in vivo insights into cardiac pathophysiology, and sought to determine the feasibility of PET and MRI for the quantification of ischemic injury in the rat model. Successful integrating information from small-animal PET and clinical MRI instrumentation allows for the quantitative assessment of cardiac function and infarct size in the rat model. The MRI measurements of scar can be complemented by metabolic imaging, addressing the extent and severity of ischemic injury and providing endpoints for therapeutic interventions (Higuchi et al., 2007).

2.2.3 Histological analysis of infarct size

In preclinical studies, still the postmortem histological analysis is considered to be the gold standard for measuring infarct size. However, there are a number of disadvantages of this technique, making a reliable non-invasive alternative highly desirable. First, histological methods leave no residual tissue for further analysis. Second, visual interpretation and planimetry of heart sections may be subjective in cases with poor viable/non-viable contrast due to hemoglobin residues within the necrotic regions or with TTC-induced geometric distortion of the sample. Finally, animals must be euthanized to measure injury, meaning longitudinal studies require separate groups of animals for each time point (Bohl et al., 2009).

Conventional TTC staining allows the quantification of infarct size much sooner than standard histological techniques, and has been shown to be equally sensitive and specific. Therefore, the direct post-sacrifice techniques such as e.g. the TTC staining, is still the most widely used, low-cost and high throughput method to assess infarct size in animal models (Skrzypiec-Spring et al., 2007).

2.2.4 Other novel methodologies

Many new methods were employed in cardiovascular functional measurement after ischemia or infarction. By using a three-axis accelerometer, researchers developed a novel technique for continuous real-time assessment of myocardial ischaemia in 14 anaesthetized open-chest pigs. Two accelerometers sutured on the left ventricle (LV) surface in the perfusion areas of the left anterior descending (LAD) and circumflex (CX) arteries, measured acceleration in the longitudinal, circumferential, and radial directions, and the corresponding epicardial velocities were calculated. The accelerometer had the ability to distinguish ischaemia from interventions altering global myocardial function, by which the myocardial ischaemia can be monitored in a continuous real-time mode (Halvorsen et al.,

2009). With the support of interventional techniques, intravascular ultrasound probe or intravascular Doppler velocimetry can be introduced into coronary artery and epicardial cross-sectional area and coronary flow velocity can be detected (Hutchison et al., 2005). Some study indicated that endocardial voltage amplitudes were closely related with sustaining myocardial ischemia or infarction. LV endocardial unipolar voltage (UpV) mapping was performed using the Biosense 3D navigation system 4 weeks after ameroid constrictor placement around the left circumflex coronary artery. Meanwhile, echocardiography was used to assess regional changes in myocardial wall thickening (MT) and fluorescent microspheres (4 x 10/injection) were used to quantify rest regional myocardial blood flow (MBF) in ischemic (left circumflex) and remote non-ischemic (left anterior descending) regions (Fuchs and Kornowski, 2005).

2.3 EECG and BS-ECG

Once a new myocardial ischemic/infarction model was to be established, validating it should be placed on the first priority. Without any doubt, traditional electrocardiogram is of first choice. Since 1970 last century, we have made much effort in developing practically modified electrocardiograms. The first one is so-called 30-point epicardial electrocardiogram (EECG), which was introduced in exposed heart. The multi-point epicardial electrodes were sutured on the ventricular surface and physiological monitor was connected to record the electrocardiogram (EECG). (Fig. 3.) ST segment elevated more than 2 mV was regarded as ischemic criterion to calculate the degree of myocardial ischemia (total mV of ST segment elevating, Σ-ST) and myocardial ischemic scope (total point number of ST segment elevating, N-ST) (Liu et al., 2007a; Liu et al., 2002; Yu et al., 2007b). (Fig. 4. and 5.)

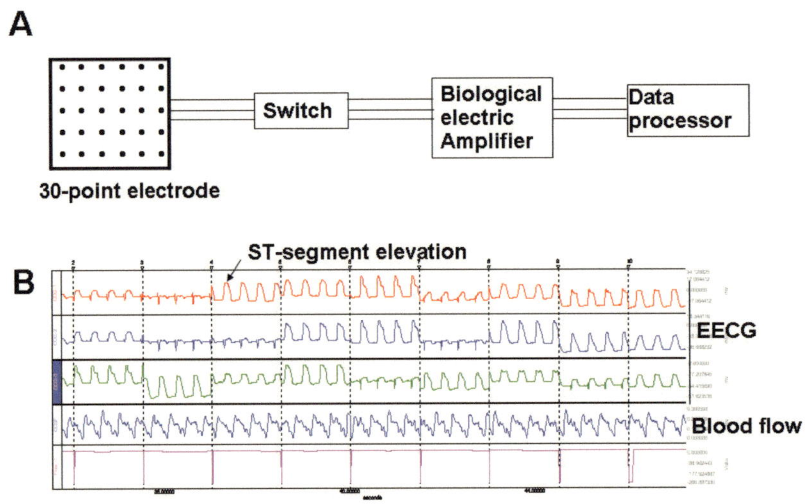

Fig. 3. Schematic components of EECG mapping system (A) and representative EECG in swine (B).

Body surface electrocardiogram (BS-ECG) is another well designed method, especially for closed chest and repeated measurement during a long period. The 30 point electrode was placed on the chest surface in the cardiac projective area and then connected to recorder

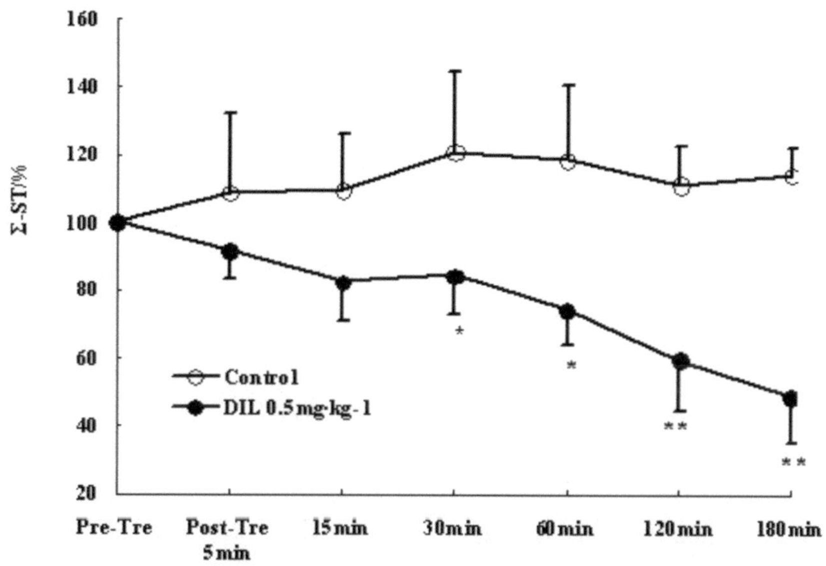

Fig. 4. The degree of myocardial ischemia (Σ -ST) determined by the epicardiogram mapping. We proposed that the percent of ischemic condition (before treatment) was 100%, Σ -ST % was obtained by the comparison with ischmemic condition. DIL, diltiazem, a classical calcium channel blocker. Pre-Tre: pre-treatment, Post-Tre: post-treatment. *P<0.05, **P<0.01 vs Control.

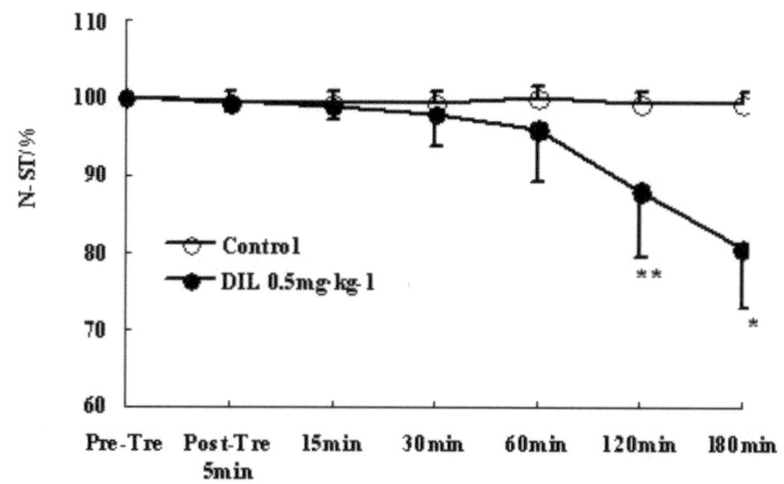

Fig. 5. The scope of myocardial ischemia (N-ST) determined by the epicardiogram mapping. We proposed that the percent of ischemic condition (before treatment) was 100%, N-ST % was obtained by the comparison with ischmemic condition. DIL, diltiazem, a classical calcium channel blocker. Pre-Tre: pre-treatment, Post-Tre: post-treatment. *P<0.05, **P<0.01 vs Control.

(Fig. 6.) (Liu et al., 2007b). Differently from EECG criteria due to relatively lower voltage on the skin, in BS-ECG, ST segment elevated to more than 0.8 mV was regarded as criterion to calculate the degree of myocardial ischemia (total mV of ST segment elevating, Σ-ST) and myocardial ischemic scope (total point number of ST segment elevating, N-ST). At the end of the protocol, the animals sacrificed and heart taken out. Under the coronary occlusion spot, the ventricle was transversely divided into 5 pieces of equal thickness. The pieces were then infiltrated with N-BT staining solution at 25 °C for 15 min. Both the ischemic area (N-BT non-stained area, white to grey) and non-ischemic area (N-BT-stained area, dark brown) were determined by histological methods.

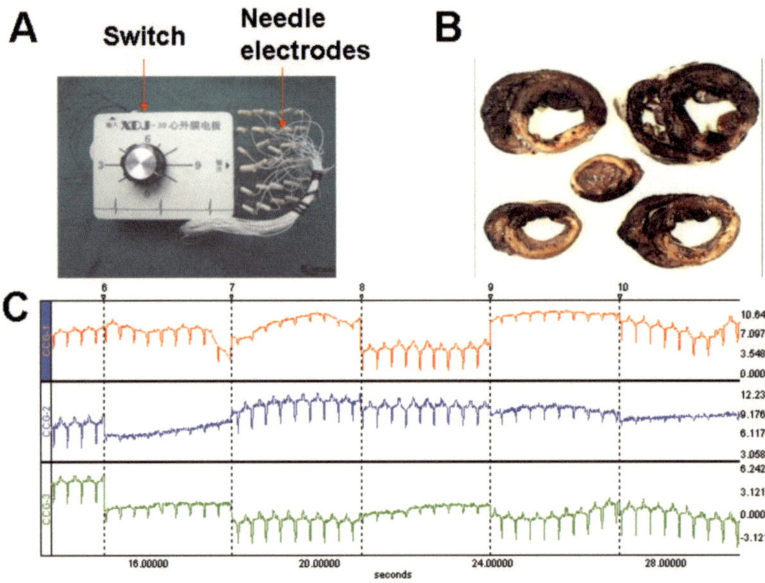

Fig. 6. BS-ECG machine (A), myocardium slices (B) (dark brown: live muscle; white: dead muscle), and BS-ECG (C).

3. Conclusion

The last few decades have seen significant advancement in the therapy of ischemic heart diseases. This is a direct outcome of the increasing knowledge of the molecular mechanisms involved during an ischemic insult of the myocardium. Another important factor is the development of animal model study, both academically and practically. The miniature swine was now widely used as research subject because of its anatomic similarity in coronary circulation to human beings (Hughes et al., 2003). Chest-closed improvement has been one of breakthroughs since birth of interventional technology. The newly introduced intervention technique avoided thoracotomy and disturbance to the environment of thoracic cavity. Moreover, cardiovascular variations could be chronically, continually and systematically observed in these models.

Despite tremendous advances in cardiovascular research and clinical therapy, ischemic heart disease remains the leading cause of serious morbidity and mortality in western society and is growing in developing countries. For researchers involving in basic science of heart diseases, one of the primary impediments to successful drug R&D is the frequent failure of successfully translating positive results obtained in animal models to human disease. To a large degree, this discrepancy is secondary to the substantial biological differences between species. We hope the information contained in this chapter will be helpful for researchers to consider prospectively their research plan regarding with myocardial ischemia/infarction animal study, which will someday bridge the gap between disease and the key molecular processes involved.

4. Acknowledgment

We thank Drs. Zhen Yu and Lei Li for their hard work with animal study. This work was supported by National Natural Science Foundation of China (30830118), National Key Scientific Program (2006BAI08B01-06, 2009ZX09303-003 and 2009ZX09502-017).

5. References

Baks, T., et al. (2006). Multislice computed tomography and magnetic resonance imaging for the assessment of reperfused acute myocardial infarction. *J Am Coll Cardiol,* Vol. 48, No. 1, pp.144-152

Bohl, S., et al. (2009). Advanced methods for quantification of infarct size in mice using three-dimensional high-field late gadolinium enhancement MRI. *Am J Physiol Heart Circ Physiol,* Vol. 296, No. 4, pp.H1200-1208

Bolukoglu, H., et al. (1992). An animal model of chronic coronary stenosis resulting in hibernating myocardium. *Am J Physiol,* Vol. 263, No. 1 Pt 2, pp.H20-29

Buecker, A., et al. (2005). A feasibility study of contrast enhancement of acute myocardial infarction in multislice computed tomography: comparison with magnetic resonance imaging and gross morphology in pigs. *Invest Radiol,* Vol. 40, No. 11, pp.700-704

Ch'en, F. F., et al. (1998). Modelling myocardial ischaemia and reperfusion. *Prog Biophys Mol Biol,* Vol. 69, No. 2-3, pp.515-538

Dogne, J. M., et al. (2005). Characterization of an original model of myocardial infarction provoked by coronary artery thrombosis induced by ferric chloride in pig. *Thromb Res,* Vol. 116, No. 5, pp.431-442

Elzinga, W. E. (1969). Ameroid constrictor: uniform closure rates and a calibration procedure. *J Appl Physiol,* Vol. 27, No. 3, pp.419-421

Falk, E., et al. (1995). Coronary plaque disruption. *Circulation,* Vol. 92, No. 3, pp.657-671

Fischell, T. A., et al. (2006). Real-time detection and alerting for acute ST-segment elevation myocardial ischemia using an implantable, high-fidelity, intracardiac electrogram monitoring system with long-range telemetry in an ambulatory porcine model. *J Am Coll Cardiol,* Vol. 48, No. 11, pp.2306-2314

Fuchs, S., Kornowski, R. (2005). Correlation between endocardial voltage mapping and myocardial perfusion: implications for the assessment of myocardial ischemia. *Coron Artery Dis,* Vol. 16, No. 3, pp.163-167

Geurts, A. M., et al. (2009). Knockout rats via embryo microinjection of zinc-finger nucleases. *Science,* Vol. 325, No. 5939, pp.433

Guth, B. D., et al. (1990). Myocardial lactate release during ischemia in swine. Relation to regional blood flow. *Circulation,* Vol. 81, No. 6, pp.1948-1958

Halvorsen, P. S., et al. (2009). Detection of myocardial ischaemia by epicardial accelerometers in the pig. *Br J Anaesth,* Vol. 102, No. 1, pp.29-37

Hennan, J. K., et al. (2001). Effects of selective cyclooxygenase-2 inhibition on vascular responses and thrombosis in canine coronary arteries. *Circulation,* Vol. 104, No. 7, pp.820-825

Higuchi, T., et al. (2007). Characterization of normal and infarcted rat myocardium using a combination of small-animal PET and clinical MRI. *J Nucl Med,* Vol. 48, No. 2, pp.288-294

Huang, Y., et al. (2004). Remodeling of the chronic severely failing ischemic sheep heart after coronary microembolization: functional, energetic, structural, and cellular responses. *Am J Physiol Heart Circ Physiol,* Vol. 286, No. 6, pp.H2141-2150

Hughes, G. C., et al. (2003). Translational physiology: porcine models of human coronary artery disease: implications for preclinical trials of therapeutic angiogenesis. *J Appl Physiol,* Vol. 94, No. 5, pp.1689-1701

Hutchison, S. J., et al. (2005). Dehydroepiandrosterone sulfate induces acute vasodilation of porcine coronary arteries in vitro and in vivo. *J Cardiovasc Pharmacol,* Vol. 46, No. 3, pp.325-332

Inou, T., et al. (1980). A newly developed X-ray transparent ameroid constrictor for study on progression of gradual coronary stenosis. *Basic Res Cardiol,* Vol. 75, No. 4, pp.537-543

Koning, M. M., et al. (1993). Intracoronary trimetazidine does not improve recovery of regional function in a porcine model of repeated ischemia. *Cardiovasc Drugs Ther,* Vol. 7, No. 5, pp.801-807

Kraitchman, D. L., et al. (2000). A minimally invasive method for creating coronary stenosis in a swine model for MRI and SPECT imaging. *Invest Radiol,* Vol. 35, No. 7, pp.445-451

Krombach, G. A., et al. (2005). Minimally invasive close-chest method for creating reperfused or occlusive myocardial infarction in swine. *Invest Radiol,* Vol. 40, No. 1, pp.14-18

Laham, R. J., et al. (2000). Intrapericardial delivery of fibroblast growth factor-2 induces neovascularization in a porcine model of chronic myocardial ischemia. *J Pharmacol Exp Ther,* Vol. 292, No. 2, pp.795-802

Leadley, R. J., Jr., et al. (2000). Contribution of in vivo models of thrombosis to the discovery and development of novel antithrombotic agents. *J Pharmacol Toxicol Methods,* Vol. 43, No. 2, pp.101-116

Li, L. (1978). The improvement of epicardial electrogram methods. *New Med Phar J,* Vol. 1, No. 11, pp.52-53

Li, X. Z., et al. (2009). Establishment of coronary heart disease model of coronary atherosclerosis in mini-swines. *Zhongguo Zhong Xi Yi Jie He Za Zhi,* Vol. 29, No. 3, pp.228-232

Lichtig, C., et al. (1975). Basic fuchsin picric acid method to detect acute myocardial ischemia. An experimental study in swine. *Arch Pathol,* Vol. 99, No. 3, pp.158-161

Liu, J. X., et al. (2007a). Effects of Corocalm (shuguan capsule) on acute myocardial ischemia in anesthetized dogs. *Chin J Integr Med,* Vol. 13, No. 3, pp.206-210

Liu, J. X., et al. (2002). Effects of recombinant staphylokinase on coronary thrombosis in Chinese experimental miniature swine. *Acta Pharmacol Sin,* Vol. 23, No. 6, pp.509-515

Liu, J. X., et al. (2007b). Cardioprotective effects of diltiazem reevaluated by a novel myocardial ischemic model in Chinese miniature swine. *Acta Pharmacol Sin,* Vol. 28, No. 1, pp.52-57

Ludemann, L., et al. (2007). Usage of the T1 effect of an iron oxide contrast agent in an animal model to quantify myocardial blood flow by MRI. *Eur J Radiol,* Vol. 62, No. 2, pp.247-256

Mahnken, A. H., et al. (2005). Assessment of myocardial viability in reperfused acute myocardial infarction using 16-slice computed tomography in comparison to magnetic resonance imaging. *J Am Coll Cardiol,* Vol. 45, No. 12, pp.2042-2047

Moreno, C., et al. (2011). Creation and characterization of a Renin knockout rat. *Hypertension,* Vol. 57, No. 3, pp.614-619

Nash, M. P., et al. (2003). Imaging electrocardiographic dispersion of depolarization and repolarization during ischemia: simultaneous body surface and epicardial mapping. *Circulation,* Vol. 107, No. 17, pp.2257-2263

Naslund, U., et al. (1992). A closed-chest myocardial occlusion-reperfusion model in the pig: techniques, morbidity and mortality. *Eur Heart J,* Vol. 13, No. 9, pp.1282-1289

Odenstedt, J., et al. (2003). Endocardial electromechanical mapping in a porcine acute infarct and reperfusion model evaluating the extent of myocardial ischemia. *J Invasive Cardiol,* Vol. 15, No. 9, pp.497-501

Park, W. H., et al. (1985). Morphological changes in the coronary circulation following experimental myocardial ischemia in swine. *Artery,* Vol. 12, No. 5, pp.286-300

Rodriguez, B., et al. (2006). Modeling cardiac ischemia. *Ann N Y Acad Sci,* Vol. 1080, No. pp.395-414

Romson, J. L., et al. (1980). Electrical induction of coronary artery thrombosis in the ambulatory canine: a model for in vivo evaluation of anti-thrombotic agents. *Thromb Res,* Vol. 17, No. 6, pp.841-853

Seta, F., et al. (2009). Renal and cardiovascular characterization of COX-2 knockdown mice. *Am J Physiol Regul Integr Comp Physiol,* Vol. 296, No. 6, pp.R1751-1760

Skrzypiec-Spring, M., et al. (2007). Isolated heart perfusion according to Langendorff---still viable in the new millennium. *J Pharmacol Toxicol Methods,* Vol. 55, No. 2, pp.113-126

Takahashi, M., et al. (2005). Effects of angiotensin I-converting enzyme inhibitor and angiotensin II type 1 receptor blocker on the right ventricular sarcoglycans and dystrophin after left coronary artery ligation. *Eur J Pharmacol,* Vol. 522, No. 1-3, pp.84-93

Tomita, S., et al. (2002). Improved heart function with myogenesis and angiogenesis after autologous porcine bone marrow stromal cell transplantation. *J Thorac Cardiovasc Surg,* Vol. 123, No. 6, pp.1132-1140

Wright, J., et al. (2009). Quantification of myocardial area at risk with T2-weighted CMR: comparison with contrast-enhanced CMR and coronary angiography. *JACC Cardiovasc Imaging,* Vol. 2, No. 7, pp.825-831

Yan, L., et al. (2006). Autophagy: a novel protective mechanism in chronic ischemia. *Cell Cycle,* Vol. 5, No. 11, pp.1175-1177

Yan, L., et al. (2005). Autophagy in chronically ischemic myocardium. *Proc Natl Acad Sci U S A,* Vol. 102, No. 39, pp.13807-13812

Yu, Y., et al. (2005). Differential impact of prostaglandin H synthase 1 knockdown on platelets and parturition. *J Clin Invest,* Vol. 115, No. 4, pp.986-995

Yu, Y., et al. (2006). Genetic model of selective COX2 inhibition reveals novel heterodimer signaling. *Nat Med,* Vol. 12, No. 6, pp.699-704

Yu, Y., et al. (2007a). Targeted cyclooxygenase gene (ptgs) exchange reveals discriminant isoform functionality. *J Biol Chem,* Vol. 282, No. 2, pp.1498-1506

Yu, Z., et al. (2007b). Protective effects of Shuangshen Ningxin capsule on miniature swine after myocardial ischemia by intervention. *Zhongguo Zhong Yao Za Zhi,* Vol. 32, No. 16, pp.1695-1699

Part 3

Autonomic Dysregulation

11

The Emergence and Development of Physiological Regulatory Systems of Newborn Infants in a Neonatal Intensive Care Unit

Motoki Bonno, Esmot Ara Begum and Hatsumi Yamamoto
Fetal – Neonatal Physiology Research, Clinical Research Institute, National Hosiptal Organization, Miechuo Medical Center, Mie, Japan

1. Introduction

In the life of a human being, the early neonatal period is the most prone to life-threatening events. After birth, following the transition from the intra- to the extra–uterine environment, babies experience dramatic hemodynamic changes. Once babies begin life in the extra-uterine environment, they must regulate their own homeostasis in order to survive. Preterm, low birth weight, newborn are even more vulnerable and require the mechanical support for proper tissue oxygenation and nutrition in order to grow and survive in the extra-uterine environment. The adaptation to extra-uterine life is a slow and difficult process for these babies because of their prematurity.

At this critical period, hypothermia, apnoea, respiratory distress, and cardiac instabilities such as bradycardia and hypotension are common features in these newborn babies (Bhatt et al., 2010; Di Fiore et al.,2001; Dransfield et al., 1983; Tirosh et al., 2010; Trevisanuto et al., 2005; Upton, et al., 1992), and the resulting hypoxia may lead to brain damage and cardiac arrest if the medical support of a special incubator equipped with a ventilator and systemic monitoring is not provided a as a "primary life support system". Therefore, the continuous monitoring of heartbeat, respiration, oxygen saturation, blood pressure and temperature has been integrated into the neonatal intensive care unit (NICU) as a mandatory tool to support the fragile clinical conditions of these infants.

Monitoring data collected using non-invasive electrocardiograms have been used to understand the physiological regulatory system of these vulnerable infants. The measurement of heart rate variability has been widely examined using various analytic methods (Ardura et al., 1997; Baldzer et al., 1989; Katona et al.,1980; Patural et al., 2004; Yiallourou et al., 2010). Among them, circadian rhythms have been documented to be a prognostic marker of physiological stability and the maturation of the physiological regulatory system, which can be defined as the long-term regulatory system. The endogenous circadian rhythm is generated by the endogenous biological clock located in the anterior hypothalamic suprachiasmatic nuclei (Panda et al., 2002) and may be modulated by exogenous factors (Reppert & Weaver, 2002). It has been documented in the growing foetus

(Patrick et al., 1982) controlled by maternal circadian signal (Seron-Ferre M et al). In full-term neonates, circadian rhythm are documented after birth, subsequently disappear and are not detectable within 3 or 4 weeks of postnatal age (Dimitriou et al., 1999; Mirmiran & Kok, 1991). However, in preterm neonates, the development of circadian rhythms is still controversial (Ardura et al., 1997; Begum et al, 2006; Bueno et al., 2001; Dimitriou et al., 1999; Korte et al., 2001; Mirmiran & Kok, 1991; Schimmel et al., 2002; Updike et al., 1985; Weinert et al., 1994) and the clinical relevance remains obscure.

Heart rate variability (HRV), derived from fast Fourier transform analysis of the R to R interval (RR interval) using an electrocardiogram, is another popular method to assess the autonomic nervous system (ANS) (Akselrod et al., 1981; Danguole et al., 2001; Finley et al., 1987; Kamen, 1996; Malik, 1996; Mazurak et al., 2010; Pontet et al., 2003; van Geijn et al., 1980). Continuous changes in sympathetic and parasympathetic neural impulses in the ANS induce changes in heart rate and cause oscillations around the mean, which is the HRV (Malik, 1996). In a frequency-based analysis of HRV, the low frequency (LF) band (0.04-0.15Hz) derived from the frequency domain analysis expresses the activity of both the sympathetic nervous system (SNS) and parasympathetic nervous system, and the high frequency (HF) band (0.15-0.5Hz) expresses the parasympathetic nervous system (PNS) activity of the ANS (Akselrod et al., 1981). The LF to HF ratio reflects the sympathovagal balances. Reports regarding the relevance of HRV to cardiac-health-related events that contribute to the ANS in the foetus, such as asphyxia (Bocking, 2003), foetal distress (Karin et al., 1993); in infants, such as respiratory distress, apnoea, sepsis, bradycardia (Bennet & Gunn, 2009; Frasch et al., 2009; Li et al., 2005; Logier et al., 2008 ; Sampson et al., 1980), and hypotension (Di Fiore et al., 2001; Dransfield et al., 1983; Fairchild & O'Shea, 2010; Frasch et al., 2009; Upton et al., 1992; Wennergren et al., 1986); and adults, such as stroke and myocardial events (Faber, 1996; Korpelainen et al., 1999; Sosnowski et al., 2002), are numerous and well-documented. In foetuses and preterm infants, the ANS is highly dependent on the SNS while the PNS is immature (Chatow et al., 1995), and the role of the PNS increases with the increase in gestational age (Van Leeuwen et al., 2003). Evidence of the effect of HRV on the adaptation of the ANS in preterm, low birth weight infants during the early neonatal period is not widely available, although it is known that an immature ANS is one of the factors contributing to the vulnerability of these infants.

In this research review, developmental and adaptation changes will be described based on heart rate records from ECG monitors. This description will provide an important perspective on the developmental physiological homeostasis of preterm infants during the early neonatal period in the intensive care unit.

2. Utilisation of the electrocardiogram - analytical methods of heart rate assessment

2.1 Monitoring and data recording through NICU local area network (LAN) system

All infants hospitalised in the NICU are monitored via electrocardiogram (ECG) for heart rate (HR) and respiration rate (RR), with a pulse oxymeter on the wrist or foot for pulse rate (PR) and oxygen saturation by pulse oxymetry (SpO_2), and arterial blood pressure (ABP) using a catheter manometer system occasionally. In our study, the monitored physiological information is transformed to measurement variables using the Wave Achieving System (WAS) or Clinical Database Engine (CDE) (Philips Electronics Japan, Tokyo, Japan) through NICU LAN system (Fig. 1) (Begum et al., 2006). In this report, we will explain the circadian rhythmicity of neonate as long-term regulatory system and HRV as short-term regulatory system of physiological homeostasis.

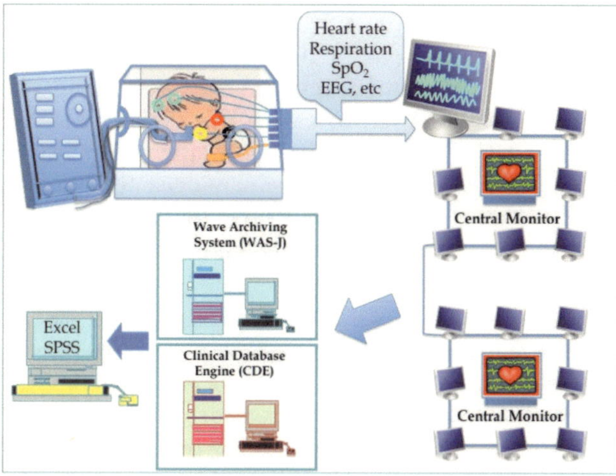

Fig. 1. NICU LAN system for recording physiological parameters.

2.2 Analysis of the heart rate circadian rhythm as a long-term regulatory system

2.2.1 Data acquisition and trend removal

For each patient, the heart rate was continuously recorded for 24 hours for the four postnatal periods (P): P1: 0-3, P2: 4-6, P3: 7-13, and P4: 14-21 postnatal days. Subjects with a continuous disruption in the data of more than 1 minute were excluded from the study. Any linear trend was removed using least square regression methods.

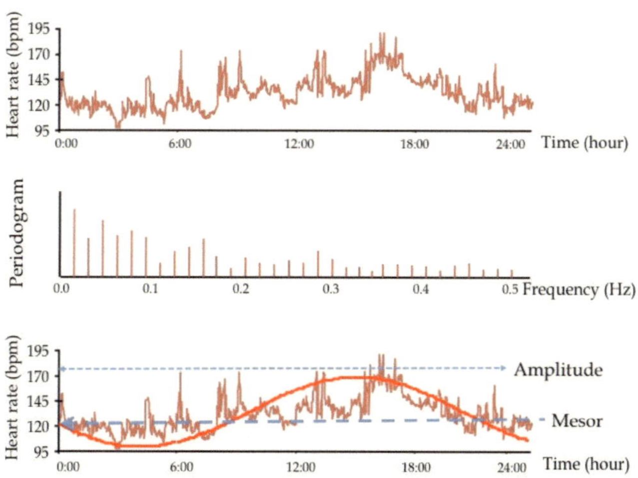

Fig. 2. Determination of the dominant cycle using spectral analysis. *A*: Plot of original data for heart rate (HR). *B*: Periodogram intensities for HR. The largest peak of the periodogram was selected as the cycle component. *C*: The intensity of the cycle corresponding to the largest peak in the periodogram was reconstructed to fit the sinusoidal function. The bold red line is the detected cycle superimposed on the original data.

2.2.2 Analysis of circadian rhythm
Circadian rhythmicity can be analyzed using various methods such as chi square periodogram, cosinor analysis.In our study, the existence of rhythmicity was analysed using power spectral analysis (periodogram) with SPSS 11.5 software (SPSS Inc. Chicago, IL) (Warner, 1998). Briefly, 24-hour sessions in 10-second intervals were run and aggregated into 1-minute time blocks. A periodogram analysis was performed using a time series of 1440 minutes. The Fisher test was used to assess the statistical significance of the cycle components ($N = 1440$, $\alpha = 0.05$) (Russell, 1985). In our study, the cycle with the largest peak in the periodogram was considered to be the dominant cycle for each time series among the significant cycles. All dominant cycles were confirmed by Fourier analysis, further circadian cycles were confirmed by cosinor analysis with a significance of $p < 0.05$ by least squares analysis (Fig. 2) (Nelson, 1993).

2.3 Analysis of heart rate variability (HRV) as a short - term regulatory system
2.3.1 Data acquisition of RR interval and the detection of outliers
To calculate R to R intervals in our study, for each patient, the heart rate wave was digitally transported to the CDE system, and the digital data for the heart rate was exported as a CSV file at a sampling rate of 500Hz. The RR interval was calculated by using MemCalc (GMS, Tokyo, Japan) which is statistical software specialised for entropy-based spectral analysis (Fig. 3).

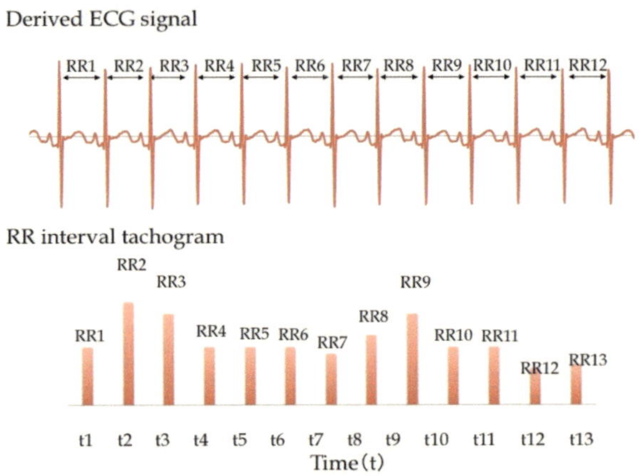

Fig. 3. Transformation of the RR interval from the waveform of a heart rate signal.

The data set obtained for the RR interval was visually inspected to identify any abnormal R - waves or artefacts. The presence of outliers in the RR interval data set can adversely effect both the time and the frequency domain analyses of HRV. Data outside of three standard deviations from the mean of RR interval data set were assumed to be statistically irrelevant and were tagged as outliers unless they were part of a trend (Niles, 2003). The missing values were replaced by the mean of the total data set.

2.3.2 Methods for HRV analysis - time domain analysis, frequency domain analysis and Poincare plot of the RR interval
Heart rate variability can be analysed in two ways: time domain and frequency domain analyses (Akselrod et al., 1981; Malik, 1996). For a geometric representation of the RR

interval, the non-linear Poincare plot can be analysed (Brennan et al., 2002). In this study, we have used the Heart Rate Variability Software (Kubios HRV, version 2.0) to analyse the time domain and frequency domain analysis as well as Poincare plot also.

2.3.2.1 Time domain analysis

Time domain measurements can be easily described using the RR interval data. From the time domain analysis, the standard deviation of RR (SDRR), and the root mean square of successive differences (RMSSD) were calculated as follows:

Standard deviation of RR interval (SDRR) $= \sqrt{\frac{1}{N-1}\sum_{n=1}^{N}(RR_n - RR)^2}$

The root mean square of successive differences (RMSSD)

$$= \sqrt{\frac{1}{N-1}\sum_{n=1}^{N-1}(RR_{n+1} - RR_n)^2}$$

2.3.2.2 Frequency domain analysis of the RR interval

For the frequency domain analysis, a spectral analysis of the RR interval was performed using fast Fourier transformation (FFT). The frequency domain analysis is widely used and is well recognised for analysing HRV. The low frequency (LF: 0.04 - 0.15 Hz) band and the high frequency (HF: 0.15 - 0.50 Hz) band were calculated.

2.3.2.3 Poincare plot of the RR interval

Poincare plots were calculated for the geometric representations of the RR intervals. The non-linear Poincare plot presents a figure with each RR interval plotted against the previous RR interval (RR_{n+1}, RR_n) and provides a detail of beat-to-beat information for the total data set (Brennan et al., 2002).

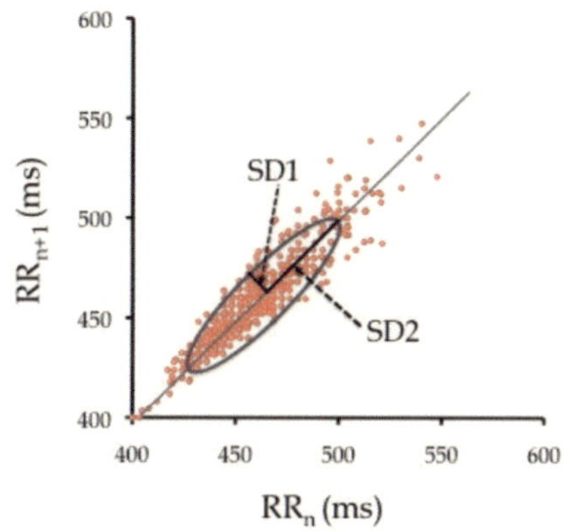

Fig. 4. An example Poincare plot: A standard Poincare plot of the R-R intervals of a healthy neonate born with 35 weeks of gestational age (GA). SD1 and SD2 represent the dispersion along the minor and major axes of the fitted eclipse.

The SD1, the width of the Poincare plot (the dispersion of points perpendicular to the line of identity), expresses the level of short-term heart rate variability, and SD2, the length (the dispersion along the line of identity), expresses the level of long-term heart rate variability (Fig. 4) (Brennan et al., 2001). The equations for SD1 and SD2 are as follows:

Width of RR_n vs. $RR_{(n+1)}$ distribution $(SD1)^2 \frac{1}{2}SDSD^2$

Length of RR_n vs. $RR_{(n+1)}$ distribution $(SD2) = 2SDSD^2 - \frac{1}{2}SDSD^2$

3. Evidence of circadian rhythmicity during the early neonatal period with clinical relevance

3.1 The development of a circadian rhythm in the neonatal period

Infants admitted in the NICU are vulnerable because of their physiological instability, and hypothermia, apnoea, respiratory distress, bradycardia and hypotension are common features for them. Frequent medical examination and therapy are common for them. Within this fragile environment, how do they adapt a physiological homeostasis? In our study, we have observed the circadian rhythmicity of preterm and full-term infants at four postnatal periods to observe their adaptation and developmental processes. The circadian rhythms of the heart rate were analysed in 187 neonates. The median GA was 34 weeks (range: 23–42 weeks). (Begum et al, 2006).

By analysing the distribution of circadian rhythmicity (Fig. 5), circadian rhythms were observed to be dominant among preterm infants (40%, < 28 wks of GA) compared to full-term infants, and a similar tendency was observed in other periods. These results partially support the previous studies (Dimitriou et al., 1999; Mirmiran & Kok, 1991).

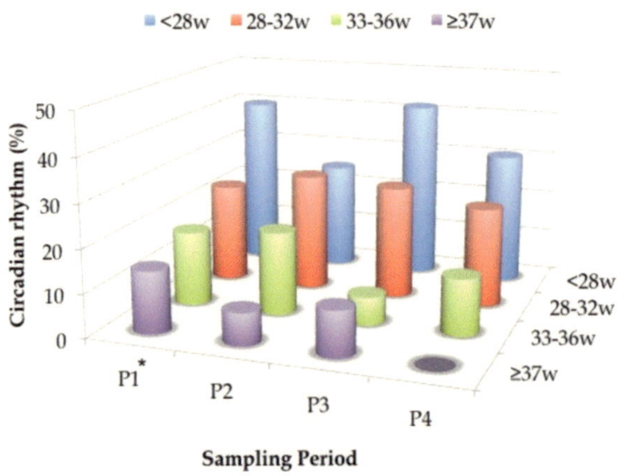

Fig. 5. The distribution of circadian cycles according to gestational age groups

In examining the relationship between circadian rhythmicity and post-conceptional age (PCA), an analysis of the correlation coefficient was performed using the amplitudes of each period. The amplitudes of the heart rate circadian rhythms were positively correlated with PCA in all four periods (Fig. 6).

The higher percentages for the existence of circadian rhythms in preterm infants compared to full-term infants suggest that the maternal influence on circadian rhythm may persist in preterm infants more strongly than in full-term infants during the neonatal period. However, the observed increase in circadian amplitude with PCA implies that the magnitude of circadian rhythmicity parallels the maturation of neonates.

Further, we analysed the heart rate circadian rhythmicity of infants born with small weight for gestational age (SGA: birth weight and height bellow < -2SDs) during 0-2 postnatal days and compared with infants born with average weight for gestational age (AGA: > -1.5 to < 1.5SDs). In the cases for which significant circadian rhythms were observed, significant differences were not observed between SGA and AGA infants, however, the amplitudes of the heart rate circadian rhythms were significantly smaller in SGA infants compared to AGA infants showed in Fig 7(Begum et al., 2010).

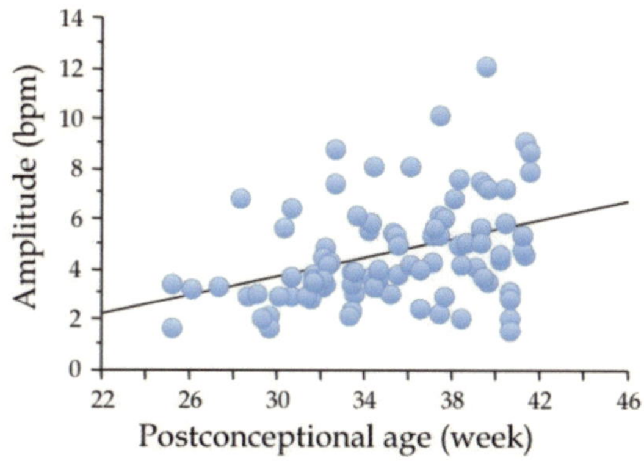

Fig. 6. The relationship between rhythmicity and PCA in P1: r = 0.38, P < 0.0001

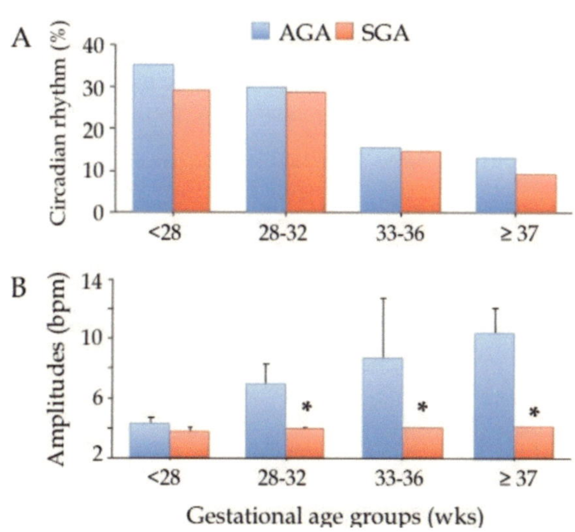

Fig. 7. The existence and amplitude of circadian rhythms in AGA and SGA neonates. A: Distribution of the infants with significant circadian rhythm and significant differences was not observed between AGA and SGA. B: Distribution of circadian amplitudes for AGA and SGA. The amplitudes were significantly smaller in SGA infants compared to AGA infants. * p <0.05, AGA vs. SGA

A decreased amplitudes in the circadian rhythm of SGA infants as shown above, intrauterine growth retardation might have influences on the quality of circadian rhythm rather than its existence.

4. Evidence of HRV in the early neonatal period and the clinical relevance

4.1 Experimental observation of alterations in HRV during the hourly neonatal period in extremely premature infants

The ANS plays an important role in the control of the physiological regulation. However, an immature ANS has been reported in the preterm infants after birth which prolongs to the later life also (De Rogalski Landrot et al., 2007). In preterm infants, particularly in extremely premature infants, the early neonatal period is a life-threatening period when cardiac failure, shock, loss of variability is frequently occurs to them. Numerous studies on ANS have been reported the GA based information with longitudinal evidences (Chatow et al., 1995; Longin et al., 2005, 2006) in preterm and full-term infants. However, the capacity and the recovery of ANS activity of extremely preterm infants immediate birth remain unclear. Thus, experimentally we observed the ANS activity of preterm infants born less than 28 weeks of GA from 3 hours after birth to 7 days to understand the changes into the capacity and recovery of ANS. For a micro-observation, ANS activity was observed at 3-hours, 6-hours, 12-hours, 24-hours, 72-hours and 7-days after birth using a dynamic analytic approach of HRV and observed the alterations in ANS through this critical period.

For analysis of HRV, a 30-minutes ECG signal data set was recorded for the calculation of RR interval from 13 extremely premature infants during a rest time at 3-hours, 6-hours, 12-hours, 24-hours, 72-hours, and 7-days after birth. From time domain analysis of HRV, mean RR, Mean HR, SDNN and RMSSD was calculated shown in Fig. 8. With the increase of time after birth, heart rates were decreased while RR intervals increased and this relation indicates the increase of the ability of the heart to function economically. Further, the increases in SDNN and RMSSD with the increase of the time after birth, might be indicated an increase in the amount of HRV. The increase in variability, which in turn indicates the significant interplay between SNS and PNS of the ANS.

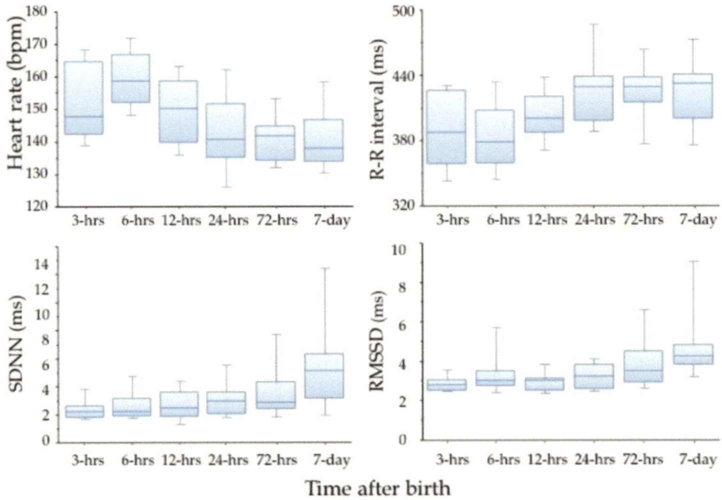

Fig. 8. Alterations in the parameters for the time domain analysis of the RR interval for HRV through the early neonatal period in extremely preterm infants (n=13). The RR interval was obtained for 30 minutes at each time point.

The power of LF region and HF region from the frequency domain analysis and SD1 and SD1 from Poincare plot analysis was calculated for each session. The power of both the LF and the HF was significantly lower at 3 hours or 6 hours after birth compared to the highest value at 7-days and the increase of LF and HF with the time after birth may indicate the maturation of the ANS. In the Poincare plot analysis, SD1 and SD2 also increased with the time after birth (Fig.9).

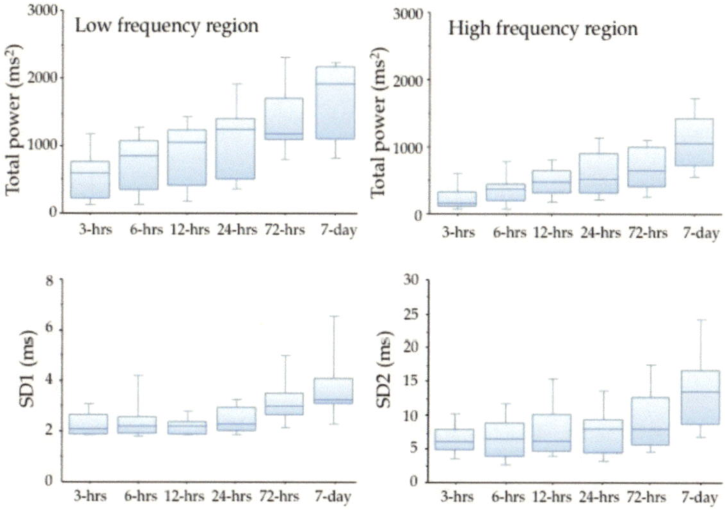

Fig. 9. Alterations in the parameters from the frequency domain analyses and Poincare plot analysis of HRV through the early neonatal period (n=13, mean gestational age = 27weeks, mean birth body weight = 875g).

The decreased HRV till 12 hours of birth may indicate the loss of variability immediate birth and transition of adaptation period for the short - term regulatory system and the increase of HRV from 24-hour to 7-days after birth might be indicated the increase in the ability of the adaptation capacity and as a sign of maturity.

4.2 Experimental observation of pain response during the early neonatal period: Three case analyses for three different gestational ages

The adverse consequences of pain response during the early neonatal period have been documented by numerous study (Grunau et al., 2006), and an emphasis has been placed on pain responses in the NICU (Brown, 2009; Johnston et al., 2010; Stevens et al., 2006, 2010). The most common pain event in NICU is blood procurement including heel lance and venepuncture (Carbajal et al., 2008). Changes in facial expression, sleep states, heart rate and SpO_2 are used as indicator of pain response in term infants, not in preterm infants (Stevens et al., 1996). The measures calculated from HRV provide sensitive indices to investigate the response of stressful stimuli. These indices are very helpful to investigate the pain response in preterm infants (Lindh et al., 1999; Morison et al., 2001; Oberlander & Saul, 2002; Padhye et al., 2009). The intensity of pain response in infants has been thought to be related with ANS activity maturation (Grunau et al., 2006). We have experimentally observed three cases with different GA (26, 31, 35 weeks) to analyse the differences in the intensity of the response to the pain stimuli during blood sampling. A heel lance episode was divided into 5 sessions as follows: A: 0-30-second (prior to needle puncture); B: 30-60 second (start of needle puncture); C: 60-90 second (squeezing for blood collection); D: 90-120 second (30 second after the end of blood collection); E: 120-150 second (after 60 second of blood collection). The RR interval data were analysed separately for each session.

Frequency domain analyses and Poincare plot analyses were applied to interpret the intensity of the response to pain. The distribution of the Fourier plot and Poincare plot is shown in Fig 10 and Fig. 11. The total spectral power increased after the pain procedure in all cases; however, it was low in the case of a 26-week GA neonate. The spectral power of the LF quickly increased following the needle puncture and gradually decreased with the cessation of the procedure in a 35-week GA infant. In contrast, the power of the HF was delayed in a 31-week GA infant and was low in a 26-week GA infant (Fig10).

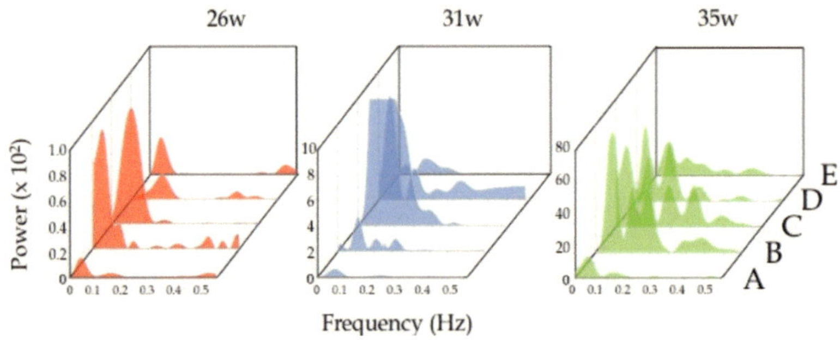

Fig. 10. A Spectral plot on the intensity of pain response during blood sampling for three different GA during early neonatal period. A: 0-30-seconds (prior to needle puncture); B: 30-60 second (start of needle puncture); C: 60-90 seconds (squeezing for blood sampling); D: 90-120 seconds (30 seconds after the end of blood sampling); E: 120-150 second (after 60 seconds of blood sampling).

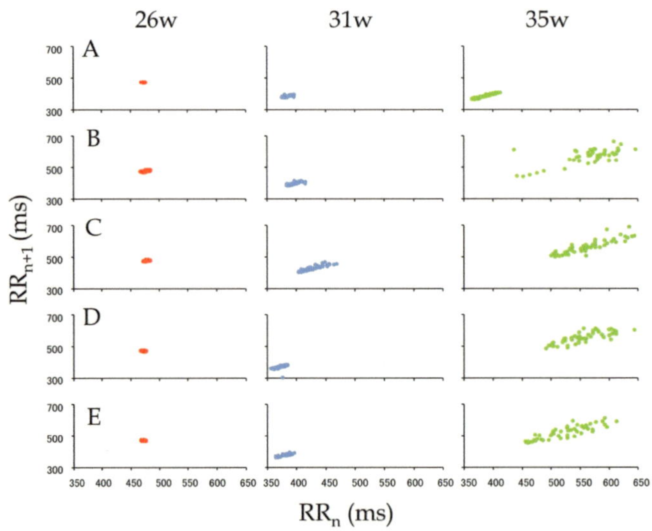

Fig. 11. Poincare plot analysis of the RR interval during blood sampling. A: 0-30 second (prior to needle puncture); B: 30-60 second (start of needle puncture); C: 60- 90 second (squeezing for blood sampling); D: 90-120 second (30 seconds after the end of blood sampling); E: 120-150 second (after 60 seconds of blood sampling).

By Poincare analysis of the RR interval, the response of the painful procedure was well recognized (Fig. 11). The Poincare plot was strongly shifted to the upper right quadrant in the 35-week GA infant, and the shift was small in the 31-week GA infant, while almost no shift was observed for the procedure in a 26-week GA infant.

Based on these findings, we suggest that an increased physiological response to painful events is related to the maturity of the ANS, and late preterm infants may be affected more strongly than extremely premature infants by painful events. Because of the immaturity of the ANS in infants <26 weeks, the response to pain was comparatively lower than that of other infants.

4.3 Kangaroo care for preterm infants as physiological relaxation

Kangaroo care (KC) has been widely practiced for preterm and low birth weight (LBW) infants in the neonatal intensive care unit (NICU). KC is now practiced not only in developing countries, but also in developed countries as developmental care because improved outcome in mortality and morbidity have been reported in infants who undergo KC. There have been many studies performed to evaluate the psychological and physiological responses during KC in preterm infants. Although still there is some contradiction on the influences of KC in infants, positive influences also reported by many literature (Bauer et al., 1997; Fohe et al., 2000; Acolet et al., 1989; Cattaneo et al., 1998; Feldman & Eidelman, 2003; Messmer et al., 1997).

In our study on the physiological responses during kangaroo care, significant differences was observed in the spectral power of heart rate within the different sessions (the %LF was significantly increased during KC, while %HF was decreased, without significant changes in the ratio of LF/HF, Fig. 12). Behavioural states were observed during kangaroo care using the Brazelton Neonatal Behaviour Assessment Scale (Brazelton, 1984). The percentage of infants with quiet sleep states remarkably increased during KC compared to those before KC. This percentage increased further at the end of KC and decreased again 30 minutes after KC (Fig. 13).

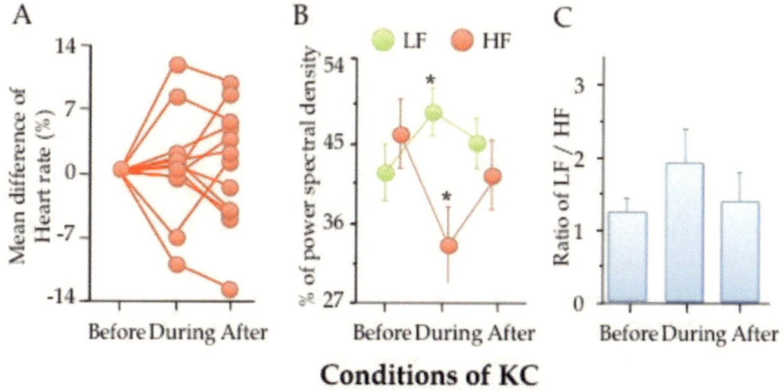

Fig. 12. Changes in heart rate variability during KC. A: mean difference in heart rate; B: power spectral density of LF and HF; C: ratio of LF/HF. *P < 0.05 (Repeated measures ANOVA)

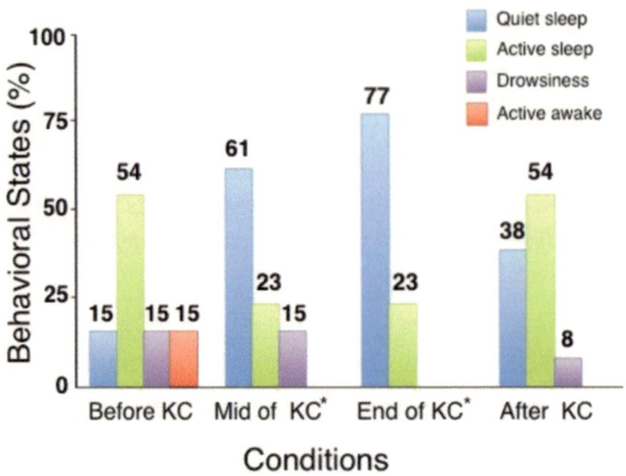

Fig. 13. Changes in the behavioural states of infants during KC. Five different behavioural states were observed: 1) Quiet sleep; 2) Active sleep; 3) Drowsiness; 4) Alert inactivity; and 5) Active awake.

As shown above, an increase in %LF during KC was observed without fluctuation of the LF/HF ratio, and infants tended to sleep deeply during KC. These findings suggest that parasympathetic nerve activity may be suppressed during KC and that decreased parasympathetic nerve activity may induce deep sleep. Improved outcome and health status with KC may be due to relaxation of vagal tone.

5. Conclusion

In this chapter, we explained the emergence and development of the ANS as physiological regulatory systems of new- born infants. Circadian rhythm, we defined it as long-term regulatory system, exist immidiate birth and persist through the neonatal period in preterm infants, while it does not persist after birth in full-term infants. On the contrary, the heart rate variability of extremely premature infants is suppressed on the day of birth and increases with time in the early neonatal period. The maternal influence on circadian rhythms may be important for extremely premature infants because the autonomic nervous system is not fully developed in these infants, as has been shown in the session on physiological response to pain.

In infants with later gestational ages, however, the physiological response to pain is stronger. During hospitalisation, infants with later gestational ages may be more sensitive to stressful stimuli. Developmental support such as Kangaroo care may offer relief from the stressful stimuli of the NICU, and relaxation during their stay in the NICU may be an important aspect for improved outcomes and later health status.

Finally, understanding the development of auto-regulation in newborn infants during the early neonatal period provides new information on the factors that influence the vulnerability of newborn infants in the NICU. Bedside monitoring of physiological hemodynamics and the implications of these monitored variables are key tools for neonatologists, not only for improving survival, but also for improving the quality of life for these vulnerable infants.

6. Acknowledgment

We thank the staff of the Department of Nursing and the Department of Paediatrics and Neonatology for their assistance in the data collection in the NICU; we also thank Ms Taeko Nakano for secretarial assistance.

7. References

Ardura J, Andres J, Revilla M, Aragon M (1997): Heart rate biorhythm changes during the first three months of life. *Biol Neonate*, 72, PP. 94-101.

Acolet D, Sleath K, Whitelaw A (1989): Oxygenation, heart rate and temperature in very low birthweight infants during skin-to-skin contact with their mothers. *Acta Paediatr Scand*, 78(2). PP. 189-193. (1989/03), ISSN: 0001-656X

Akselrod S, Gordon D, Ubel FA, Shannon DC, Berger AC, Cohen RJ (1981): Power spectrum analysis of heart rate fluctuation: a quantitative probe of beat-to-beat cardiovascular control. *Science*, 213(4504). PP. 220-222., (1981/07), ISSN: 0036-8075

Bueno C, Diambra L, Menna-Barreto L (2001): Sleep-Wake and Temperature Rhythms in Preterm Babies Maintained in a Neonatal Care Unit. *Sleep Research Online*, 4(3). PP. 77-82.

Bocking AD (2003): Assessment of fetal heart rate and fetal movements in detecting oxygen deprivation in-utero. *Eur J Obstet Gynecol Reprod Biol*, 110 Suppl 1. PP. S108-112. (2003/09), ISSN: 0301-2115,

Brazelton TB (1984): Neonatal Behavioral Assessment Scale 2nd Edition. *London: Heinemann.*

Brennan M, Palaniswami M, Kamen P (2002): Poincare plot interpretation using a physiological model of HRV based on a network of oscillators. *Am J Physiol Heart Circ Physiol*, 283(5). PP. H1873-1886., (2002/11), ISSN: 0363-6135

Brennan M, Palaniswami M, Kamen P (2001): Do existing measures of Poincare plot geometry reflect nonlinear features of heart rate variability? *IEEE Trans Biomed Eng*, 48(11). PP. 1342-1347. (2001/11), ISSN: 0018-9294

Bennet L, Gunn AJ (2009): The fetal heart rate response to hypoxia: insights from animal models. *Clin Perinatol*, 36(3). PP. 655-672., (2009/09), ISSN: 1557-9840

Begum E, Bonno M, Obata M, Yamamoto H, Kawai M, Komada Y (2006): Emergence of physiological rhythmicity in term and preterm neonates in a neonatal intensive care unit. *J Circadian Rhythms*, 4:11. (2006/09), ISSN: 1740-3391

Begum E, Bonno M, Omori Y, Sugino N, Sasaki N, Yamamoto H (2010): Blunted Circadian Rhythms in Heart Rate of Small for Gestational Age Infants in Early Neonatal Period, Conference: Asian Society for Prdiatric Research (ASPR). *Taipei, Taiwan*, April, 2010

Begum EA, Bonno M, Ohtani N, Yamashita S, Tanaka S, Yamamoto H, Kawai M, Komada Y (2008): Cerebral oxygenation responses during kangaroo care in low birth weight infants. *BMC Pediatr* , 8:51, (2008/11), ISSN: 1471-2431

Bauer K, Uhrig C, Sperling P, Pasel K, Wieland C, Versmold HT (1997): Body temperatures and oxygen consumption during skin-to-skin (kangaroo) care in stable preterm infants weighing less than 1500 grams. *J Pediatr*, 130(2). PP. 240-244. (1997/02), ISSN: 0022-3476

Bhatt DR, White R, Martin G, Van Marter LJ, Finer N, Goldsmith JP, Ramos C, Kukreja S, Ramanathan R (2010): Transitional hypothermia in preterm newborns. *Adv Neonatal Care*, 10(5 Suppl). PP. S15-17. (2010/10) ISSN: 1536-0911

Baldzer K, Dykes FD, Jones SA, Brogan M, Carrigan TA, Giddens DP (1989): Heart rate variability analysis in full-term infants: spectral indices for study of neonatal cardiorespiratory control. *Pediatr Res*, 26(3). PP. 188-195. (1989/09), ISSN: 0031-3998

Brown G (2009): NICU noise and the preterm infant. *Neonatal Netw*, 28(3).PP. 165-173. (2009/05), ISSN: 1539-2880

Carbajal R, Rousset A, Danan C, Coquery S, Nolent P, Ducrocq S, Saizou C, Lapillonne A, Granier M, Durand P *et al* (2008): Epidemiology and treatment of painful procedures in neonates in intensive care units. *JAMA*, 300(1). PP. 60-70. (2008/07), ISSN: 1538-3598

Cattaneo A, Davanzo R, Bergman N, Charpak N (1998): Kangaroo mother care in low-income countries. International Network in Kangaroo Mother Care. *J Trop Pediatr*, 44(5). PP. 279-282. (1998/10), ISSN: 0142-6338

Chatow U, Davidson S, Reichman BL, Akselrod S (1995): Development and maturation of the autonomic nervous system in premature and full-term infants using spectral analysis of heart rate fluctuations. *Pediatr Res*, 37(3). PP. 294-302. (1995/03), ISSN: 0031-3998

Dransfield DA, Spitzer AR, Fox WW (1983): Episodic airway obstruction in premature infants. *Am J Dis Child*, 137(5). PP. 441-443. (1983/05), ISSN: 0002-922X

Dimitriou G, Greenough A, Kavvadia V, Mantagos S (1999) : Blood pressure rhythms during the perinatal period in very immature, extremely low birthweight neonates. *Early Hum Dev*, 56(1). PP. 49-56. (1999/9), ISSN: 0378-3782

De Rogalski Landrot I, Roche F, Pichot V, Teyssier G, Gaspoz JM, Barthelemy JC, Patural H (2007): Autonomic nervous system activity in premature and full-term infants from theoretical term to 7 years. *Auton Neurosci*, 136(1-2). PP. 105-109. (2007/10), ISSN: 1566-0702

Di Fiore JM, Arko MK, Miller MJ, Krauss A, Betkerur A, Zadell A, Kenney SR, Martin RJ (2001): Cardiorespiratory events in preterm infants referred for apnea monitoring studies. *Pediatrics*, 108(6). PP. 1304-1308. (2001/12), ISSN: 1098-4275

Finley JP, Nugent ST, Hellenbrand W (1987): Heart-rate variability in children. Spectral analysis of developmental changes between 5 and 24 years. *Can J Physiol Pharmacol*, 65(10). PP. 2048-2052. (1987/10), ISSN: 0008-4212

Frasch MG, Muller T, Weiss C, Schwab K, Schubert H, Schwab M (2009): Heart rate variability analysis allows early asphyxia detection in ovine fetus. *Reprod Sci* , 16(5). PP. 509-517. (2009/05), ISSN: 1933-7205

Feldman R, Eidelman AI (2003): Skin-to-skin contact (Kangaroo Care) accelerates autonomic and neurobehavioural maturation in preterm infants. *Dev Med Child Neurol*, 45(4). PP. 274-281. (2003/04), ISSN: 0012-1622 (Print)

Fairchild KD, O'Shea TM (2010): Heart rate characteristics: physiomarkers for detection of late-onset neonatal sepsis. *Clin Perinatol,* 37(3). PP. 581-598. (2010/09), ISSN: 1557-9840

Faber TS, Staunton A, Hnatkova K, Camm AJ, Malik M (1996): Stepwise strategy of using short- and long-term heart rate variability for risk stratification after myocardial infarction. *Pacing Clin Electrophysiol,* 19(11 Pt 2). PP. 1845-1851. (1996/11), ISSN: 0147-8389

Fohe K, Kropf S, Avenarius S (2000): Skin-to-skin contact improves gas exchange in premature infants. *J Perinatol,* 20(5). PP. 311-315. (2000/08), ISSN: 0743-8346

Grunau RE, Whitfield MF, Fay T, Holsti L, Oberlander T, Rogers ML (2006): Biobehavioural reactivity to pain in preterm infants: a marker of neuromotor development. *Dev Med Child Neurol,* 48(6). PP. 471-476. (2006/06), ISSN: 0012-1622

Johnston CC, Fernandes AM, Campbell-Yeo M (2010): Pain in neonates is different. *Pain,* 152(3 Suppl). PP. S65-73. (2010/03), ISSN: 1872-6623

Korpelainen JT, Sotaniemi KA, Myllyla VV(1999): Autonomic nervous system disorders in stroke. *Clin Auton Res,* 9(6). PP. 325-333. (1999/12), ISSN: 0959-9851

Kamen P (1996): Heart rate variability. *Aust Fam Physician,* 25(7). PP. 1087-1089, 1091-1085. (1996/07), ISSN: 0300-8495

Karin J, Hirsch M, Akselrod S (1993): An estimate of fetal autonomic state by spectral analysis of fetal heart rate fluctuations. *Pediatr Res,* 34(2). PP. 134-138. (1993/08). ISSN: 0031-3998

Korpelainen JT, Sotaniemi KA, Makikallio A, Huikuri HV, Myllyla VV (1999): Dynamic behavior of heart rate in ischemic stroke. *Stroke,* 30(5). PP. 1008-1013. (1999/05), ISSN: 0039-2499

Korte J, Wulff K, Oppe C, Siegmund R (2001): Ultradian and circadian activity-rest rhythms of preterm neonates compared to full-term neonates using actigraphic monitoring. *Chronobiol Int,* 18(4). PP. 697-708. (2001/7), ISSN: 0742-0528

Logier R, De Jonckheere J, Jeanne M, Matis R (2008): Fetal distress diagnosis using heart rate variability analysis: design of a high frequency variability index. *Conf Proc IEEE Eng Med Biol Soc.* PP. 4728-4731. (2009/01, EPUB), ISSN: 1557-170X

Li X, Zheng D, Zhou S, Tang D, Wang C, Wu G (2005): Approximate entropy of fetal heart rate variability as a predictor of fetal distress in women at term pregnancy. *Acta Obstet Gynecol Scand,* 84(9). PP. 837-843. (2005/09), ISSN: 0001-6349

Lindh V, Wiklund U, Hakansson S (1999): Heel lancing in term new-born infants: an evaluation of pain by frequency domain analysis of heart rate variability. *Pain,* 80(1-2). PP. 143-148. (1999/03), ISSN: 0304-3959

Longin E, Schaible T, Lenz T, Konig S (2005): Short term heart rate variability in healthy neonates: normative data and physiological observations. *Early Hum Dev,* 81(8). PP. 663-671. (2005/08), ISSN: 0378-3782

Longin E, Gerstner T, Schaible T, Lenz T, Konig S (2006): Maturation of the autonomic nervous system: differences in heart rate variability in premature vs. term infants. *J Perinat Med,* 34(4). PP. 303-308. (2006/07), ISSN: 0300-5577

Morison SJ, Grunau RE, Oberlander TF, Whitfield MF (2001): Relations between behavioral and cardiac autonomic reactivity to acute pain in preterm neonates. *Clin J Pain,* 17(4). PP. 350-358. (2001/12), ISSN: 0749-8047

Mirmiran M, Kok JH (1991): Circadian rhythms in early human development. *Early Hum Dev,* 26(2). PP. 121-128. (1991/08), ISSN: 0378-3782

Malik M (1996): Heart rate variability. Standards of measurement, physiological interpretation, and clinical use. Task Force of the European Society of Cardiology and the North American Society of Pacing and Electrophysiology Heart rate variability. Standards of measurement, physiological interpretation, and clinical use. *Eur Heart J,* 17(3). PP. 354-381. (1996/03), ISSN: 0195-668X

Mazurak N, Enck P, Muth E, Teufel M, Zipfel S (2010): Heart rate variability as a measure of cardiac autonomic function in anorexia nervosa: A review of the literature. *Eur Eat Disord Rev* . (2010/12), ISSN: 1099-0968

Messmer PR, Rodriguez S, Adams J, Wells-Gentry J, Washburn K, Zabaleta I, Abreu S (1997): Effect of kangaroo care on sleep time for neonates. *Pediatr Nurs,* 23(4). PP. 408-414. (1997/07), ISSN: 0097-9805

Nelson W, Tong YL, Lee JK, Halberg F (1979): Methods for cosinor rhythmometry. *Chronobiologia* , 6. PP. 305-323. (1979/10), ISSN: 0390-0037

Niles R: http://www.robertniles.com/stats/stdev.shtml,Accessed 5/4/2003. 2003.

Oberlander T, Saul JP (2002): Methodological considerations for the use of heart rate variability as a measure of pain reactivity in vulnerable infants. *Clin Perinatol* , 29(3). PP. 427-443. (2002/09), ISSN: 0095-5108

Ozdemir OM, Ergin H, Sahiner T (2009): Electrophysiological assessment of the brain function in term SGA infants. *Brain Res,* 1270:33-38. (2009/05), ISSN: 1872-6240

Pontet J, Contreras P, Curbelo A, Medina J, Noveri S, Bentancourt S, Migliaro ER (2003): Heart rate variability as early marker of multiple organ dysfunction syndrome in septic patients. *J Crit Care* , 18(3). PP. 156-163. (2003/9), ISSN: 0883-9441

Padhye NS, Williams AL, Khattak AZ, Lasky RE (2009): Heart rate variability in response to pain stimulus in VLBW infants followed longitudinally during NICU stay. *Dev Psychobiol,* 51(8). PP. 638-649. (2009/12), ISSN: 1098-2302

Panda S, Hogenesch JB, Kay SA (2002): Circadian rhythms from flies to human. *Nature,* 417(6886). PP. 329-335. (2002/05), ISSN: 0028-0836

Patrick J, Campbell K, Carmichael L, Probert C (1982): Influence of maternal heart rate and gross fetal body movements on the daily pattern of fetal heart rate near term. *Am J Obstet Gynecol,* 144(5). PP. 533-538. (1982/11), ISSN: 0002-9378

Patural H, Pichot V, Jaziri F, Teyssier G, Gaspoz JM, Roche F, Barthelemy JC (2008): Autonomic cardiac control of very preterm newborns: a prolonged dysfunction. *Early Hum Dev,* 84(10). PP. 681-687. (2008/10), ISSN: 0378-3782

Russell R (1985): Significance table for the result of first Fourier transformations. *British J of Mathematical and statistical psychology,* 38. PP. 116-119.

Reppert SM, Weaver DR (2002): Coordination of circadian timing in mammals. *Nature,* 418(6901). PP. 935-941. (2002/08), ISSN:0028-0836

Stevens B, McGrath P, Ballantyne M, Yamada J, Dupuis A, Gibbins S, Franck L, Allen Finley G, Howlett A, Johnston C *et al (2010)*: Influence of risk of neurological impairment and procedure invasiveness on health professionals' management of procedural pain in neonates. *Eur J Pain*, 14(7). PP. 735-741. (2010/08), ISSN: 1532-2149

Stevens B, McGrath P, Yamada J, Gibbins S, Beyene J, Breau L, Camfield C, Finley A, Franck L, Howlett A *et al (2006)*: Identification of pain indicators for infants at risk for neurological impairment: a Delphi consensus study. *BMC Pediatr*, 6(1). (2006/02), ISSN: 1471-2431

Stevens B, Johnston C, Petryshen P, Taddio A (1996): Premature Infant Pain Profile: development and initial validation. *Clin J Pain*, 12(1). PP. 13-22. (1996/03), ISSN: 0749-8047

Schimmel M, Waterhouse J, Marques M, Weunert D (2002): Circadian and Ultradian Rhythmicity in Very Premature Neonates Maintained in Incubators. *Biol Rhythm Res*, 33. PP. 83-112.

Sosnowski M, MacFarlane PW, Czyz Z, Skrzypek-Wanha J, Boczkowska-Gaik E, Tendera M (2002): Age-adjustment of HRV measures and its prognostic value for risk assessment in patients late after myocardial infarction. *Int J Cardiol*, 86(2-3). PP. 249-258. (2002/12), ISSN: 0167-5273

Trevisanuto D, Doglioni N, Ferrarese P, Zanardo V (2005): Thermal management of the extremely low birth weight infants at birth. *J Pediatr*, 147(5). PP. 716-717; author reply 717. (2005/11), ISSN: 0022-3476

Tirosh E, Ariov-Antebi N, Cohen A (2010): Autonomic function, gastroesophageal reflux in apparent life threatening event. *Clin Auton Res*, 20(3). PP. 161-166. (2010/06), ISSN: 1619-1560

Updike PA, Accurso FJ, Jones RH (1985): Physiologic circadian rhythmicity in preterm infants. *Nurs Res* , 34(3). PP. 160-163. (1985/05), ISSN: 0029-6562

Upton CJ, Milner AD, Stokes GM (1992): Episodic bradycardia in preterm infants. *Arch Dis Child* 1992, 67(7 Spec No). PP. 831-834., (1992/07), ISSN: 1468-2044

Van Leeuwen P, Geue D, Lange S, Hatzmann W, Gronemeyer D (2003): Changes in the frequency power spectrum of fetal heart rate in the course of pregnancy. *Prenat Diagn*, 23(11). PP. 909-916. (2003/11) ISSN: 0197-3851

van Geijn HP, Jongsma HW, de Haan J, Eskes TK (1980): Analysis of heart rate and beat-to-beat variability: Interval difference index. *Am J Obstet Gynecol*, 138(3). PP. 246-252. (1980/10), ISSN: 0002-9378

Wennergren M, Krantz M, Hjalmarson O, Karlsson K (1986): Fetal heart rate pattern and risk for respiratory disturbance in full-term newborns. *Obstet Gynecol*, 68(1). PP. 49-53. (1986/07), ISSN: 0029-7844

Warner RM (1998): Spectral Analysis of Time - Series Data. *The Guilford Press, New York, London . PP.* 49-96.

Weinert D, Sitka U, Minors DS, Waterhouse JM (2005): The development of circadian rhythmicity in neonates. *Early Hum Dev*, 36(2). PP. 117-126. (2005/07), ISSN: 0742-0528

Weinert D, Sitka U, Minors DS, Waterhouse JM(1994): The development of circadian rhythmicity in neonates. *Early Hum Dev*, 36(2). PP. 117-126. (1994/02), ISSN: 0378-3782

Yiallourou SR, Sands SA, Walker AM, Horne RS (2010): Postnatal development of baroreflex sensitivity in infancy. *J Physiol*, 588(Pt 12). PP. 2193-2203. (2010/06), ISSN: 1469-7793

12

Automated Detection and Classification of Sleep Apnea Types Using Electrocardiogram (ECG) and Electroencephalogram (EEG) Features

Onur Kocak[1], Tuncay Bayrak[1], Aykut Erdamar[1],
Levent Ozparlak[2], Ziya Telatar[3] and Osman Erogul[4]
[1]*Baskent University, Biomedical Engineering Department,*
[2]*Baskent University, Electrical Electronics Engineering Department,*
[3]*Ankara University, Electronics Engineering Department,*
[4]*GATA, Gulhane Military Medicine Academy, Biomedical Engineering Center,*
Turkey

1. Introduction

1.1 Sleep and sleep disorders

Sleep, which is defined as a passive period in organic physiology until the mid-20th century, is accepted to be an indispensable period of life cycle with today's technological advances. While wakefulness is associated with the active excitation of Central Nervous System (CNS), sleep has been recognized as a passive period by the elimination of excitation. However, recent studies have shown that sleep is independent of wakefulness, generated by a sequence of changes in CNS, and a combination of five periods with clear boundaries. Sleep is not the disruption of daily life for a period of time or a waste of time. It is an active period which is important to renew our mental and physical health everyday and is covering one-third of our lives. Sleep activity is important for resting during the working period of basal metabolism of human body.

The advances in technology enabling the measurement and quantification of brain activity make possible the micro and macro analysis of brain during both sleep and wakefulness states. With the studies investigating the CNS, it is observed the existence of some centrals causing the sleep by inhibiting the other regions of brain. As a result, sleep, which is an active and other state of consciousness, is a brain state of high coordination (Erdamar, 2007).

Since breathing is established autonomously during sleep, it is affected by many anatomical and physiological parameters. Depending on this situation, various sleep disorders occur. There are more than eighty known sleeping diseases. Most of them cause person's health to deteriorate and a decrease in life quality. As a result of the research carried out for many years, a list of sleep disorders, which are generally occurring, can be seen as in Table 1. Sleep disorders can be examined in two classes, parasomnia and dissomnia.

SLEEP DISORDERS	
DISSOMNIAS	PARASONMINAS
Insomnias	Dream Disorders
Hypersomnias	Somnambulism
Sleep Disorders in Sleep - Awake Cycle	
Sleep Disorders in Respiration	

Table 1. Sleep Disorders

1.2 Sleep respiration disorders

A significant portion of the sleep disorders are the respiratory disorders during sleep. It is thought that sudden deaths during sleep, daytime sleepiness, fatigue and snoring at night are caused by respiratory disorders in sleep. Therefore, regular breathing during sleep has vital importance for human health (Aksahin, 2010). The most important one of the sleep breathing disorders is the *sleep apnea*. Identification and monitoring of apnea during sleep is of great importance. As a result, in order to help physicians during the process of diagnosis and treatment of apnea, there are many studies on the topics of the detection and quantitative characteristics of sleep apnea using analytical methods from sleep records in literature.

The most important work on sleep in the field of engineering is the measurement and recording of physiological signals during sleep.

The device used for measuring and recording physiological signals during sleep is called as polysomnograph and the signals retrieved from the device are called as polysomnography (PSG). By the use of PSG, it is possible to observe the physiological changes in humans during sleep.

Various physiological signals of the patients are recorded simultaneously by the PSG device, which has an embedded multi-channel data acquisition system. The recording process made as analog recordings in the 90s has left its place to digital recorders after the development of digital systems. Thus, the prevention of errors caused by the hardware chaos of analog systems is provided (Erogul, 2008). By the use of these devices, Electroencephalogram (EEG), Electrocardiogram (ECG), Electromyogram (EMG), Electrooculogram (EOG), breathing, Pulseplethysmograph (PPG) and various desired or necessary signals of patients in sleep are recorded. In this way, the patients' statuses are determined during the night sleep and their diagnosis and treatment outcomes can be delineated. The classification of sleep apnea is also realized by the investigation of these physiological signals obtained from the PSG device.

The first time application of PSG by Gastaut in 1965 has increased the interest in research of breathing disorders in sleep. Sleep Apnea Syndrome defined as a separate disease by Guilleminault in 1973 is renamed as "Sleep Apnea-Hypopnea Syndrome" in 1988 by the identification of hypopneas with polysomnography (Erdamar, 2007).

In 1997, ASDA (American Sleep Disorder Association) has defined obstructive sleep apnea syndrome as "A syndrome characterized by recurrent obstructions in upper respiratory tract (URT) during sleep and seen often with a decrease in oxygen saturation". The prevalence of the disease is 1-5%. Even generally knowing the risk factors during the beginning of this disease, which has no less than prevalence of Diabetes (Diabetes Mellitus) and Bronchial Asthma, the physiopathology of the obstructions are not totally explained.
By a general evaluation, the stopping of breathing during sleep for at least 10 seconds is defined as '*sleep apnea*'. Due to stopping of breathing during sleep, sleep qualities of such patients are disturbed since they often wake up at night. Additionally, they become sleepy during most of the day and have promoted degrees of pulmonary artery pressure and arterial P_{CO_2}. Sleep apnea is mostly observed amongst premature infants, adult males and post-menopausal women (Firat, 2003).
The frequency of occurrence of apneas is high in obese and snoring individuals with narrow URT. Apneas can be observed in the stages of sleep other than rapid eye movement (REM) and non-REM (NREM) stages. The apnea types occurring during sleep and respiratory parameters related to these types can be defined as follows.

1.3 Sleep apnea and its types

In literature, there are three types of sleep apnea. These are listed as central, obstructive and mixed apnea. Obstructive sleep apnea (OSA) has the highest prevalence. Together with the absence of respiratory effort in the lungs, the absence of air flow inside the mouth and nose is defined as central sleep apnea. Despite the respiratory effort, the lack of air flow in the nose and mouth is obstructive sleep apnea. The situation starting with central sleep apnea and continuing as obstructive sleep apnea is defined as mixed sleep apnea. Mixed apnea patients can be treated by the methods applied to the patients with obstructive sleep apnea. Obstructive sleep apnea is the most common sleep apnea syndrome (Aydin et al., 2005).
Obstructive sleep apnea is the state of absence of oral and nasal air flow despite the respiratory effort. Although the diaphragm and intercostal muscle activity continued, exchange of air through the nose and mouth stands (Aydin et al., 2005). In this case, it Is thought to be an obstruction at the URT of patient. In order to prevent the blockage, an intense activity in the chest and abdomen is observed.
Central sleep apnea (CSA) is the state in the absence of both respiratory effort and air flow together. Central apneas grow by the corruption of the central regulation of respiration.
Mixed sleep apnea is the state starting with central sleep apnea and continuing the absence of oral and nasal air flow when the respiratory effort begins. How the respiratory effort after the central sleep apnea starts is still a unresolved research topic. In the new terminology, mixed apneas are discussed as obstructive apneas.

1.4 Sleep respiratory parameters

There are a few basic definitions of sleep respiratory parameters in literature. *Hypopnea* is the 50% reduction of air flow during sleep for at least 10 seconds, 3% decrease in blood oxygen saturation or the staging of arousal. *Arousal* is defined as sudden sleep state transition to lighter sleep stages or wakefulness. Arousal terminates the apnea or hypopnea. *Apnea Index (AI)* is defined as the number of apneas per hour during sleep *Apnea+Hypopnea Index (AHI)* is defined as the number of apneas and hypopneas per hour during sleep. It is also called as *Respiratory Distress Index (RDI)*. *Respiratory Arousal Index (RAI)* is defined as the number of arousals per hour during sleep. *Obstructive Sleep Apnea* is the situation AHI>5 during sleep. *Obstructive Sleep Apnea Syndrome* is the clinical situation that AHI>5 and major symptoms (snoring, witnessed apnea, excessive daytime sleepiness or drowsiness) met together.

Central Sleep Apnea Syndrome is the situation where more than 50% of detected apneas are central type. The physician examining the patients with sleep respiratory parameters suggest the diagnosis of sleep apnea syndrome.

Therefore, the scoring process performed over the PSG data obtained after sleep recording operations is extremely critical, specialized work, time consuming and inferential process (Roche et al. 1999; Firat, 2003; Aydin et al., 2005).

1.5 Previous studies for the detection and classification of sleep apnea

In sleep analyzing studies, there are a lot of approaches which are about detection and classification of sleep apnea. In recent years, the popular studies contain automated detection and classification of sleep apnea. The newly developed techniques have given an increased speed to the classification and detection of sleep apnea. However, these new techniques are usually built over the detection over a data scored by a health authority. Few works have tried to construct an automated system which will detect or classify the measured data and score by itself. Most of the automated systems developed in this manner have used only one bio-signal to detect or classify the apnea. However, a fusion of features extracted from the multiple bio-signals (ECG and EEG synchronization) can be expected to give better success rates for the detection and classification.

Another interesting issue for the previously studied works is the classifier selection. Most of the works are designed to work on neural networks. Thoroughly, sleep EEG series recorded from patients are classified by using Feed Forward Neural Network (FFNN). The NN architecture has several numbers of neurons and hidden layers. This method shows that the degree of central EEG synchronization during night sleep is closely related to CSA and OSA (Aksahin et al., 2010). However, neural networks are very unstable structures when the design constraints are not selected carefully. In contrasting, very few of the works use well-known stable classifier such as support vector machines (SVM). Additionally, it is possible to use a feature selection scheme to observe the effects of the features to the success rates.

Khandoker et al. (Khandoker, 2009a) proposed an SVM based algorithm to identify Obstructive Sleep Apnea Syndrome (OSAS) over 125 patients by using their 8-hour-long ECG recordings. They achieved high success rates to classify OSAS and non-OSAS patients. Their method covers determining the class of a patient. However, they do not mention where the apnea occurs. In the same year, Khandoker et al. (Khandoker, 2009b) tried to differentiate between OSAS and hypopnea patient in a similar methodology. Mendez et al. (Mendez, 2008) have developed an autoregressive model to screen sleep apnea from a single ECG lead. They used RR intervals and the area of QRS complex as their features for the analysis. According to Xu et al. (Xu, 2009), it is possible classify the sleep apnea by monitoring the variations on heart rate variability (HRV) signal.

Another approach to detect the OSAS patient is to use EEG signal as a source to generate features from Liu et al. (Liu, 2008) have proposed a neural network based detection method for OSAS and narcolepsy patients. They used the energy of EEG signal, theta and beta wave activities as features to detect patients correctly.

In literature, there are no previous works combining the detection and classification procedures. In this context, an automated system can be constructed to detect apnea regions and classify them as obstructive, central or mixed apnea as a new approach.

This shows it is a new area in biomedical engineering and it needs some good research to reveal the relationships between bio-signals and sleep apnea. In order to detect apnea, this chapter presents a methodology over ECG recordings, which contains time and frequency domain features. Moreover, EEG recordings are used to verify the detection of sleep apnea. The basic frequency domain features of ECG are very low frequency (VLF), low frequency (LF), high frequency (HF), the ratio of LF and HF (LF/HF) over HRV information. To obtain true HRV information, we will use Teager's energy operator to detect R-R durations. The Teager energy operator (Hamila et al., 1999) was first defined over real-valued signals and then defined for multidimensional continuous-domain signals and used for image demodulation. From the first appearance of the Teager energy operator, it has been used in several applications such as one dimensional (1-D) signal processing, image processing, and color image processing.

There are previously very few works about Teager energy operator for detection of RR intervals. We will also use wavelet information to find the exact positions for P, Q-R-S and T complexes. In addition, TEO is used for other physiological signals (speech, EEG etc.). For EEG signals, short time period correlations and power spectral densities will reveal the apnea regions and help us to find the type of apnea. Power spectral densities are calculated by a few methods for example Pyulear, Welch, Burg (Stoica, 1997). These features will have valuable information for the classification of apnea types. In extent, the change in frequency features of HRV information will help us to detect the apnea regions. The consideration of this change can be determined by using statistical methods such as Annova-Mannova, and types of t-test (Gula et al., 2003). These analyze methods can be used over the considerable measurements. Their logical validation is determined by using the reliability consistency test which is a statistical analysis method and measures how much accurate is a measurement set. For example, if a scale can give the same result with the measurement process repeated n times and statistical reliability factor is close to the value $\alpha= 1$, then we conclude that the *measurements of the scale are reliable*. The presence of the nonparametric variables in the physiological signals obtained from the patient shows the idea that the reliability test cannot be applied to these types of measurements.

2. Sleep recording and scoring

Sleep records began in the 1960s for the first time, took its final form with the addition of respiratory recordings and their final definition, which is still valid, is issued by Holland and his colleagues in 1974.

Holland used the term polysomnography to indicate the simultaneous recording, analysis and interpretation of various physiological parameters during the sleep through the night.

2.1 Polysomnograph and recording system

Polysomnography is mainly investigating the structure and physiological changes of sleep during sleep. This investigation provides reviewing sleep structure, psychological, biological and pathological changes in sleep by relating them with the sleep stages. Furthermore, it enables to investigate the sleep changes in human physiology under the conditions of sleep itself. During these investigations, whether a physiological event can be addressed alone, or multiple event and their implications can be explicated (Aydın et al., 2005).By examining data collected during sleep, the turn-up form, characteristics, the process and the response to the treatment of various diseases can be examined. In Fig. 1, output records for a sample polysomnogram are shown.

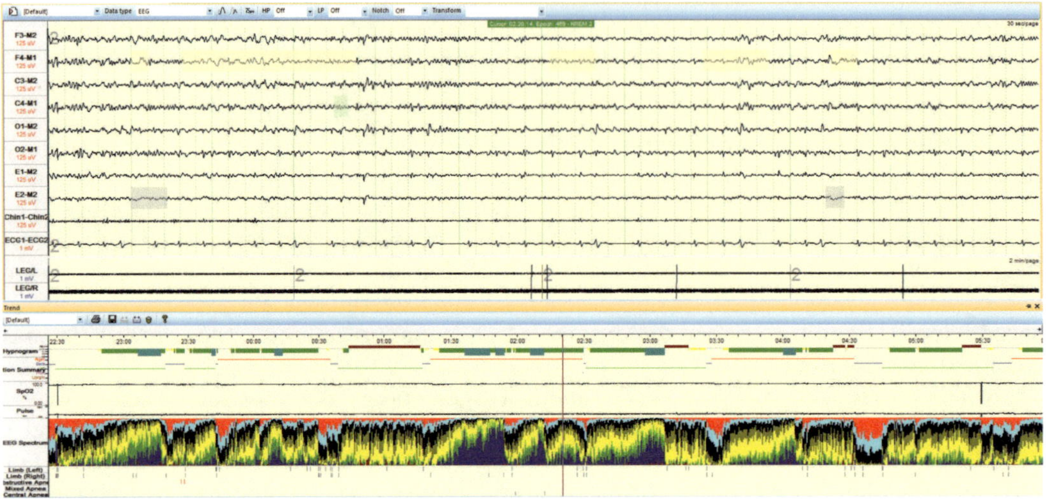

Fig. 1. Output records for a polysomnogram

Simultaneous recording of the sleep parameters should be able to give sufficient information about both the sleep and breathing pattern in sleep. In order to do staging of sleep, at least 2-channel EEG, EOG, chin EMG, oro-nasal air flow, arterial oxygen saturation, respiratory effort and ECG or pulse recordings must be done. In many cases, the anterior tibial EMG recording can be useful to detect periodic motion disorder.

Polysomnogram is used, in general, for the investigation, diagnosis and following up the treatment of sleep related breathing disorders.

2.2 Electrocardiogram (ECG) recordings

The technology interpreting the changes in electrical potential during heart activity is called as electrocardiography and the recorded by the device are called as electrocardiogram (ECG). Fig. 2 shows a normal ECG recording.

The duration of P wave and QRS complex is 0.1 seconds while the average wave amplitude (peak R) is around 1 mV. This peak value rarely rises up to 5 mV. These nominal values can change from one person to another by the patient's heart and body size and body conductivity.

2.3 Electroencephalography (EEG) recordings

EEG is the system used to measure and record the electrical activity of the brain. The brain waves obtained from EEG system have delta, theta, alpha, and beta wave bands.

Delta waves have 0.5-4 Hz frequency band with 20-400 µV amplitudes and are encountered in the situations of very low activity of brain, such as deep sleep and general anesthetic state.

Theta waves have 4-8 Hz frequency band with 100-500 µV amplitudes and are encountered in the situations of low activity of brain, such as dreaming sleep and medium anesthetic state.

Alpha waves have 8-13 Hz frequency band with 2-10 µV amplitudes and they are closest ones to the sinusoidal form between EEG waves. They are observed at awake individuals with closed eyes in a physically and mentally full resting condition.

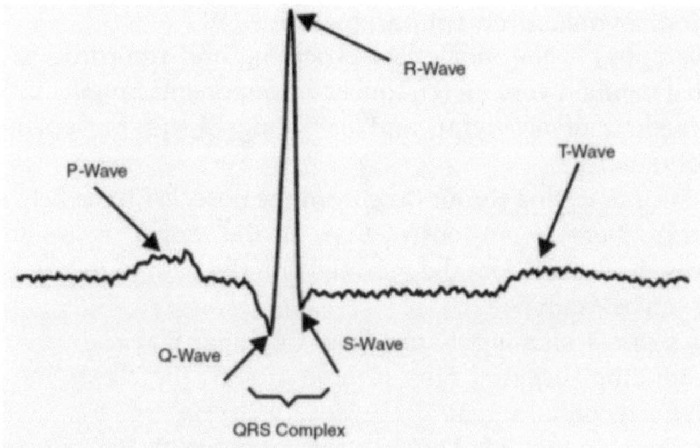

Fig. 2. QRS complex of a ECG signal (Köhler et al., 2002)

Beta waves are observed at the frequencies higher than 13 Hz and their amplitudes change in the range of 1-5 μV. They are observed at focused attention, mental working states, and rapid eye movement stages of sleep. These waves correspond to the level of the highest activity of the brain waves (Pehlivan, 2004).

By using EEG signals, sleep stages during the sleep period can be distinguished. These stages are divided into 5 classes. In general, as the sleep gets deeper, a frequency decrease in EEG signals. In sleep, there are two change stages following each other periodically. These are REM (Rapid Eye Movement - Paradoxical Sleep) and NREM (Non-Rapid Eye Movement) stages. The period between eyes shut to sleep and full sleep stage is called as the latent period of diving into sleep. After latent period, the exchange periods start.

NREM sleep is occasionally divided into 5 phases based on the electroencephalographic changes occurring during the course of sleep. Phase 0 is wakefulness stage, Phase 1 and 2 is the shallow sleep period, Phase 3 and 4 are the periods of deep sleep. It is possible to observe high amplitude low frequency waves and spindles in EEG. In this stage, there is no eye movements, muscle tones are decreased, pulse and respiratory are slowed. In Table 2, the phases of NREM sleep and their characteristics are given (Park, 2000).

REM sleep is the dream stage of sleep or the dreams seen in this stage can be remembered in wakefulness state. This stage is interspersed between the other phases of the sleep. It is connected with a large number of different features.

NREM Sleep Phases	Characteristics
Phase 0 (Wakefulness)	The stage before diving into sleep.
Phase I	The state one individual who is diving into sleep has faced. If the individual is forced to wake up in this phase of sleep, he will say he was usually awake even he was not aware of the events around him.
Phase II	In this phase of sleep, consciousness is in a state that he will be aware of he was in sleep when he was forced to wake up. EEG patterns can be seen. K- complex and sleep spindles are expected to be seen.
Phase III and IV	Low frequency deep sleep.

Table 2. NREM Sleep Phases and their characteristics.

2.4 Other physiological measurement parameters

EMG (Electromyography) is the method of observing and recording of skeletal electrical activity. EMG signals contain very high frequency components ranging between 10 and 5000 Hz. *EOG* is the method of observing and recording of eye movements resulting from electrical activity of muscles.

Thermistor is the sensor detecting the air flow from the nose. With the help of thermistor, it is determined whether there is an obstruction at the upper respiratory tract or not. Microphone records the sound from the mouth. With the help of microphone, the recorded sounds of snoring can be examined.

Thoracic respiratory signal, which is obtained from the expansion and narrowing of the chest, is recorded by wounding a special type of tape around the chest. The breathing can be examined through the recorded signal.

SpO_2 is the signal showing the blood oxygen saturation. With the signal recorded through PPG device, amount of change of oxygen in the blood after breathing is analyzed.

3. The sleep apnea features based on electrocardiogram (ECG) and electroencephalogram (EEG) biosignals

Sleep apnea detection approach over ECG and EEG physiological signals taken from polysomnograph recently appears to be a popular study. The methods apart from the classical methods followed by the physician to detect sleep apnea is based on the examination of features correlated with the sleep apnea from ECG and EEG signals to construct an automatic decision support mechanism.

3.1 Sleep apnea features based on electrocardiogram biosignals

Heart rate variability (HRV) information takes the first place amongst the researchers conducted on ECG physiological signals. Heart rate variability is related to the nature and the presence of sleep apnea. While many commercial medical equipments measure the automatically, they cannot bring a fully automated approach on detection and diagnosis of disorders such as sleep apnea.

Heart rate variability includes many features in both time and frequency domains and needs different methods in calculation of these features. ECG raw data, which is analyzed statistically in both time and frequency domains, is separated as short term and long term by the length of data (Camm et al., 1996).

3.1.1 Calculation of heart rate variability

In order to perform the calculation of heart rate variability from the ECG signal, first of all, R-wave detection needs to be done as much as possible. There are many approaches in detection of R-wave in the literature. Some of these methods are summarized in Table 3.

For example, there are methods based on wavelet transform and digital filtering for R-wave detection. In order to remove noise from ECG signal, it is passed through a wavelet transform block and QRS complex is emphasized in contrast to P and T waves by the moving average based low pass filter given in Eq. 1. In Eq. 1, y1 is the output signal, x[n] is the input signal and M is regarded as the length of the filter. Later, the processed ECG signal, which is passed through a nonlinear amplifier, is applied to an adaptive thresholding block (Chen et al., 2006).

$$y_1 = \frac{1}{M}\sum_{m=0}^{M-1} x[n-m] \tag{1}$$

Teager Energy Operator (TEO)
Wavelet Transform
Support Vector Machines
Pan- Tompkins Algorithm
Filtering in Frequency Domain
Zero Crossing Rate

Table 3. R-wave Detection Methods

From Table 3, it can be said that the most commonly used method is the Teager energy operator based on derivative operation. Teager energy operator is a very convenient method for studying over a single component in both continuous and discrete domains. It carries a lot of attributes together and is derived from the signal energy. In continuous domain, Teager energy operator is defined as:

$$\Psi[x(t)] \triangleq \left(\frac{dx(t)}{dt}\right)^2 - x(t)\frac{d^2x(t)}{dt^2} \tag{2}$$

Teager energy operator is applied off-line over the signal on the basis of discrete time domain. Sampled at a particular frequency, ECG signal is applied to the discrete version of the Teager energy operator given below:

$$\Psi[x(n)] = x^2(n) - x(n+1)x(n-1) \tag{3}$$

Teager energy operator covering the three samples of the signal side by side, shows a very local feature of the signal (Kaiser, 1993). In Fig. 3, an exemplary sequence of the ECG signal and the corresponding output of the Teager energy operator is given.

Before applying the Teager energy operator, ECG signal must be freed from noise. These noises are usually seen as baseline drift and motion artifact. In both time and frequency domains, there are algorithms used to eliminate these types of noises. For example, if there is a low frequency noise on ECG signal, a "moving average filter" in time domain (Rangayyan, 2002) or high-pass filters in frequency domain are applied.

After the TEO algorithm is applied to ECG signal, a threshold value comparison should be made to determine the R-wave peak points. 60% of the maximum value of the output signal from TEO block can be chosen as the threshold value. If the output of TEO exceeds the threshold at time t0 and no greater value in the next 0.25 seconds is observed, t0 is marked as R-wave peak point (Erdamar, 2007). TEO output of a sample ECG signal and detected R wave peaks after the threshold comparison is shown in Fig. 4.

Heart rate variability is defined as the time differences between the two consecutive R-wave peak points and are expressed in units of milliseconds or seconds. Heart rate variability data given in Fig. 5 is examined in both time and frequency domains. In case of missing R wave or finding extra R waves, we can observe upside or downside peaks on the HRV data. In order to eliminate this situation, an adaptive thresholding algorithm must be applied to detect R-wave peak points.

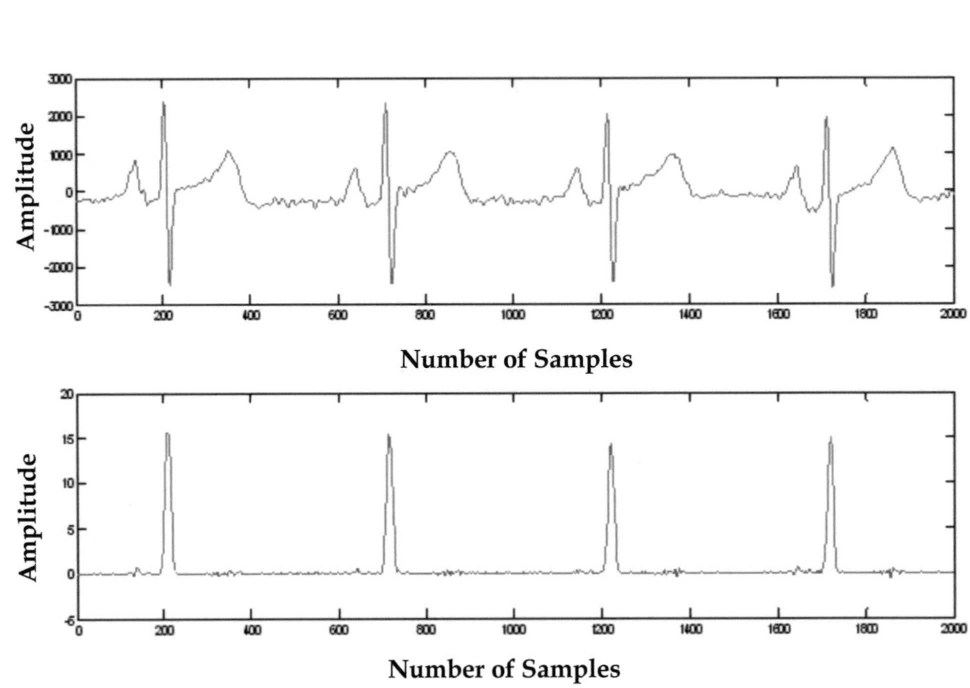

Fig. 3. ECG signal (top) and TEO output (bottom)

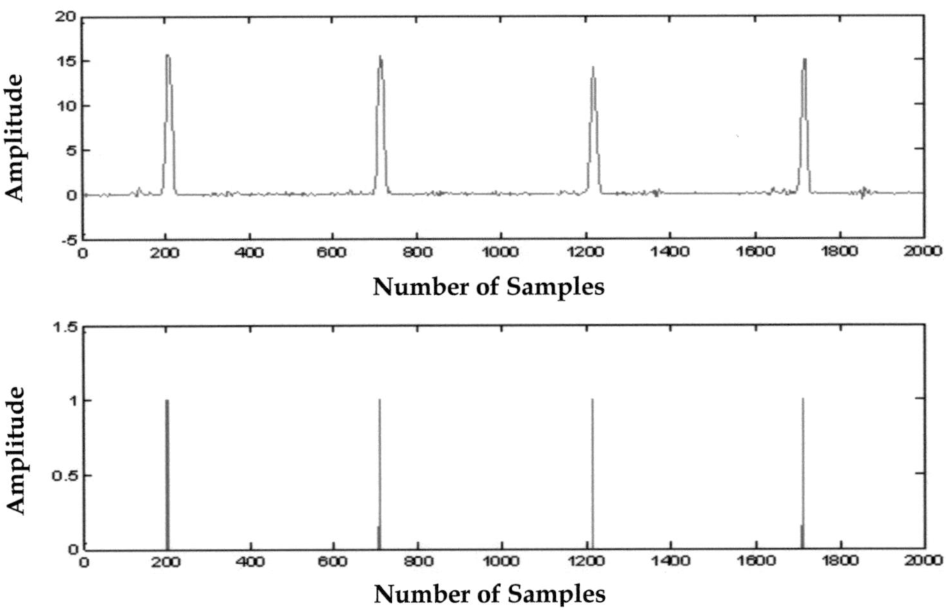

Fig. 4. TEO output of ECG signal (top) and detected R-wave peak points(bottom)

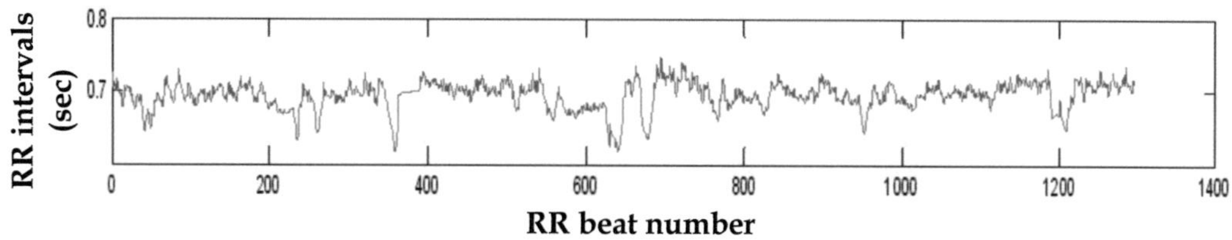

Fig. 5. Heart rate variability obtained from ECG signal

HRV parameter can be used to obtain the time and frequency domain features given in Table 4. Time domain features are calculated over 24 hours (long term) recordings and frequency domain features are calculated over 2-5 minutes (short term) recordings (Camm et al., 1996; Roche et al., 2002). The difficulty of the long term analysis is the impossibility of finding 24 hours noiseless raw data.

Time Domain Features		
SDNN	Standard deviation of all normal RR intervals	long term
SDANN	Standard deviation of the mean of all consecutive 5 minute segments of normal RR intervals	long term
SDNN index	Mean of the standard deviation of consecutive 5 minute segments	long term
r-MSSD	Root mean square of successive differences between adjacent normal RR intervals	long term
NN50 count	Number of pairs of adjacent NN intervals differing by more than 50 ms in the entire recording. Three variants are possible counting all such NN intervals pairs or only pairs in which the first or the second interval is longer.	long term
pNN50	NN50 count divided by the total number of all NN intervals.	long term
Frequency Domain Features		
VLF	Very low frequency 0.015- 0.04 Hz	short term
LF	Low frequency 0.04-0.15 Hz	short term
HF	High frequency 0.15- 0.4 Hz	short term
LF/HF		Short term

Table 4. Time and Frequency Domain Features of HRV

While the time domain analyses are calculated through HRV itself, the frequency domain analyses are calculated through the power spectral density of HRV. In order to do a frequency domain analysis, HRV must be freed from its DC component and resampled at 2 Hz.

In most studies, it is observed that the power spectral densities obtained from the signals containing the sleep apnea syndrome have more intense low frequency (LF) components than that of the normal signals. After the treatment of sleep apnea it is usually seen that low frequency density has decreased and converged to the nominal values of normal individuals (Roche et al., 1999).

Table 5 exhibits the time and frequency domain feature values of a normal individual (Camm et al., 1996). On the other hand, it is possible to obtain different feature values over data gathered from different patient groups and different polysomnography devices. The reasons for these differences are the resolution of the device and patients having different characteristics of physiological parameters affecting AHI values. We suggest creating simultaneously a control group of healthy subjects as a reference in HRV analysis procedures.

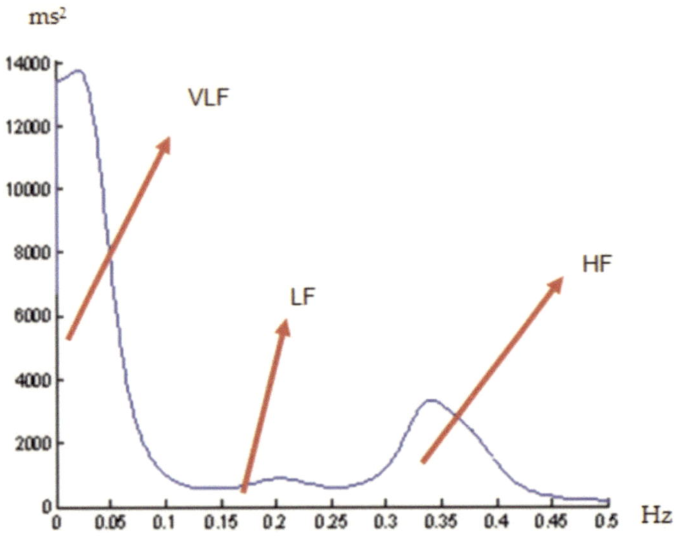

Fig. 6. Power Spectral Density of HRV

Choosing the created control group as a reference and analyzing the other patient groups will be useful to obtain statistically significant results.
Statistical methods, such as Anova-Manova, student's t test, multi variable regression and correlation, are used for scientific analysis of the features obtained from the spectral analysis of HRV. For instance, ANOVA test can be applied to show the statistical difference between groups of patients with sleep apnea. Within the scope of this test, it is clarified as a result that two groups are different when $P<0.05$ between the groups is achieved (Gula et al., 2001).

Variables	Units	Normal Values (mean ± SD)
Time Domain Analysis of 24 h		
SDNN	ms	141±39
SDANN	ms	127±35
RMSSD	ms	27±12
Spectral analysis of stationary supine 5-min recording		
Total power	ms^2	3466±1018
LF	ms^2	1170±416
HF	ms^2	975±203
LF/HF ratio	nu	

Table 5. Normal values of HRV features

Another statistical methods based parameter is Form Factor. This parameter is a statistical value depending on the exchange of activity amongst one-second-long signals (Hjorth, 1973; Rangayyan, 2002).
In form factor calculation, σ_x^2 (activity-variance) and μ_x (variability) are used. In Eq. 4, the formula for variability and in Eq. 5, form factor formula is given.

$$\mu_x = \left(\frac{\sigma_{x'}^2}{\sigma_x^2}\right)^{1/2} \tag{4}$$

$$FF = \left(\frac{\mu_{x'}}{\mu_x}\right) \tag{5}$$

3.2 The features based on electroencephalogram biosignals

EEG signals are another physiological signal type used in the detection and classification of sleep apnea. Due to the morphological properties separating from the ECG signals, they are applied to different analyses. Since sleep apnea is a ten second long event, they can usually be detected by an examination of epochs before and after sleep apnea. If the analyses cover 20-30 seconds part, they contain macro structure. The processes such as spindle scaling, slow wave activities, and arousal detection are included in macro structure analysis (Malinowska et al., 2006).
In Fig. 7, a regular part of the respiratory system and the corresponding sub-band representation of the EEG signal in that epoch are shown. The horizontal axis represents the time and the vertical axis represents amplitude. In occurrence of sleep apnea, changes observed at the corresponding sub-band range.

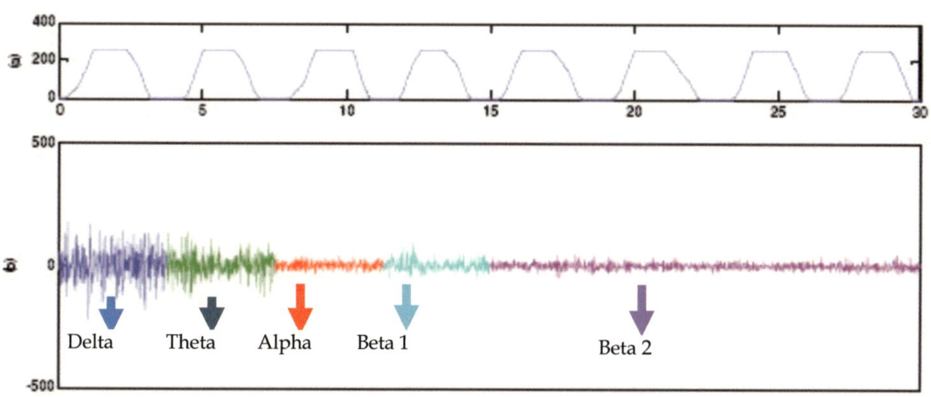

Fig. 7. a) Thermistor signal b) EEG sub-bands

In Fig. 8, respiratory signal with apnea and the corresponding sub-bands of EEG signal are shown. In this representation, change in the sub-bands of the EEG section corresponding to the respiratory signal with apnea is observed. The existence and amount of this change can be proved by calculating power spectral density. The analyses are made over 10 second portions within the scope of micro structure (Erdamar, 2007).
Some approaches are based on the EEG arousal detection of micro-structures. This is because the EEG signal of a patient diagnosed with OSA contains arousal structures during

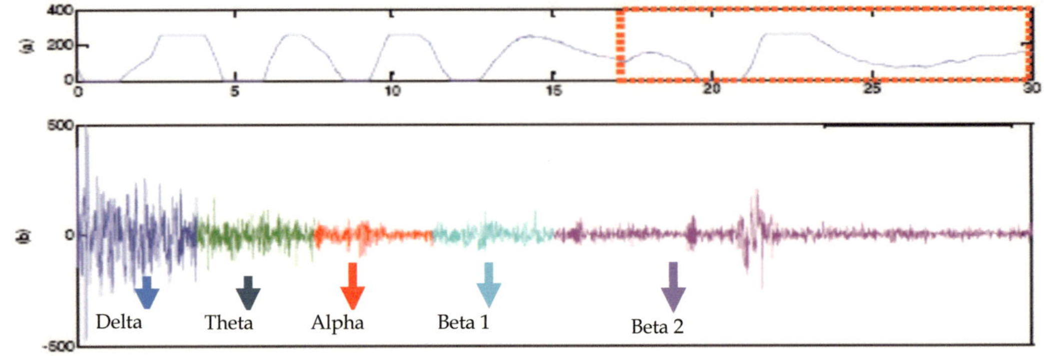

Fig. 8. a) Thermistor signal b) EEG sub-bands

sleep apnea. In detection of arousal structures, data from EEG, pressure and temperature of thermistor, chin-EMG, and tibialis EMG are used.

In order to detect the status that arousal response is longer than 3 seconds, the PSG data is examined in 1.28-second segments with a 0.4 Hz frequency resolution. Chin-EMG and tibialis EMG records are important for the detection of pathological events. Since arousal events inside the EEG signal generates rapid changes in all frequency components, direct analysis methods give no results (Sugi, 2008).

In addition, the important alterations are observed on previous divisions of sleep apneas. In sleep apnea events, the most significant alternations are observed in alpha and beta waves. These alterations cannot be realized in whole EEG spectrum because of their sizes. Therefore, EEG signals can be analyzed by using short time fouirer transform of narrow windows (Erdamar, 2007).

4. Results

The R detection algorithm based on TEO and adaptive thresholding (Fig.3 and Fig 4.) was applied over 600 epochs (200 epochs normal patients, 200 epochs OSA, 200 epochs CSA). The LF/HF rates calculated from HRV of these patients are shown in Table 6.

											mean LF/HF
Normal Patient 1	0.73	0.49	0.3	0.81	0.3	0.73	0.671	0.7	0.21	0.89	0.58
Normal Patient 2	0.4	0.64	1.126	0.45	0.66	0.82	0.9	0.86	0.23	1.52	0.76
OSA 1	0.87	0.97	1.45	1.15	1.46	1.28	1.42	1.81	1.03	2.6	1.4
OSA 2	1.1	3.4	1.1	5.3	1.58	3.5	1.1	1.87	5	2.5	2.7
CSA 1	2.03	5.21	0.520	1.21	0.59	0.74	2.149	0.35	0.71	2.747	1.63
CSA 2	3.09	1.13	0.73	1.06	1.62	1.15	3.12	0.49	1.22	1.33	1.5

Table 6. LF/HF rates of three different patients

In Table 6, it is shown that the LF/HF rates of OSA and CSA are higher than normal patients' values. This difference is visible on Table 6 but, we need to do a statistical test to prove the difference. In this context, the statistical data of the LF / HF rates obtained from 600 epochs (300 minutes) ECG recordings is gathered in Table 7.

		Number of Epoch	
Normal	OSA	200 - 200	P=0.000 (<0.05)*
Normal	CSA	200 - 200	P=0.004 (<0.05)*
OSA	CSA	200 - 200	P=0.001 (<0.05)*

*Statistically significant

Table 7. Independent samples T-test between the patients groups

In independent samples T-test, P value less than 0.05 means that analyzed two groups are statistically different from each other. The results show that OSA, CSA and normal diagnosed patients can be separated by a statistical analysis on change of LF / HF rates of each other.

In order to observe the ability to separate between the epochs with and without apnea, paired sampled t-test analysis method is used. In Table 8, it is shown that 10 epochs with apnea and 10 epochs without apnea of an OSA patient are statistically different from each other (P = 0.006 <0.05).

This statistical result scientifically indicates that the parts with apnea have different morphological features than the ones without apnea even for the same patient's 24 hours (long term) ECG recordings.

		Paired Differences					t	df	Sig. (2-tailed)
					95% Confidence Interval of the Difference				
		Mean	Std. Deviation	Std. Error Mean	Lower	Upper			
Pair 1	apnea osa18 - non-apnea osa18	3.89091	3.74696	1.12975	1.37367	6.40815	3.444	10	**.006**

Table 8. Paired Samples Test Outputs

On the other hand, form factor (FF) calculation can be shown as a different approach for the detection of sleep apnea and different approach from literature. FF calculations made for a segment from 160 msec before to 240 msec after of each detected R-wave of the ECG signal can be thought as a determining factor for predicting the sleep apnea. In experimental works, a threshold FF value was determined in ECG recordings to identify apnea. In this context, apnea is appeared for 4 and upper FF values in ECG recordings. Fig. 9 corresponds to the FF series of an ECG recording with apnea.

In Fig. 10, the thermistor signal with 256 Hz sampling frequency of non-apnea patient and corresponding FF values calculated on ECG signal are given. When a number of FF values obtained from apnea and non-apnea patient recordings with equal length are examined, a decrease in heart rate in case of apnea is found.

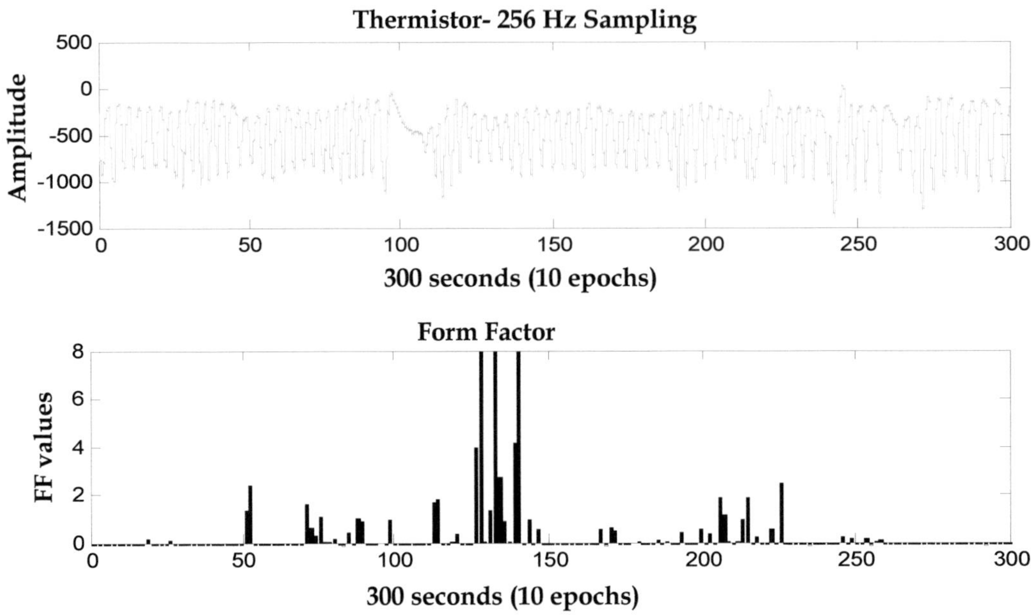

Fig. 9. Thermistor signal with apnea and corresponding FF values

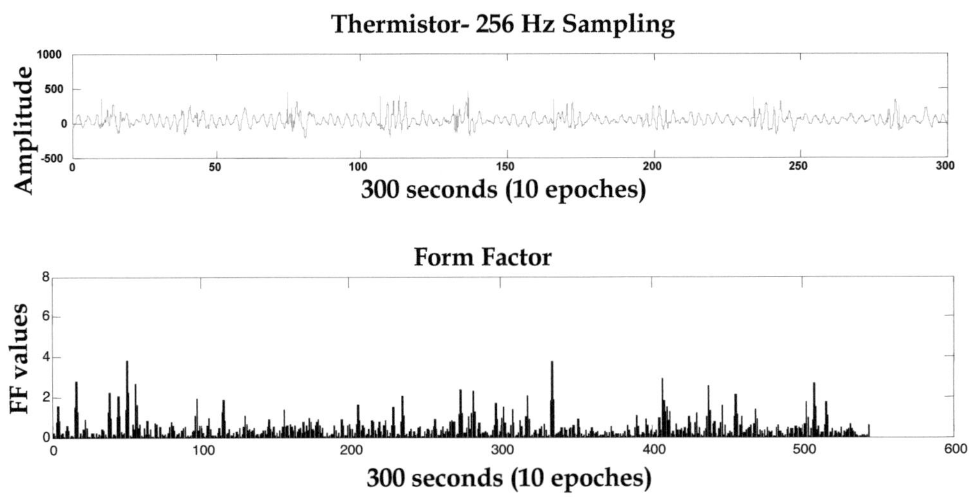

Fig. 10. Thermistor signal without apnea and corresponding FF values

In the ECG signal without apnea, more R-waves is found and as a result of that phenomena, it is understood that power spectral density of HRV has shifted to HF area. Thus, FF values are closely related to apnea events over ECG recordings.

5. Conclusion

Due to the fact that human physiology do not continuously respond in the same way to the same stimulus, both automated and adaptive analysis procedures over biosignals are limited. Thus, the sections, that have negative effect on variance and cause the algorithm to work inaccurately, are removed from the ECG signal and then the HRV analysis is done. When an automated system is requested, a general algorithm that can remove these corrupted fields from the ECG signal can be written at most. For this purpose, it is possible to find approaches in both time and frequency domains.

In detection and classification of sleep apneas, usage of support vector machines (SVM) instead of neural network based algorithms may be a better and more original approach. SVM, similar to neural networks, uses a part of the data for training purposes and the rest of data to testing purposes. On contrary, by its structure, it can present a more determined working strategy in contrast to neural networks.

It is possible to obtain a very good HRV curve with the help of an algorithm that does not miss R-peaks as much as possible. In order to investigate the frequency domain attributes of HRV, the frequency characteristics are obtained from the HRV after the fast fourier transform (FFT) of it calculated. Thus, the features obtained from healthy patients and patients with sleep apnea can be easily differentiated.

With a quite smooth algorithm, the obtained HRV curves from the healthy patients fluctuate around a constant value in the amplitude range. In the fourier domain, we get the results in discrete time series.

For the detection of QRS complex, finding many adaptive approaches are possible. From the output of Teager energy operator, 60% of the average of the magnitudes of previous detected consecutive n (<6) R-peaks can be used as the threshold value for the detection of current R-peak. Thus, it will be possible to detect signal with slowly changing magnitude threshold value will be adaptive to catch the magnitudes correctly. However, the signal loss due to the misplacement of electrodes on the surface of body cannot be recovered with this adaptive structure. Actually, there is possibly no way to get the signal from nothing.

Another approach in design of an automated system can be a template matching algorithm. The basic requirement for this algorithm is the selection of a good clean QRS complex. There are numerous methods to decide a clean signal. If the cross correlation between the signal and the selected QRS complex, we get normalized outputs peaking at the R-peaks. In order to improve the results, this operation can be applied before the TEO operator and adaptive thresholding. This approach will give a more precise and an automated result. This operation is done by the normalized cross-correlation formulation given as:

$$\text{Normalized Cross Correlation Function} = \frac{\sum_{i=0}^{N-1}(\text{temp}_i - \overline{\text{temp}}) * (\text{ecg}_i - \overline{\text{ecg}})}{\sqrt{\sum_{i=0}^{N-1}(\text{temp}_i - \overline{\text{temp}})^2 * \sum_{i=0}^{N-1}(\text{ecg}_i - \overline{\text{ecg}})^2}} \quad (6)$$

temp= chosen template QRS complex
ecg_i = windowing of raw ECG (size of temp)
ecg=raw data

The critical point of this methodology is that the correct choice of the QRS template should be done automatically. Selections can lead to incorrect outputs with a wrong template, and this may lead other analyses converge to an erroneous point.

During a decrease in the respiratory frequency, physiological systems of human body also reduce heart rhythm in order to provide homeostasis. In this way, oxygenated blood to spill all the biological system is more efficient.

A slowdown in heart rhythm causes observing the HRV power spectral density to shift to VLF-LF region. In the normal case, an opposite loop is provided, and the HRV power spectrum density increases towards HF band.
Within the scope of sleep apnea detection processes, it is needed to use statistical analysis softwares to make sense in the scientific manner from the results. For example, for two different groups of independent samples, it is possible to prove that they different from each other in statistical sense by t-test.
Pulse Transit Time (PTT), which will constitute the basis of the study, is thought to be a very strong microstructure for the detection of sleep apnea and obtained from ECG, EEG and PPG signals. PTT analyses can rarely be seen in the literature (Smith et al. 1999). PTT is the duration of arterial pulse pressure occurring during the instance of pumping of blood from aortic leaflet to peripherals (limbs). PTT can be detected by reference to R-peaks on ECG signals.
After the ventricle depolarization corresponding to a R-peaking, PTT can be taken as the time of transmission of blood pressure to the fingers. For this purpose, the PPG signal from the oxygen plethysmograph probe is needed. The PPG located inside the PSG system with the name PLETH provides this data. By looking at the average duration of PTT, we can make a correlation analysis on respiratory effort. As a result of this analysis, the features to detect sleep apnea can be obtained (Pitson et al., 1995).
The experimental studies show that HRV power spectral densities in patients with OSA and CSA shift towards the low frequency (VLF-LF) band while a dense nature in high frequency (HF) band is observed for normal patients. In this extent, the statistical analyses before and after uvulopalatofarengoplasti (UPPP) surgical operation, one of the methods used in treatment of sleep apnea, can be a good approach to measure the performance of the surgical operation. Another study conducted by our group is the evaluation of statistical analysis methods on the preoperative and postoperative sleep time and frequency domain parameters.
It is thought that a prediction to sleep apnea and an implementation of indirect diagnosis system to help the physician are possible by investigating the cases called microstructures, which are impossible to see on ECG signals and EEG sub-bands, in the 1-2 epochs before and after the parts that contain sleep apnea in the EEG and ECG signals. This approach can provide more specific and original results.

6. References

Aksahin, M.F. (2010). *Classification of Sleep Apnea Types*, Baskent University PhD Thesis, Ankara, Turkey

Aydin, H.; Ozgen, F.; Yetkin, S. & Sütcügil, L. (2005). *Sleep and Respiratory Disorders in Sleep*, GATA Printing House, Ankara, Turkey

Camm, A. J.; Malik, M.; Bigger, J. T.; Breithardt, G.; Cerutti, S.; Cohen, R. J.; Coumel, P.; Fallen, E. L.; Kennedy, H. L.; Kleiger, R. E.; Lombardi, F.; Malliani, A.; Moss, A. J.; Rottman, J. N.; Schmidt, G.; Schwartz, P. J. & Singer, D. H. (1996). *Heart rate variability-Standards of measurement, physiological interpretation, and clinical use*, European Heart Journal, Vol. 17, No.3, (March 1996), pp.354-381

Chen, S-W.; Chen H-C. & Chen H-C. (2005). A real time QRS detection method based on moving- averaging incorporating with wavelet denosing, *Elsevier Computer Methods and Programs in Biomedicine,* Vol. 82, No. 3, (November 2005), pp.187-195, ISSN 0169-2607

Erdamar, A. (2007). *A model development for prediction of sleep apnea and stimulation of genioglossus muscle,* Hacettepe University PhD Thesis, Ankara, Turkey

Erogul, O. (2008). Engineering Approaches in Sleep Studies, *Proceedings of 9th Sleep Medicine Congress,* Aydin, Turkey, 2008

Firat, H. (2003). Sleep apnea syndrome diagnosis (definition, physiopathology, clinic, diagnosis methods, scores), *Turkish Thoracic Society Second Winter School,* (January 2003), Lecture Notes

Gula,L.J.; Krahn, A.D.; Skanes, A.; Kathleen, A. F.; George, C.; Yee, R. and Klein G.J. (2003). Heart rate variability in obstructive sleep apnea: a prospective study and frequency domain analysis, *A.N.E, Vol. 8, No. 2,* (april 2003), pp. 144-149, ISSN 1542-474X

Hamila, R.; Astola, J.; Alaya Cheikh, F.; Gabbouj, M.; & Renfors, M. (1999). Teager energy and the ambiguity function, *IEEE Transactions on Signal Processing,* Vol. 47, No. 1, (January 1999), pp. 260-262, ISSN 1053–587X.

Hjorth, B. (1973). Physical significance of time domain descriptors in EEG analysis, *Electroencephalography and Clinical Neurophysiology,* Vol. 34, No. 3, (March 1973), pp. 321-325, ISSN 0013-4694

Kaiser, J. F., (1993). Some useful properties of teager's energy operators, *acoustics, speech and signal processing, ICASSP-93, IEEE International Conference,* Vol.3, Issue April 1993, pp.149-152, ISSN 1520-6149

Khandoker, A. H.; Palaniswami, M.; & Karmakar, C. K. (2009a), Automated scoring of obstructive sleep apnea and hypopnea events using short-term electrocardiogram recordings, *IEEE Transactions On Information Technology In Biomedicine,* Vol. 13, No. 6, (November 2009), pp. 1057-1067, ISSN 1089-7771.

Khandoker, A. H.; Gubbi, J.; & Palaniswami, M. (2009b), Support vector machines for automated recognition of obstructive sleep apnea syndrome from ECG recordings, *IEEE Transactions On Information Technology In Biomedicine,* Vol. 13, No. 1, (January 2009), pp. 37-48, ISSN 1089-7771.

Köhler, B-U.; Henning, C. & Orglmeister, R. (2002). The Principles of Software QRS Detection-Reviewing and Comparing Algorithms for Detecting this Important ECG Waveform, IEEE Engineering In Medicine And Biology, Vol. 21, No. 1, (January 2002), pp.42-57, ISSN 0739-5175

Liu, D.; Pang, Z.; Lloyd, S. R. (2008). Neural Network Method for Detection of Obstructive Sleep Apnea and Narcolepsy Based on Pupil Size and EEG, *IEEE Transactions on Neural Networks,* Vol. 19, No. 2, (February 2008), pp. 308-318, ISSN 1045-9227.

Malinowska, U.; Durka, P-J.; Blinowska K-J.; Szelenberger W. & Wakarow A. (2006). Micro and Macrostructure of Sleep EEG, *IEEE Engineering Medicine and Biology Magazine,* Vol. 25, No. 4, August 2006, pp. 26-31, ISSN 0739-5175

Mendez, M. O.; Bianchi, A. M.; Matteucci, M.; Cerutti, S.; & Penzel, T. (2008) Sleep Apnea Screening by Autoregressive Models From a Single ECG Lead, *IEEE Trans. on Biomed. Eng.,* Vol. 56, No. 12, ISSN 0018-9294.

Park, H. (2000). *Automated Sleep Stage Analysis Using Hybrid Rule-Based and Case-Based Reasoning,* Interdisciplinary Program of Medical and Biological Engineering Major Seoul National University PhD Thesis, Seoul, Korea

Pehlivan, F. (2004). Biophysics, Hacettepe Tas Printing, ISBN 975-7731-45-5

Pitson, D.J., Sandell, A., Hout, R.V., Stradling, J.R., 1995. Use of Pulse Transit Time as a Measure of Inspiratory Effort in Patients with Obstructive Sleep Apnoea, *European Respiratory Journal*, Vol.8, No.10, (October 1995), pp.1669-1674.

Rangayyan, R. M. (2002). *Biomedical Signal Analysis: A Case-Study Approach*, IEEE Press, ISBN 0-471-20811-6, USA

Roche, F.; Gaspoz, J-M.; Fortune, I.; Minini, P.; Pichot, V.; Duverney, D.; Costes, F.; Lacour J-R. & Barthelemy, J-C. (1999). Screening of Obstructive Sleep Apnea Syndrome by Heart Rate Variability Analysis, *Journal of the American Heart Assocation-Circulation*,Vol. 100, (June 1999), pp.1411-1415, 1524-4539

Roche F.; Duverney D.; Gortune-Court I.; Pichot V.; Costes F.; Lacour J-R.; Antonladis A.; Gaspoz J-M. & Barthelemy J-C. (2002). Cardiac Interbeat Interval Increment for the Identication of Obstructive Sleep Apnea, *Journal of Pacing and Clinical Electrophysilogy*, Vol. 25, No.8, (August 2002), pp.1192-1199, 10504-0418

Smith, P.R.; Argod, J.; Pepin, J.L. & Levy, P.A. (1999). Pulse Transit Time: An Appraisal of Potential Cliniccal Applications, *Journal of Throax*, Vol.54, No.5, (May 1999), pp.452 - 457,

Stoica, P. & Moses , R.L. (1997), *Introduction to spectral analysis*, Prentice Hall, ISBN: 0-13-258419-0, New Jersey, U.S.

Sugi, T.; Kawana, F. & Nakamura M. (2009). Automatic EEG Arousals Detection for Obstructive Sleep Apnea Syndrome, *Biomedical Signal Processing and Control,* Vol. 4, No. 4, (October 2009), pp. 329-337

Xu, W., & Liu, X. (2009), Sleep Apnea Assessment by ECG Pattern, *2nd International Congress on Image and Signal Processing, 2009. CISP '09*, ISBN: 978-1-4244-4129-7, Tianjin, China, October 2009.

13

Low Heart Rate Variability in Healthy Young Adult Males

Richard M. Millis, Stanley P. Carlyle, Mark D. Hatcher and Vernon Bond
Department of Physiology & Biophysics, College of Medicine, Howard University, Washington, DC, USA

1. Introduction

The autonomic nervous system coordinates a person's responsiveness to physiological and environmental stressors. Attenuated respiratory sinus arrhythmia (RSA) with small standard deviation of the normal-normal electrocardiogram RR intervals (SDNN) is found in subjects with low heart rate variability (HRV) by time domain analysis (Montano et al., 2009). Low HRV is also characterized by sympathovagal balance shifted toward sympathetic predominance observed as an increase in the low frequency/high frequency ratio by frequency domain (fast Fourier transform) spectral analysis (Montano et al., 2009). However, inter- and intra-individual spectral changes are highly variable (Taverner et al., 1996) and the physiological significance is not always clear. Paced breathing at 0.2 Hz normally shifts sympathovagal balance toward greater vagal and less sympathetic activity (Driscoll and Dicicco, 2000) because of increased tidal volume and/or minute ventilation (Pinna et al., 2006). Sympathovagal imbalance related to low HRV is a risk factor for hypertension and various other cardiovascular and non-cardiovascular diseases (Kuch et al., 2001; Montano et al., 2009). Epidemiological studies estimate that the prevalence of hypertension ranges from 8% in an urban adolescent population (Rabinowitz et al., 1993) to 43% in black physicians twenty-two years after medical school (Gillum, 1999). However, no studies have determined the incidence and behavioral significance of sympathovagal imbalance in healthy young adult African-Americans. Abnormal autonomic responsiveness to environmental stressors is thought to be an important factor in the evolution of essential hypertension (Fauvel et al., 1996; Mezzacappa et al., 2001; Lucini et al., 2002a; 2002b) and African-American males are a subpopulation at high risk for such hypertension (Gillum, 1979; Kaplan, 1994; Gillum, 1999). The present study was, therefore, designed to determine whether sympathovagal imbalance related to low HRV occurs in a population of healthy young adult African-American males and whether it is an indicator of abnormal responsiveness to environmental stressors.

2. Materials and methods

2.1 Study participants and design

The study protocol was approved by the Howard University Human Participants Institutional Review Board, and each subject provided informed consent. A study population of 52 healthy normotensive 18-26 year-old African-American male university students was included in the study. Criteria for inclusion in the study were: non-smoking status, absence of alcohol abuse (less than two standard alcohol drinks a day), absence of use of medication that could interfere with autonomic modulation, resting systolic/diastolic blood pressure <140/90 mm Hg and body mass index less than 28 kg m^{-1}.

2.1.1 Paced breathing

After entering the laboratory subjects were instrumented and instructed as to the experimental procedures. Subjects breathed normally while seated and at rest and 5 min of this resting data was recorded. Following the normal breathing protocol subjects were instructed to perform 5 min of paced breathing in such a manner that each respiratory cycle was 5 s in duration or 12 breaths per min (0.2 Hz). The subject observed a visual tracking image on a computer monitor for periodic durations of inspirations and expirations. Each subject practiced paced breathing for a period of 1 min and was then instructed to perform the paced respiration for 5 min during which time the electrocardiogram signal was recorded using a Biopac MP100 data acquisition system (Biopac Systems, Santa Barbara, CA). The electrocardiogram electrodes were placed on the subject's chest in a standard three-lead position with recordings obtained from lead II.

2.1.2 Group assignment

Two groups of subjects were a priori classified as either "broadband" or "narrowband". The criterion for the "narrowband" group was that the maximum SDNN value, a time-domain marker of vagal modulation, was more than one standard deviation below the mean SDNN for the study population during the 5 min trial of paced breathing. The "broadband" group, thereby, consisted of the subjects exhibiting SDNN one standard deviation less than that of the mean SDNN of the study population. Figure 1 shows cardiotachogram tracings of representative broadband and narrowband subjects.

2.1.3 Heart rate variability analyses

Heart rate was measured in beats · min^{-1} and vagal modulation of HRV in the time domain was measured as the standard deviation of all normal-to-normal standard electrocardiogram inter-beat intervals (SDNN). Time domain HRV, measured as standard deviation of the RR intervals, was expressed in ms and was computed using data acquisition and analysis software specifically designed to measure HRV in the time and frequency domain (Nevrokard, Version 6.3.1, Ljubljana, Slovenia). All time domain HRV data were reported herein as mean SDNN ± standard error. Fast Fourier transform analysis of the electrocardiogram RR intervals was used to spectrally decompose HRV in the frequency domain. For the frequency domain analysis, vagal modulation was represented by the area under the high-frequency power spectrum (HF: 0.14-0.4 Hz) expressed as the power in ms^2. We also included the LF/HF ratio of heart rate variability as a measure of sympathetic modulation according to the Task Force of the European Society of Cardiology and the North American Society of Pacing and Electrophysiology (1996). However, this concept has received great criticism (Eckberg, 1999). All time and frequency domain analyses were carried out in accordance with the guidelines put forth by the Task Force of the European Society of Cardiology and the North American Society of Pacing and Electrophysiology (1996).

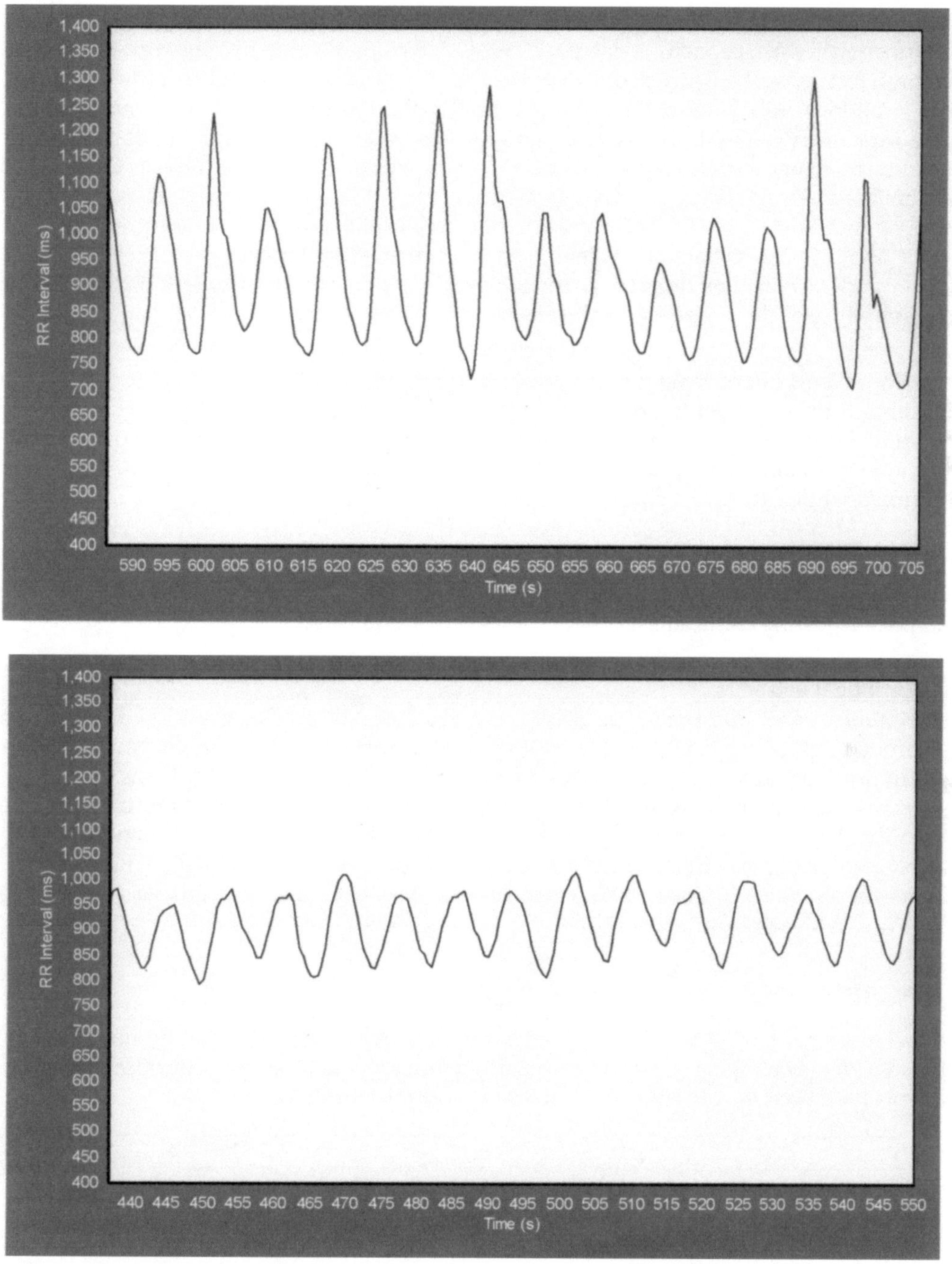

Fig. 1. **Electrocardiogram RR intervals for broadband and narrowband subjects.** Representative cardiotachogram tracings showing electrocardiogram RR intervals (ms) on the ordinate and time (s) on the abscissa for a representative subject exhibiting characteristics for assignment to the broadband group (Top Panel) and to the narrowband group (Bottom Panel).

2.1.4 Aerobic capacity (VO_{2peak})

The functional work capacity measure of VO_{2peak} was performed during a graded exercise treadmill test using the Bruce protocol with stage 1 beginning at an incline of 10% at a speed of 1.7 mph for 3 min. After stage 1, the treadmill incline was increased by 2% and the speed by 0.8 mph every 3 min until voluntary fatigue. Respiratory measures of ventilation and gas fractions of oxygen and carbon dioxide were performed using a Physio-Dyne Max I metabolic system (Physio-Dyne Inc., Quogue, NY). VO_{2peak} was defined as the VO_2 value achieved during the last min of the graded treadmill exercise test. Before the graded exercise test of VO_{2peak}, the metabolic system was calibrated with known gas concentrations of oxygen and carbon dioxide. The participants performed the VO_{2peak} test during the first laboratory visit at the beginning of the study.

2.1.5 Paced and uncontrolled spontaneous breathing conditions

The subjects were trained to breathe at 0.2 Hz by following an analog signal generated by a computer for timing the inspiratory and expiratory phases of respiration. Measurements of heart rate variability made during paced and uncontrolled spontaneous breathing were performed while sitting in a chair.

2.1.6 Mental and nociceptive stress conditions

Mental stress was produced by Stroop word-color conflict testing and physical stress by cold pressor testing using single foot immersion in an ice bath.

2.2 Statistical analysis

The significance of differences in SDNN, the absolute HF power, the LF/HF power was determined by comparing the paced breathing control to the spontaneous breathing condition using Student's t-test for paired samples. Linear regression analysis was used to verify the correlation between SDNN and HF power. The significance of intergroup ("broadband" vs. "narrowband") differences was determined using Student's t-test for independent samples. Probability for all analyses was set at $P<0.05$. Significance of differences in SDNN across testing conditions was evaluated by analysis of variance (ANOVA), with significance at $P<0.05$.

3. Results

Table 1 presents the physiological characteristics of the study population showing that it consisted of a healthy group of 18-26 year-old healthy male African-American university students measured during the paced breathing control condition.

Age (years)	20.92 ± 2.48
Weight (kg)	76.03 ± 10.89
Height (cm)	179.44 ± 7.06
Resting Systolic Blood Pressure (mm Hg)	130.08 ± 8.64
Resting Diastolic Blood Pressure (mm Hg)	76.36 ± 9.33
Resting Heart Rate (beats $\cdot$ min^{-1})	75.48 ± 9.65
Peak Oxygen Consumption (mL $\cdot$ kg^{-1} $\cdot$ min^{-1})	35.30 ± 7.28

* Mean ± standard deviation

Table 1. Physiological characteristics of the study population*

The heart rates of the study population measured during the normal spontaneous breathing condition were found to be lower than those measured during the paced breathing control condition (67.9 ± 1.8 vs. 70.1 ± 1.7, P=0.01); this difference was extremely small (3%) and, therefore, not of physiological significance. On the other hand, the heart rates measured during the Stroop word color conflict and cold pressor testing were 16% higher (81.3 ± 2.3 and 81.3 ± 2.3 vs. 70.1 ± 1.7, P<0.01, respectively) and the heart rates during exercise at 30%-50% of peak oxygen consumption were 34%-77% higher (94.5 ± 2.1 and 124.6 ± 3.5 vs. 70.1 ± 1.7, P<0.01, respectively) than those measured during the paced breathing control condition; these differences were considered to be physiologically significant.

The study group of 52 subjects was characterized by a maximum SDNN of 249.70 ms, a minimum SDNN of 39.15 ms and a mean ± standard deviation of 108.40 ± 40.95 ms during the paced breathing control condition. A subgroup of subjects met the criterion for low HRV (6/52, 12%) and, by experimental design, exhibited a very small SDNN, more than one standard deviation below the mean of the study population, during paced breathing at a fixed frequency (0.2 Hz). This subgroup was differentiated from the larger study group by a minimum SDNN of 39.15 ms, a maximum of 64.55 and a mean ± standard deviation of 49.40 ± 7.15 ms (P<0.0001).

Figure 1 demonstrates the range of SDNN values measured in this study and shows a significantly greater SDNN of the study population for the paced breathing control condition than for the two conditions of exercise at 30% and 50% of peak oxygen consumption (P<0.0001). SDNN measured during the periods of normal spontaneous breathing, at 0.18-0.48 Hz while at rest sitting in a chair and on a cycle ergometer, and Stroop word color conflict testing (mental stress) were smaller than the SDNN measured during the paced breathing control period and intermediate between the largest SDNN during paced breathing and the smallest SDNN measured measured during aerobic exercise (P<0.001). The SDNN measured during cold pressor testing (cold stress) was not significantly different that that during the paced breathing control (P>0.1).

Figure 2 shows that the SDNN of the study group during the control paced breathing was significantly greater than that during the uncontrolled spontaneous breathing, both measured while sitting in a chair (P<0.05). Figure 3 demonstrates that the group of 6 subjects ("narrowband" group) found to have significantly smaller SDNN of the remaining group of 46 subjects ("broadband" group) during normal spontaneous breathing (0.18-0.4 Hz), both measured at rest while sitting in a chair (P<0.05). Figure 4 shows that, between the normal spontaneous breathing and paced breathing conditions, the SDNN of this "low HRV, narrow heart rate bandwidth" or "narrowband" group of 6 subjects increased by 1.58 ± 13.59%; whereas, that of the remaining group of 46 "normal HRV, broad heart rate bandwidth" subjects ("broadband" group) increased by 30.41 ± 2.29% (P=0.0006) during paced breathing at 0.2 Hz.

Figure 5 presents a comparison of the SDNN of the broad and narrow heart rate bandwidth groups across all of the physiological states studied. By experimental design, the SDNN measured during the paced breathing control condition differentiated between the narrow and broad heart rate bandwidth groups which were also found to be differentiated by the SDNN measured during the normal spontaneous breathing state. These groups were not differentiated by the SDNN measured during the experimental conditions of Stroop word color conflict testing (mental stress), cold pressor testing (cold stress) and exercise at 30% and 50% of peak oxygen consumption.

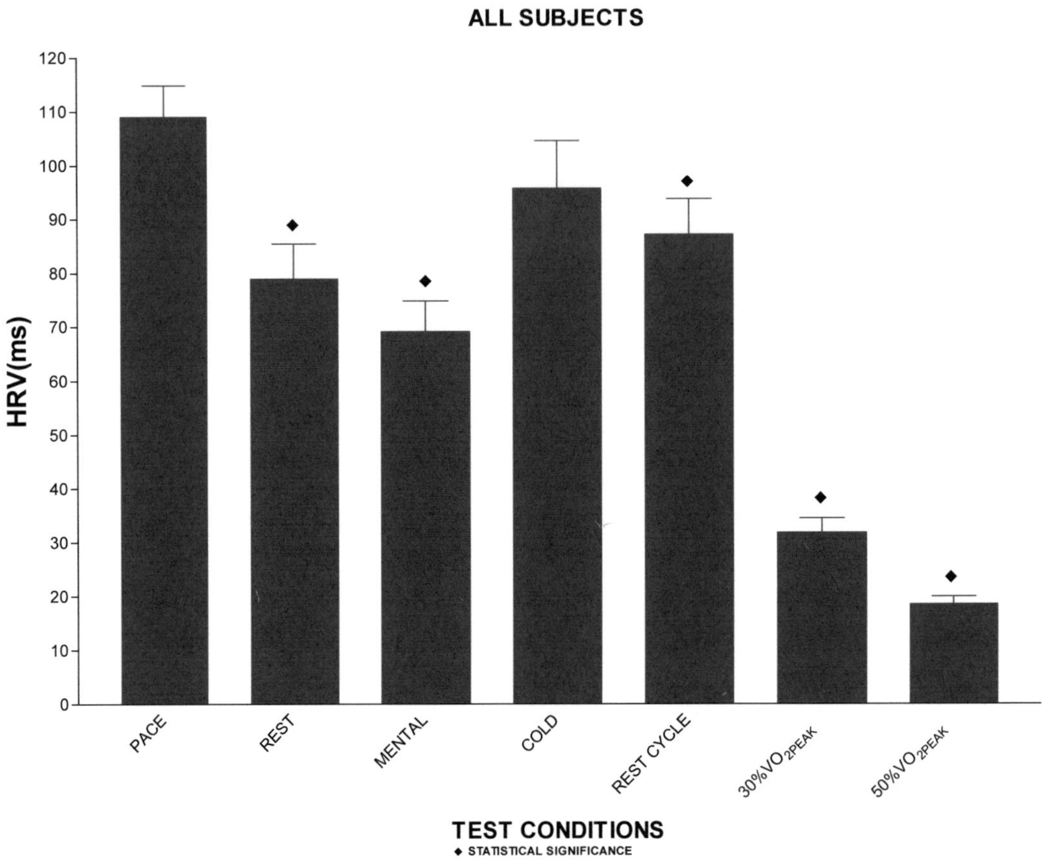

Fig. 2. **Heart rate variability across various testing conditions.** Bars represent heart rate variability (HRV, ms) expressed as time domain measure of mean standard deviation of normal-normal electrocardiogram RR intervals (SDNN) during paced breathing at 0.2 Hz (pace), normal uncontrolled spontaneous breathing at rest sitting in a chair (rest), Stroop word-color conflict testing of mental stress (mental), cold pressor testing of nociceptive stress (cold), normal uncontrolled spontaneous breathing at rest sitting on a cycle ergometer (rest cycle) and aerobic exercise stress at 30% and 50% of peak oxygen consumption (30% VO_{2peak}, 50% VO_{2peak}). Subjects are 52 healthy young adult African-American males. Data in mean ± standard error. ♦ SDNN different from paced breathing control (pace) at $P<0.05$.

The "broadband" group's total spectral power was significantly greater than the "narrowband" group's total HRV spectral power for paced but not for spontaneous breathing (16,600 ± 1,842 vs. 2,858 ± 176 ms^2, P=0.01 and 7,807 ± 1,224 vs. 2,106 ± 424 ms^2, P=0.1, respectively). The "broadband" versus "narrowband" intergroup difference in absolute LF power was not significant for spontaneous breathing. The "broadband" group's absolute LF power was significantly higher than the "narrowband" group's absolute LF power (12,830 ± 1,461 vs. 1,981 ± 296 ms^2, P=0.01) for paced breathing. The "broadband" group's absolute HF power was not significantly different than the "narrowband" group's absolute HF power for both paced and spontaneous breathing (P=0.12). The "broadband" versus "narrowband" intergroup difference in the percentages of total LF and HF power was also not significant.

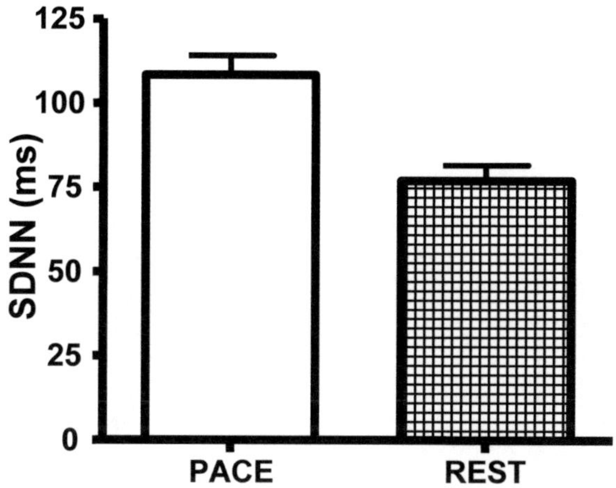

Fig. 3. **Heart rate variability for paced and uncontrolled breathing conditions.** Bars represent heart rate variability (HRV, ms) expressed as time domain measure of mean standard deviation of normal-normal electrocardiogram RR intervals (SDNN) during paced breathing at 0.2 Hz (pace) and normal uncontrolled spontaneous breathing at rest sitting in a chair (rest). Subjects are 52 healthy young adult African-American males. Data in mean ± standard error. The rest condition is different from paced breathing control (pace) at $P<0.05$.

Figure 6 shows that the LF/HF ratio of HRV spectral power, a measure of cardiac sympathovagal balance, was significantly higher during paced breathing at 0.2 Hz than during uncontrolled spontaneous breathing for the study group of 52 subjects ($P<0.01$) and, during paced breathing at 0.2 Hz, was significantly higher for the narrowband band group of 6 subjects than for the broadband group of 46 subjects ($P<0.05$).

4. Discussion

Humans vary in their responsiveness to environmental stressors and HRV measurements may serve as physiological markers for such variation (DeBecker et al., 1998). HRV in the time domain, measured as standard deviation or standard error, estimates the range of differences in the time intervals between heartbeats (Lucini et al., 2002c). HRV has been used as a measure of autonomic balance that emanates from endogenous sympathetic and parasympathetic rhythms which are partly modulated by respiratory sinus arrhythmia (Hayano et al., 1990; Hrushesky, 1991). Fast Fourier transform (FFT) analysis of HRV differentiates the frequency components of the heart's inter-beat intervals and yields more detailed information about autonomic tone than time domain analysis (Petretta et al., 1995). Such analysis makes it possible to differentiate conditions with physiological features in common. For example, common autonomic contributions to HRV have been evaluated by examining specific FFT frequency bands. This frequency domain analysis is useful under diverse physiological states such as dynamic exercise (Pichon et al., 2004), hypertension associated with sleep apnea (Vanninen et al., 1996; Narkiewicz et al., 1998; Salo et al., 2000) and optic neuropathy (Gutierrez et al., 2002). In this study, we found that healthy young adult African-Americans exhibit greater SDNN, a time domain measure of HRV, during conditions of paced breathing and cold stress than during conditions of normal breathing

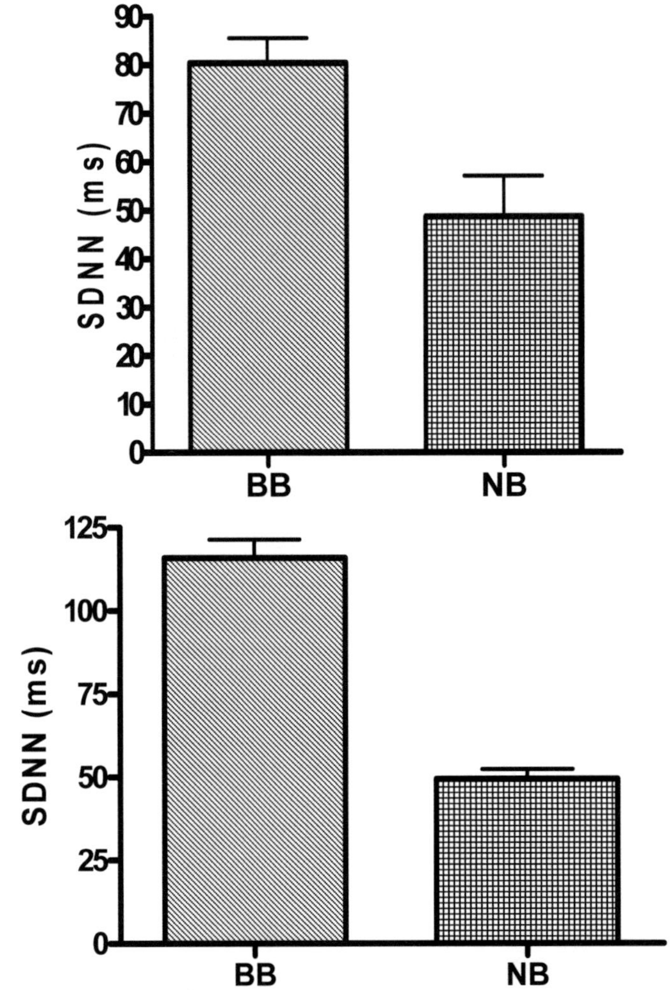

Fig. 4. **Heart rate variability for broadband and narrowband groups.** Bars represent heart rate variability (HRV, ms) expressed as time domain measure of mean standard deviation of normal-normal electrocardiogram RR intervals (SDNN) during paced breathing at 0.2 Hz (Bottom Panel) and normal uncontrolled spontaneous breathing at rest sitting in a chair (Top Panel). Subjects are 46 broadband (BB) healthy young adult African-American males with normal HRV compared to a similar group of 6 narrowband (NB) subjects with low HRV defined as exhibiting SDNN during paced breathing more than one standard deviation from the mean SDNN of the study group of 52 subjects. Data in mean ± standard error. The rest condition is different from paced breathing control (pace) at $P<0.05$.

and mental stress. We also identified a small subpopulation (12%) of subjects exhibiting SDNN more than one SD below the mean SDNN of the larger study population of 52 males during the paced breathing condition. It was beyond the scope of this part of the study to measure HRV spectral power. Because of the high variability of frequency domain measurements during short time intervals (Taverner et al., 1996), we limited a part of this study to the time domain measurement of SDNN.

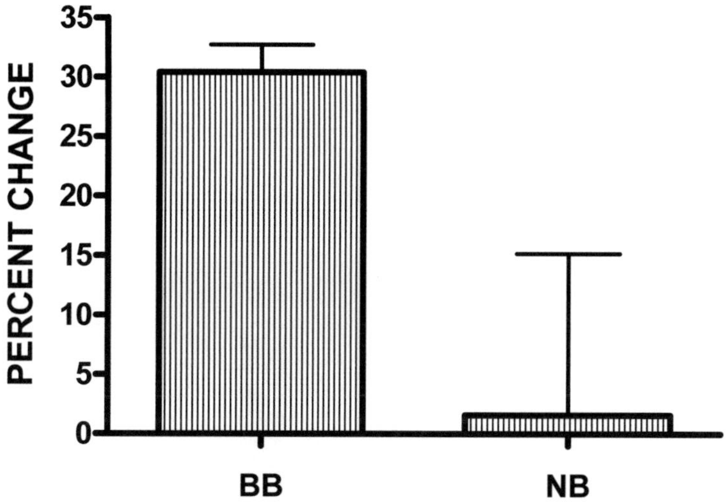

Fig. 5. **Percent change in heart rate variability for broadband and narrowband groups.** Bars represent percent increase in heart rate variability expressed as time domain measure of mean standard deviation of normal-normal electrocardiogram RR intervals (SDNN) during paced breathing at 0.2 Hz. Subjects are 46 broadband (BB) healthy young adult African-American males with normal HRV compared to a similar group of 6 narrowband (NB) subjects with low HRV defined as exhibiting SDNN during paced breathing less than one standard deviation from the mean SDNN of the study group of 52 subjects. Data in mean ± standard error. The percent increase in SDNN of the BB group is different from that of the NB group at $P<0.05$.

Respiratory sinus arrhythmia is thought to be the main source of HRV. However, there may be other non-autonomic contributions to respiratory sinus arrhythmia and to the high frequency (HF) components of HRV which may distort the signal-to-noise ratio and estimates of capacity for vagal modulation of heart rate (Pichon et al., 2004). HF HRV may mostly reflect noise if breathing shifts a substantial amount of HRV power to the low frequency (LF) range. The low time domain HRV occurring in subjects with apnea syndromes (Vanninen et al., 1996; Narkiewicz et al., 1998; Salo et al., 2000) could also be an effect of respiratory rate and/or tidal volume (Pinna et al., 2006). Low time domain HRV has been found in subjects exhibiting pre-hypertensive (Lucini et al., 2002a) and obesity (Salo et al., 2000) risk factors. Acetylcholine, when released from the vagus nerve, appears to act synergistically with vasoactive intestinal peptide to increase respiratory sinus arrhythmia (Markos and Snow, 2001). Higher HRV spectral frequencies and greater inter-beat intervals have been associated with a high capacity for vagal modulation of heart rate which occurs in normotensive healthy adults breathing at rest (Gutierrez et al., 2002). The peak HRV spectral frequency occurs in the range of HF in normotensive healthy adults breathing at rest and shifts to the range of LF during periods of exercise and stress, as well as, during disease states such as hypertension (Murakami et al., 1996)

Because of the respiration-related variability of electrocardiogram inter-beat (RR) intervals, the necessity of controlling respiratory frequency during measurements of HRV has been demonstrated (De Meersman et al., 1995). We used the frequency of 0.2 Hz during the paced breathing trial because this frequency produced the most reproducible conditions across subjects. As expected, the time domain HRV during paced breathing was significantly greater than during spontaneous breathing in the same subjects. This breathing pattern was

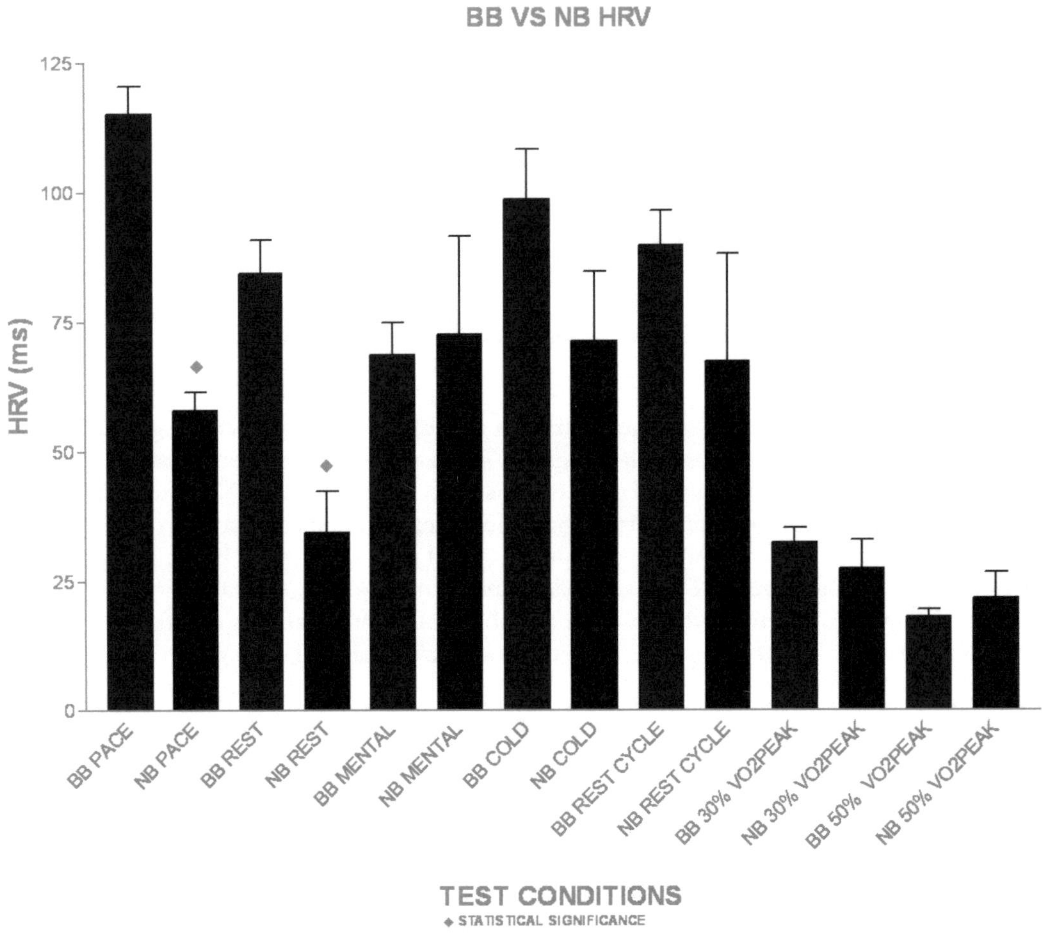

Fig. 6. **Heart rate variability across various testing conditions for broadband and narrowband subjects.** Bars represent heart rate variability (HRV, ms) expressed as time domain measure of mean standard deviation of normal-normal electrocardiogram RR intervals (SDNN) during paced breathing at 0.2 Hz (pace), normal uncontrolled spontaneous breathing at rest sitting in a chair (rest), Stroop word-color conflict testing of mental stress (mental), cold pressor testing of nociceptive stress (cold), normal uncontrolled spontaneous breathing at rest sitting on a cycle ergometer (rest cycle) and aerobic exercise stress at 30% and 50% of peak oxygen consumption (30% VO_{2peak}, 50% VO_{2peak}). Subjects are 46 broadband (BB) healthy young adult African-American males with normal HRV compared to a similar group of 6 narrowband (NB) subjects with low HRV defined as exhibiting SDNN during paced breathing more than one standard deviation from the mean SDNN of the study group of 52 subjects. Data in mean ± standard error. ♦ NB different from BB at $P<0.05$.

under technical supervision and in the low range of normal respiratory rate. Breathing in the range of 3-9 breaths per minute (0.05-0.15 Hz) may produce higher amplitude respiratory sinus arrhythmia because of more complete acetylcholine metabolism during exhalation (Song and Lehrer, 2003). Respiratory sinus arrhythmia might also be maximized if subjects breathe at frequencies controlled by other physiological processes. For example, when breathing between 4-7 breaths per minute (0.07-0.12 Hz), the baroreceptor reflex might be stimulated; thereby, causing a resonance effect and an increase in HRV (Vaschillo et al., 2002). In the present study, paced breathing was associated with significantly lower SDNN (0.2 Hz) than the spontaneous breathing trials (0.18-0.48 Hz) and we did not measure tidal volume which has been shown to positively modulate the high frequency (vagal) component of HRV spectral power (Pinna et al., 2006). At a high respiratory frequency paced breathing has been shown to produce predominance of the HF power of HRV in normal healthy adult subjects during meditation (Cysarz and Bussing, 2005). HRV studied during paced breathing in subgroups of pre-hypertensive and hypertensive middle-aged men and women has been shown to produce greater HF power in the pre-hypertensive than in the hypertensive subgroups (Prakash et al., 2005).

HRV in a subgroup of healthy normotensive middle-aged persons whose natural spontaneous respiratory frequency ranged 9-27 breaths per minute (0.15-0.45 Hz) with predominance of the HF power of HRV was compared to another subgroup whose natural respiratory frequency was less than 9 breaths per min (0.15 Hz) (Pinna et al., 2006). In that study, paced breathing at 15 breaths per min (0.25 Hz) failed to alter either the time domain or the frequency domain HRV parameters. In a study population of healthy adults, data sets matching respiratory frequencies at rest with those during dynamic exercise demonstrated that the LF and HF powers of HRV were not changed by controlled breathing in the absence of dynamic exercise but were significantly decreased at the same respiratory frequencies during exercise (Bartels et al., 2004). Because of the expected transients and uncertainties about the role of respiration and significance of changes in frequency domain HRV, we limited this part of the study to use of a time domain measure of HRV that, based on the current knowledge, would be more easily interpreted.

5. Conclusions

This study has demonstrated a wide range of SDNN measurements performed under various experimental conditions from the largest SDNN measured during paced breathing at 0.2 Hz to the smallest during exercise at 30%-50% of peak oxygen consumption in a group of 52 healthy young adult African-American males. The SDNN measured during short periods of normal spontaneous breathing at 0.18-0.48 Hz while at rest sitting both in a chair and on a cycle ergometer, cold stress and mental stress were intermediate, between those of paced breathing and aerobic exercise. SDNN was used to differentiate a "narrowband" subgroup (6/52 subjects, 12%) on the basis of a much smaller observed difference in SDNN between paced and normal spontaneous breathing and, despite an increase in the heart rate, the absence of a decrement in SDNN during a state of mental stress. These findings suggest that mental stress, elicited by Stroop word conflict testing, seems to have a differentiating effect on SDNN, an easily performed and interpreted time domain measure of heart rate variability. In the frequency domain, higher LF/HF heart rate variability spectral power, a reliable measure of sympathetic modulation of the heart rate, differentiated the paced from the uncontrolled spontaneous breathing condition and the same "narrowband" subgroup, as demonstrated in figures 7 and 8.

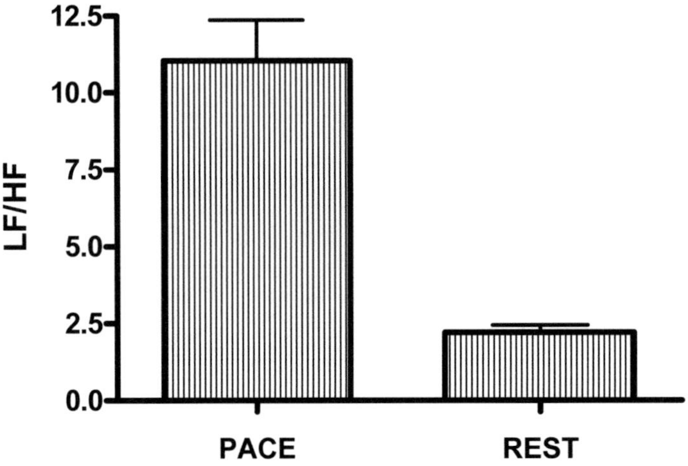

Fig. 7. **Heart rate variability spectral power measure of sympathovagal balance for paced and uncontrolled breathing conditions.** Bars represent low frequency/high frequency ratio (LF/HF) of heart rate variability spectral power measured by fast Fourier transform analysis of electrocardiogram RR intervals during paced breathing at 0.2 Hz (pace) and normal uncontrolled spontaneous breathing at rest sitting in a chair (rest). Subjects are 52 healthy young adult African-American males. Data in mean ± standard error. The rest condition is different from paced breathing control (pace) at $P<0.01$.

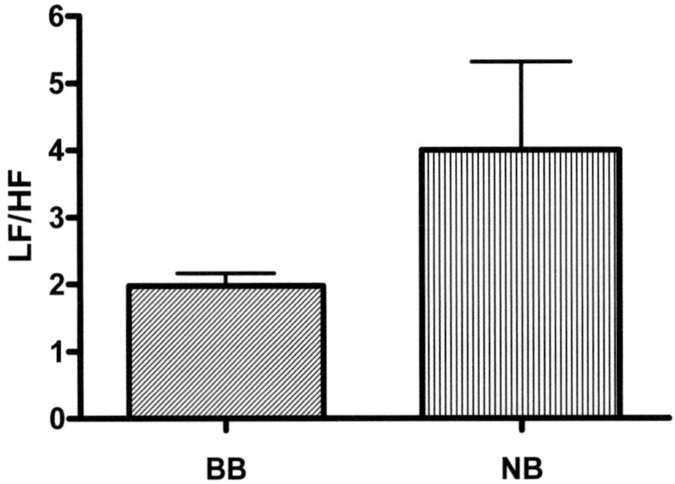

Fig. 8. **Heart rate variability spectral power measure of sympathovagal balance for broadband and narrowband groups.** Bars represent low frequency/high frequency ratio (LF/HF) of heart rate variability spectral power measured by fast Fourier transform analysis of electrocardiogram RR intervals during paced breathing at 0.2 Hz. Subjects are 46 broadband (BB) healthy young adult African-American males with normal HRV compared to a similar group of 6 narrowband (NB) subjects with low HRV defined as exhibiting SDNN during paced breathing more than one standard deviation from the mean SDNN of the study group of 52 subjects. Data in mean ± standard error. LF/HF of the BB group is different from that of the NB group at $P<0.05$.

6. References

Bartels, M.N., Jelic, S., Ngai, P., et al (2004). The effect of ventilation on spectral analysis of heart rate and blood pressure variability during exercise. *Respir Physiol Neurobiol.* 144, 91-98.

Burutcu, I., Esen, A.M., Kaya, D., et al (2005). Cigarette smoking and HRV: dynamic influence of parasympathetic and sympathetic maneuvers. *Ann Noninvasive Electrocardiol.* 10, 324-329.

Cysarz, D., and Bussing, A (2005). Cardiorespiratory synchronization during Zen meditation. *Eur J Appl Physiol.* 95, 88-95.

De Becker, P., Dendale, P., De Meirleir, K., et al (1998). Autonomic testing in patients with chronic fatigue syndrome. *Am J Med.* 105, :22S-26S.

De Meersman, R.E., Reisman, S.S., Daum, M., et al (1995). Influence of respiration on metabolic, hemodynamic, psychometric, and R-R interval power spectral parameters. *Am J Physiol.* 269(4 Pt 2), H1437-H1440.

Delaney, J.P., and Brodie, D.A (2000). Effects of short-term psychological stress on the time and frequency domains of heart-rate variability. *Percept Mot Skills.* 91, 515-524.

Driscoll, D., and Dicicco, G (2000). The effects of metronome breathing on the variability of autonomic activity measurements. *J Manipulative Physiol Ther.* 23, 610-614.

Fauvel, J.P., Bernard, N., Laville, M., et al (1996). Reproducibility of the cardiovascular reactivity to a computerized version of the Stroop stress test in normotensive and hypertensive subjects. *Clin Auton Res.* 6, 219-224.

Gillum, R.F (1979). Pathophysiology of hypertension in blacks and whites. A review of the basis of racial blood pressure differences. *Hypertension.* 1, 468-475.

Gillum, R.F (1999). Risk factors for stroke in blacks: a critical review. *Am J Epidemiol.* 150, 1266-1274.

Gutierrez, J., Santiesteban, R., Garcia, H., et al (2002). High blood pressure and decreased HRV in the Cuban epidemic neuropathy. *J Neurol Neurosurg Psychiatry.* 73, 71-72.

Hayano, J., Sakakibara, Y., Yamada, M., et al (1990). Decreased magnitude of heart rate spectral components in coronary artery disease. Its relation to angiographic severity. *Circulation.* 81, 1217-1224.

Hrushesky, W.J (1991). Quantitative respiratory sinus arrhythmia analysis. A simple noninvasive, reimbursable measure of cardiac wellness and dysfunction. *Ann NY Acad Sci.* 618, 67-101.

Kaplan, N.M (1994). Ethnic aspects of hypertension. *Lancet.* 344, 450-452.

Kuch, B., Hense, H.W., Sinnreich, R., et al (2001). Determinants of short-period HRV in the general population. *Cardiology.* 95, 131-138.

Lucini, D., Mela, G.S., Malliani, A., et al (2002a). Impairment in cardiac autonomic regulation preceding arterial hypertension in humans: insights from spectral analysis of beat-by-beat cardiovascular variability. *Circulation* 106, 2673-2679.

Lucini, D., Norbiato, G., Clerici, M., et al (2002b). Hemodynamic and autonomic adjustments to real life stress conditions in humans. *Hypertension.* 39, 184-188.

Lucini, D., Guzzetti, S., Casiraghi, S., et al (2002c). Correlation between baroreflex gain and 24-h indices of HRV. *J Hypertens.* 20, 1625-1631.

Markos, F. and Snow, H.M (2001). The potentiation of sinus arrhythmia by vasoactive intestinal polypeptide (VIP) in the anaesthetized dog. *Neuropeptides.* 35, 238-243.

Mezzacappa E.S., Kelsey, R.M., Katkin, E.S., et al (2001). Vagal rebound and recovery from psychological stress. Psychosom Med. 63, 650-657.

Montano, N., Porta, A., Cogliati, C., et al (2009). Heart rate variability explored in the frequency domain: a tool to investigate the link between heart and behavior. *Neurosci Biobehav Rev*. 33, 71-80.

Murakami, E., Matsuzaki, K., Sumimoto, T., et al (1996). Clinical significance of pressor responses to laboratory stressor testing in hypertension. *Hypertens Res*. 19, 133-137.

Narkiewicz, K., Montano, N., Cogliati, C., et al (1998). Altered cardiovascular variability in obstructive sleep apnea. *Circulation*. 98, 1071-1077.

Petretta, M., Marciano, F., Bianchi, V., et al (1995). Power spectral analysis of heart period variability in hypertensive patients with left ventricular hypertrophy. *Am J Hypertens*. 8(12 Pt 1), 1206-1213.

Pichon, A.P., De Bisschop, C., Roulaud, M., et al (2004). Spectral analysis of HRV during exercise in trained subjects. *Med Sci Sports Exerc*. 36, 1702-1708.

Pinna, G.D., Maestri, R., La Rovere, M.T., et al (2006). Effect of paced breathing on ventilatory and cardiovascular variability parameters during short-term investigations of autonomic function. *Am J Physiol Heart Circ Physiol*. 290, H424-H433.

Pinna, G.D., Maestri, R., La Rovere, M.T., et al (2006). Effect of paced breathing on ventilatory and cardiovascular variability parameters during short-term investigations of autonomic function. *Am J Physiol Heart Circ Physiol*. 290, H424-H433.

Prakash, E.S., Madanmohan-Sethuraman, K.R., Narayan, S.K (2005). Cardiovascular autonomic regulation in subjects with normal blood pressure, high-normal blood pressure and recent-onset hypertension. *Clin Exp Pharmacol Physiol*. 32, 488-494.

Rabinowitz, A., Kushner, H. and Falkner, B (1993). Racial differences in blood pressure among urban adolescents. *J Adolesc Health*. 14, 314-318.

Salo, T.M., Jula, A.M., Piha, J.S., et al (2000). Comparison of autonomic withdrawal in men with obstructive sleep apnea syndrome, systemic hypertension, and neither condition. *Am J Cardiol*. 85, 232-238.

Song, H-S. and Lehrer, P.M (2003). The effects of specific respiratory rates on heart rate and HRV. *Appl Psychophysiol Biofeedback*. 28, 13-23.

Taverner, D., Nunan, T.A., Tonkin, A.L et al (1996). Reproducibility of conventional and power spectral measurements of cardiovascular sympathetic activation in normal subjects. *Clin Exp Pharmacol Physiol*. 23, 804-806.

Vanninen, E., Tuunainen, A., Kansanen, M., et al (1996). Cardiac sympathovagal balance during sleep apnea episodes. *Clin Physiol*. 16, 209-216.

Vaschillo, E., Lehrer, P., Rishe, N., et al (2002). HRV biofeedback as a method for assessing baroreflex function: a preliminary study of resonance in the cardiovascular system. *Appl Psychophysiol Biofeedback*. 27, 1-27.

14

The Role of Exercise Test After Percutaneous Coronary Intervention

Iveta Mintale et al.*
Paul Stradins Clinical University Hospital, Latvian Centre of Cardiology
Latvia

1. Introduction

Cardiovascular diseases is the most common cause of death worldwide and coronary artery disease (CAD) still remains the leading cause of death in Latvia. The incidence of CAD in Europe is 20-40 thousands per one million people (Fox et al., 2006). According to the data of Health Statistics and Medical Technology Agency in Latvia 16 079 individuals died due to cardiovascular disease in 2009 (54% of total mortality rate). Mortality rate due to CAD is three times higher in Latvia than average in European Society in individuals group younger than 64 years. The loss of productive years of life has negative influence neither to private, nor public economical sector.

The common electrocardiographic finding on exercise stress test, which can be evident for CAD, is recurrent, load-induced ST-segment depression. It points to myocardial ischemia in patient with significantly narrowed coronary arteries in status of progressive oxygen demand, while at rest blood flow is not limited. The sensitivity of the stress test increases along with severity of disease. It is possible correctly to identify the patients with proximal several arteries disease or left main artery stenosis performing a standard exercise stress test, nevertheless it gives unsufficient prognostic information in patient with less severe obstructive disease.

Progression of coronary artery restenosis after percutaneous coronary intervention (PCI) is a clinical "final" result, which reflects complex pathophysiological process, including different combinations of residual coronary stenosis and neointimal proliferation. Unfortunately, the set of clinical symptoms is uncertain criteria for detection of coronary artery restenosis, patient's complaints could be similar to non-coronary pain post revascularization ('false-positive' symptoms), at the same time - "silent" ischemia may be present in many patients ('pseudo-negative' symptoms). Restenosis is observed in 25% of cases (data of balloon angioplasty) in asymptomatic patients with documented ischemic changes on exercise test (Bengston et al., 1990).

Discussions are still extended, whether early performed strategy of exercise test is with prognostic value for clinical events in patients after PCI. There are no conclusive results about association of complaints' limited exercise tests and long-term prognosis early after PCI.

---

*Milana Zabunova, Dace Lurina, Inga Narbute, Sanda Jegere, Ilja Zakke, Vilnis Taluts Dzerve and Andrejs Erglis

CAD patients with left main coronary artery (LM) stenosis is another one group of interest, and there is stable introduced invasive PCI treatment and stent implantation for this patients' group. It is important to evaluate the efficacy of new treatment, outcomes and following risk of cardiovascular events. Patients after LM PCI are at higher risk of thrombosis and restenosis, angiographic follow-up of these patients is expensive enough, with additional radiation dose and contrast amount for patients. Thus, high attention is focused on non-invasive investigation methods in patients with CAD.
The results of recent studies should be taken into account, that the higher risk of cardiovascular events is observed in patients with unstable atheromatous plaque, even in case if stenosis of coronary artery is not significant (in segment of this plaque location). Exercise test in this situation should be evaluated more precisely and seriously in order to improve the prognostic value of the method. The question is - whether exercise test (with electrocardiogramm (ECG)) can be used in evaluation of prognostic criteria for patient along with possibility to detect obstructive lesion of coronary arteries with a goal to decrease effectively the risk of sudden death and serious coronary events?

2. Objective of the study

The aim of the study was to evaluate effectiveness of medical and invasive treatment in patients with CAD after PCI by performing physical test and proving test prognostic value of cardiovascular events - clinical (myocardial infarction, recurrent hospitalization, cardiac death) and angiographic (restenosis and/or new stenosis of coronary arteries) events.
The main goals were defined:

1. to define specific criteria of exercise stress test for possible restenosis diagnostics;
2. to develop the algorhythm for the patients' functional status evaluation after PCI, as well as for evaluation the possibility of coronary artery stenosis correction (intervention);
3. to create the prognostic model, which can help to evaluate and reveal the patients with unfavorable long-term outcomes or unsatisfactory treatment results timely;
4. to integrate targeted follow-up patients' programme.

3. Materials and methods

The follow-up programme was developed in 1990 in the Latvian Centre of Cardiology and surveyed patients with CAD which underwent PCI treatment method.
The programme has been proceeded since the first patient was treated with the method of coronary angioplasty in Latvia.
The study was implemented from January, 2004 till January, 2009. The patients with established CAD (based on coronary angiography data) were included in the study. The patients underwent invasive treatment - PCI in the Latvian Centre of Cardiology. The number of performed PCIs during mentioned period of time - 16 109. All patients were informed about possibility to be included in the follow-up programme.
The data of 7 300 patients with CAD and complete 24-months follow-up after PCI were included in the study.
The patients were observed in defined follow-up periods of time after PCI by performing exercise stress test (veloergometry – bicycle ergometer exercise test):

- 1-3 months after invasive treatment - immediate risk evaluation and correction of medical treatment;
- 3-6 months after PCI - distant period - determination of possibility of restenosis and correction of medical treatment;
- 12-24 months after PCI - late period - determination of possibility of restenosis and correction of medical treatment.

Control coronary angiography was performed based on indications, which included following patients groups:

- patients with new-onset angina proved by ischemic changes on ECG during exercise stress test;
- patients without typical coronary complaints, but with registered ischemic changes on exercise test ECG;
- patients with non-sufficient information on exercise test in order to evaluate indications for coronary angiography, therefore exercise test with additional visualization method was performed - myocardial perfusion scintigraphy.
- Patients without indications for control coronary angiography underwent the correction of medical treatment (if it was needed) and were included in the next scheduled exercise test control.

Large patients group was revealed during the follow-up process - patients without typical coronary chest pain but with registered ischemic changes on ECG during exercise test. These patients were defined like „silent" ischemia patients group which has the higher risk of cardiovascular events and worse prognosis.

All the patients of this group underwent control coronary angiography and were divided into different groups according to angiographic finding:

- patients with restenosis of coronary artery (in previously repaired segment);
- patients with new stenosis of coronary artery;
- patients without restenosis or new stenosis on angiographic finding.

Patients with restenosis or new stenosis underwent PCI and were included in consequent follow-up plan and medical treatment correction. Patients without restenosis or new stenosis continued previously defined follow-up plan.

The analysis of used medications groups was performed because of medical treatment correction during follow-up process. It was dependent on obtained data during exercise test (e.g., arterial blood pressure and/or heart rate, compliance of these parameters changes to physical load, etc.). Medications after performed PCI (recommended on discharge) and in one year follow-up period were compared.

Very high risk patients were included into the separate group analysis (400 patients) with LM stenotic lesion. All patients were informed about possibility to be included in the 24 months follow-up plan. 133 patients have accomplished complete follow-up programme (1, 3, 6, 12 and 24 months after PCI). In order to define precise indications for control coronary angiography, myocardial perfusion scintigraphy with physical or pharmacological test was performed in this patients group (94 examinations). This examination was performed in 12-24 months period after PCI in patients without indications for control angiography.

Phone follow-up survey was also performed in this patients group in order to clarify possible coronary events - hospitalization, myocardial infarction or death. Patients groups with and without performed follow-up programme were compared.

SPSS 12.0.1. version was used for statistical analyses. Baseline characteristics were summarized as frequencies and percentages for categorical variables and as means and SDs for continuous variables. Analyses were performed using χ^2/Fisher exact test for categorical variables and Student *t* test/ *ANOVA* method for continuous variables. The correction with *Tukey* test was performed in *post hoc* analysis for multiple comparisons correction. Differences were considered statistically significant at $p<0.05$.

3.1 Exercise test – veloergometry

Exercise stress test - veloergometry was performed in sitting or reclining position in patients of the study, depending on used bicycle ergometer (in sitting position - veloergometer „Ergometrs 900" and since April, 2008 - veloergometer „e-bike" for test performing in reclining position). Modified Bruce protocol was used during exercise test - standardized load grading programme according to the protocol accepted by Latvian Cardiology Society:

- first degree - three minutes with 50 Watt (W) load;
- second degree - three minutes with 100 W load;
- third degree - three minutes with 150 W load;
- fourth degree - three minutes with 200 W load;
- fifth degree - three minutes with 250 W load.

Maximal allowed load was defined as 250 W. In specific cases (if it was necessary) or according to patient condition (patients with chronic heart failure) the protocol was accommodated individually - the load was increased for 25 W every three minutes with the beginning of second degree of the test protocol.

ECG was monitored continuously during the test time, increasing the load till the goal heart rate was achieved - 85 % of maximal heart rate according (appropriate) to concrete age or the load was limited by symptoms of ischemia.

Following indications were defined for the test discontinuation:

a. typical increasing chest pain and/or ST-segment changes on ECG (ST-segment depression > 2 mm - as a relative indication for the test interruption, ST-segment depression > 3 mm - as a absolute indication for the test interruption);
b. ST-segment elevation > 1 mm (if pathologic Q-wave is not present on ECG at rest);
c. arrhythmias (supraventricular tachycardia, multiple politope and pair premature beats (extrasystoles));
d. systolic blood pressure decrease (> 10 mmHg compared with onset blood pressure level), despite of the load increase;
e. hypertension (> 250 mmHg systolic and > 115 mmHg diastolic blood pressure);
f. central nervous system symptoms (ataxy, weakness, syncope);
g. signs of decreased perfusion (cyanosis);
h. fatigue, dyspnoe, leg cramps, claudication;
i. complete left His bundle branch block;
j. achieved submaximal heart rate;
k. patient's request to terminate the test;
l. technical problems.

Exercise test was defined as positive, if there were registered changes on ECG associated with myocardial ischemia:

- horizontal or downslopping ST-segment depression or elevation, greater than or equal with 1 mm 60 msec after QRS complex;

- especially, if these changes were associated with chest pain, appeared at lower load (< 75 W) and lasting for more than 3 minutes after load was finished.

Following parameters were analized:

a. Electrocardiographic parameters:
   - maximal ST-segment depression;
   - maximal ST-segment elevation;
   - configuration (shape) of ST-segment depression (horizontal, downslopping, upslopping);
   - the number of leads ST-segment changes registered in;
   - duration of ST-segment changes at the test phase of rest (after load discontinued);
   - ST/pulse index;
   - ventricular arrhythmias induced by exercise;
   - the time to ST-segment changes appeared at.

b. Hemodynamic parameters:
   - maximal heart rate;
   - maximal systolic blood pressure;
   - maximal double rate-pressure product (Robinson index) (maximal heart rate multiply by maximal systolic arterial pressure, divided by 100)
   - total exercise (load) time;
   - hypotension (arterial pressure decrease under the blood pressure level before load was started);
   - chronotropic incompetence.

c. Symptomatic parameters:
   - angina provoked by load;
   - load-limiting symptoms;
   - time to the onset of angina.

Following information was included in the protocol of veloergometry (accordingly the methodological guidelines):

- maximal load;
- total time of the load;
- heart rate at the beginning;
- initial systolic and diastolic blood pressure;
- maximal heart rate;
- maximal systolic and diastolic blood pressure;
- double rate-pressure product;
- the intensity and quantity of ECG changes;
- recovering period after load;
- patient's complaints;
- test termination reasons;
- tolerance of the exercise (load) (high, satisfactory, lowered, low);
- load-limiting factors.

The data mentioned above (collected from veloergometry test protocols) were included into the total database of the study.

There were no any complications registered during exercise test perfoming - myocardial infarction, life-threating arrhythmias or death.

Myocardial perfusion scintigraphy was perfomed in patients at the case of embarrassing interpretation of ECG, and in order to evaluate the indications for control coronary angiography.
Myocardial perfusion scintigraphy was also performed in patients after LM PCI.

3.2 Coronary angiography and PCI

The information about atherosclerotic lesions degree of coronary arteries was collected and included into the total database of the study (based on coronary angiography finding). Follow-up period results were included – data of coronary angiography finding (restenosis and/or new stenosis of coronary artery(-ies)), acute coronary events (recurrent hospitalization, myocardial infarction, coronary artery bypass grafting, recurrent coronary angiography and/ or PCI).
The result of revascularization was defined, basing on the data of coronary angiography finding:

- successful PCI defined as a dilatation of coronary artery stenosis with complete revascularization, if residual stenosis of coronary artery(-ies) does not exceed 50 % (Wenaweser et al., 2008);
- incomplete revascularization defined as a residual stenosis (narrowing of the lumen of artery after performed PCI) greater than or equal with 50 % in any coronary artery (Chalela et al., 2006).

Restenosis of coronary artery at the follow-up period was defined as a narrowing of coronary artery(-ies) lumen greater than or equal with 50 % and progression of coronary artery disease, if new stenosis of coronary artery was diagnosed (Chalela et al., 2006).

4. Results

4.1 Data registry of the patients with coronary artery disease treated with PCI

In total 7300 patients with established CAD and performed treatment with PCI, with complete follow-up programme - 1, 3, 6 and 12 months follow-up visits, were included into the study. The patients underwent physical stress test, correction of used medications plan and doses of drugs, if it was necessary, and the control of risk factors. Control coronary angiography was performed in 2583 patients accordingly the indications.
Indications for performance of control coronary angiography were determined basing on exercise test (13% of cases), restenosis on angiography was detected in 6.4% of the total patients' group.
In the patients' group with left main artery stenosis (LM group) 400 patients were observed, 133 of them worked out complete follow-up program and underwent control coronary angiography. Myocardial perfusion scintigraphy was performed in 98 LM-patients in order to evaluate more precisely the indications for coronary angiography.
In total patients' group 1226 patients (17%) showed coronary complaints, and ST-segment changes on ECG, which could be associated with myocardial ischemia, were observed in 975 patients (13% of total number of patients). According to the indications these patients underwent coronary angiography. In general, angiographically confirmed coronary artery restenosis was diagnosed in 470 patients (6.4%) of all controlled patients' group (7300) (Figure 1.).

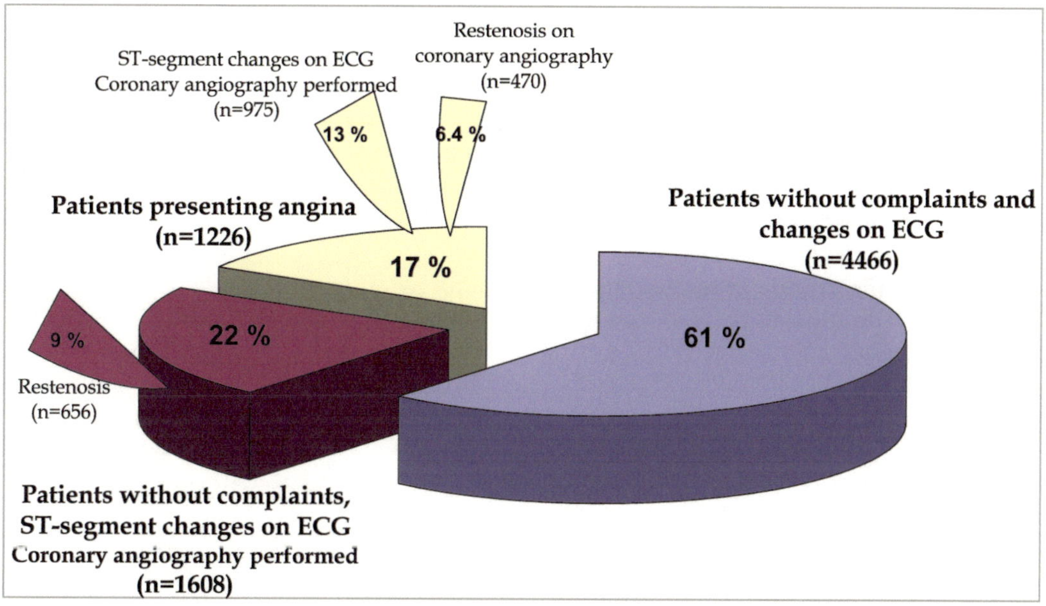

Fig. 1. Results of the follow-up programme (the total number of the patients - 7300).

Exercise test is useful in detection of patients with „silent" ischemia (22%), which have the indications for control angiography; restenosis is found in 9% of this patients group.

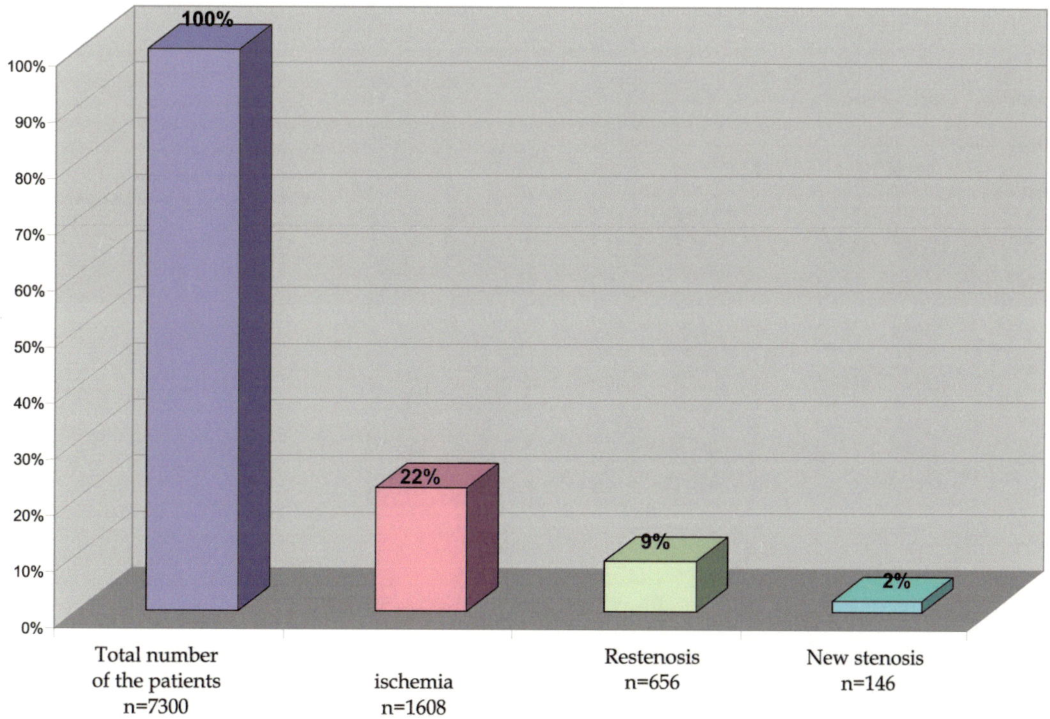

Fig. 2. Patients with „silent" ischemia.

It was observed during patients follow-up, that a separate group of the patients is forming, which is characterized by no complaints of chest pain, but significant ST-segment changes on exercise test ECG (so-called, silent ischemia, poor prognostic factor). These are 22% of the patients (1608 patients), all of them underwent coronary angiography. Restenosis of coronary artery was detected in 656 patients (9% of the total number of patients) and new hemodinamically significant stenosis in coronary artery (> 50% of artery lumen) - in 146 patients (2%) of this patients group (Figure 2.).

4.2 New specific criteria in restenosis diagnostics

Several new specific criteria were found in restenosis diagnostics field additionally to ST-segment ischemic changes on ECG during exercise stress test - reduced load tolerance, decreased maximal heart rate and maximal systolic blood pressure, maximal rate-pressure product (double product) - Robinson index, also increased ST/pulse index (ST/p index). Differences in parameters derived from exercise tests in patients with restenosis, new stenosis and in patients without restenosis/new stenosis on coronary angiography are shown in Figure 3.

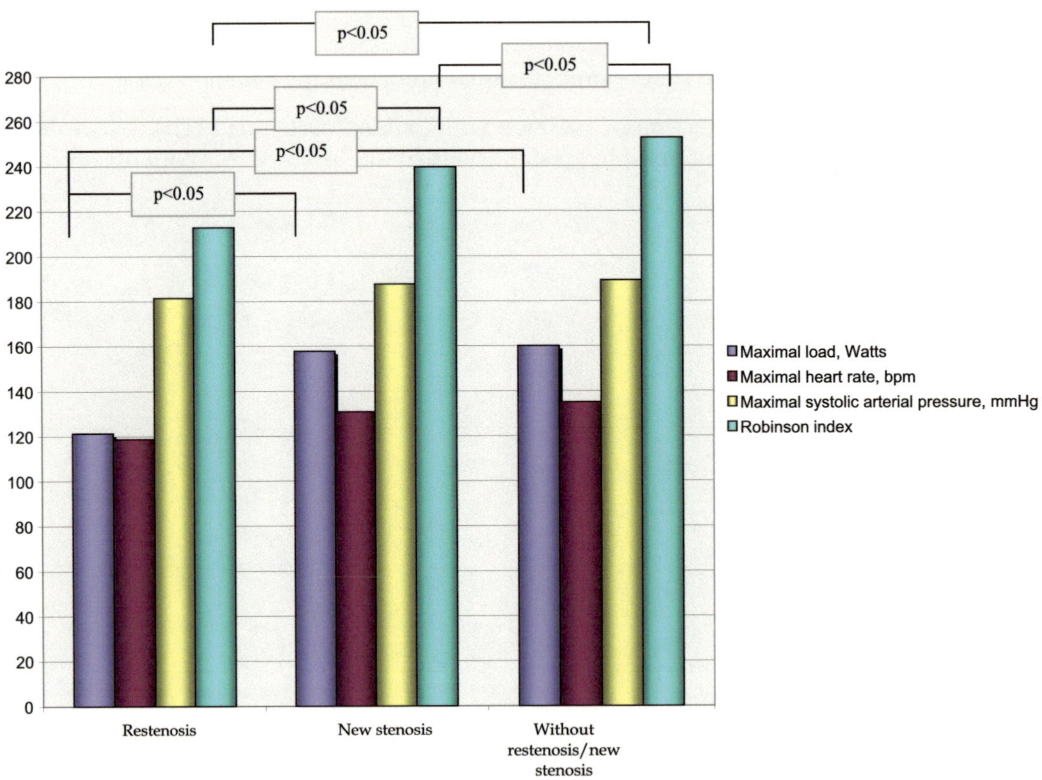

Fig. 3. Results of exercise test in „silent" ischemia patients' group.

Patients with restenosis on coronary angiography (first group) showed definitely ischemic changes on exercise ECG at lower physical load 121.4±33.2 W compared with those patients' group with neither restenosis, nor new stenosis on coronary angiography (third group) - 160.0±25.8 W ($p<0.05$). Achieved maximal heart rate and systolic blood pressure during physical load also showed lower parameters in the first group, which is characterized by double rate-pressure product compared in both groups - 212.8±42.9 and 252.62±36.9, accordingly, in the first and third patients' group ($p<0.05$) (Figure 4.).

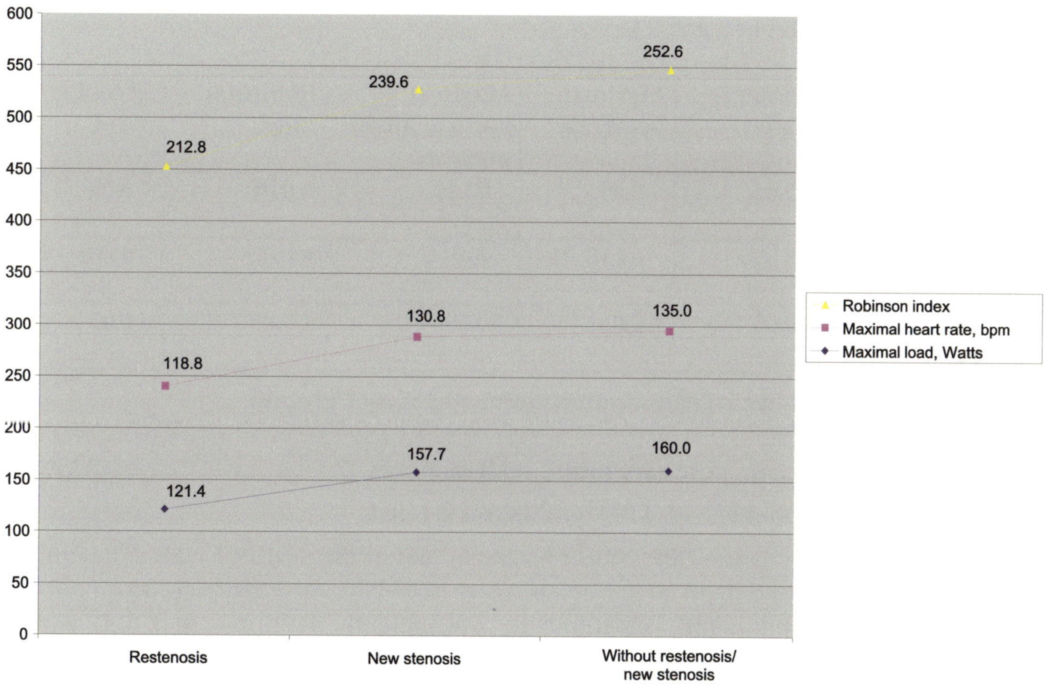

Fig. 4. Analysis of average parameters of veloergometry data (maximal heart rate, maximal systolic arterial pressure, maximal rate-pressure product - Robinson index).

Patients' groups/ Parameter on veloergometry	Maximal physical load, W	Maximal heart rate (when ECG changes appear)	Maximal systolic blood pressure	Robinson index (rate-pressure product)	ST/pulse index
1. Restenosis (n=656)	121.4±33.2	118.8±14.6	181.5±28.3	212.8±42.9	1.3±0.5
2. New stenosis (n=146)	157.7±38.5	130.8±14.9	187.6±30.7	239.6±46.9	1.0±0.3
3. Without restenosis/ new stenosis (n=806)	160.0±25.8	135.0±40.1	189.2±23.3	252.62±36.9	0.9±0.2

Table 1. Analysis of average parameters of veloergometry data (achieved physical load, maximal heart rate, maximal systolic blood pressure, Robinson index, ST/pulse index).

Parameters of neither maximal heart rate, nor maximal systolic arterial blood pressure, and so Robinson index, accordingly, are significantly lower in patients' group witht coronary artery restenosis. The most important parameter, which can reflect patient's risk of restenosis more precisely is ST/pulse index. In restenosis group this parameter is the highest one (1.3±0.5) (Table 1. and 2.).

p value (between patients' groups)	**Load, Watts**	**Maximal heart rate**	**Maximal systolic blood pressure**	**Robinson index**	**ST/pulse index**
First and second group	**< 0.05**	**< 0.05**	**0.012**	**< 0.05**	**< 0.05**
Second and third group	0.396	0.118	0.48	**< 0.05**	**0.004**
First and third group	**< 0.05**	**< 0.05**	**< 0.05**	**< 0.05**	**< 0.05**

Table 2. Statistical analysis in comparison of different patients' groups.

4.3 Patients with left main coronary artery (LM) stenosis

The database of the patients with LM stenosis was created.

The group of the patients (n=400) with LM stenosis and performed PCI with drug-eluting stents (DES) was analyzed. In a period of years 2005-2010, 133 patients accomplished complete follow-up programme. Veloergometry was regularly performed in 3, 6, 12 and 24 months after PCI, also control coronarography was performed in 6-12 months after PCI.

Clinical characteristics of the patients:

LM patients group – 80% of the patients are males, with mean age 61.3 ± 9.8 years. The most part of the patients is characterized with most important risk factors of coronary artery disease: in 96% of cases – dyslipidemia, in 77% of cases – arterial hypertension, smoking habits – active smokers (18%) or ex-smokers (30.8%). Previous myocardial infarction – in 45.1% of patients, positive family history (first-line relatives at young age with CAD) in 36.1% of cases (Table 3.).

All the patients underwent LM PCI: 47 patients (38%) underwent solely LM PCI and 86 patients (65%) – also PCI additionally in other artery (Table 4.).

The changes of the parameters registered on exercise test (maximal heart rate, maximal systolic blood pressure and Robinson index) in every follow-up period (independently of the follow-up data on coronary angiography) are showed in Table 5.

4.3.1 Association of veloergometry results with clinical events

Recurrent hospitalization was ascertained for 14 patients (8.3%) in analysis of clinical events in follow-up period. The reasons for recurrent admission to the hospital: in two cases – myocardial infarction, in four cases – chest pain (angina) (three of these patients underwent recurrent coronary angiography), in two cases – next step PCI, in two cases – heart rhythm disorders (in one case – implantation of permanent pacemaker), in one case – stroke, in one case – elevated arterial blood pressure, in two cases – non-coronary reasons for hospitalization.

Characteristics	Prevalence
Gender (males), n (%)	107 (80.5)
Age, mea(±SD)	61.3 (± 9.8)
Dyslipidemia, n (%)	96 (72.2)
Arterial hypertension, n (%)	77 (57.9)
Diabete mellitus, n (%)	11 (8.3)
Smoking status:	
Active smoker, n (%)	24 (18.0)
Ex-smoker, n (%)	41 (30.8)
Non-smoker, n (%)	51 (38.3)
Positive family history, n (%)	48 (36.1)
Prior myocardial infarction, n (%)	60 (45.1)
Prior PCI, n (%)	26 (19.5)
Prior coronary artery bypass grafting, n (%)	7 (5.3)

Table 3. Clinical characteristics of the patients (demographic parameters and risk factors of coronary artery disease) (n=133).

Characteristics	**Prevalence**
Coronary artery disease:	
One-vessel disease, n (%)	51 (38.3)
Two- vessel disease, n (%)	54 (40.6)
Three- vessel disease, n (%)	28 (21.1)
Complete/incomplete revascularization, %	40/27
PCI LM only, n (%)	47 (38.0)
PCI LM and other artery:	
PCI LAD, n (%)	47 (35.3)
PCI LCx, n (%)	26 (19.5)
PCI RCA, n (%)	14 (10.5)
PCI RIM, n (%)	4 (3.0)
PCI D_1, n (%)	3 (2.3)
PCI M_1, *RPL*, *RPD*, n (%)	1 (0.8)

LM-left main coronary artery; *LAD*-left anterior descending artery; *LCx*-left circumflex artery; *RCA*-right coronary artery; *RIM*-ramus intermedius; D_1-first diagonal branch; M_1-first marginal branch; *RPL*-right posterolateral branch; *RPD*-right posterodiaphragmal branch.

Table 4. Caracteristics of angiographic and PCI data of the patients (n=133).

Data of exercise test/ follow-up period	1-3 months	3-6 months	6-12 months	12-24 months	>24 months
Maximal heart rate (bpm ± SD)	118 ± 16	122 ± 17	121 ± 16	119 ± 15	119 ± 15
Maximal systolic blood pressure (mmHg ± SD)	180 ± 31	181 ± 29	182 ± 29	183 ± 31	184 ± 32
Robinson index(max heart rate x max systolic blood pressure/100) ± SD	213.27±51.02	220.93±52.55	221.55±45.9	217.84±47.68	219.32±48.46

Table 5. Mean values of parameters analyzed on exercise test follow-up (maximal heart rate, maximal systolic blood pressure, Robinson index).

Indications for control angiography were defined according to ST-segment ischemic changes on ECG and/or typical patients' complaints during exercise test.
Control angiography in follow-up period was performed in 33.8% of cases - 3-6 months after PCI, in 36.8% and in 10.5% of cases - 6-12 months and 12-24 months after PCI, respectively.

4.3.2 Analysis of the results of control exercise tests (1-3 and 3-6 months after PCI) and coronary angiography

There was no significant difference between patients group with LM restenosis and/or other coronary artery restenosis on control coronary angiography and patients group without diagnosed restenosis, analyzing maximal achieved physical load in early follow-up period (control exercise test performed 1-3 and 3-6 months after PCI).
Statistically significant difference (in maximal achieved physical load analysis) was observed comparing with the patients group with new coronary artery stenosis on control coronary angiography: these patients achieved lower maximal load on 1-3 months control exercise test - 90 ± 17 W vs. 129 ± 26 W, accordingly ($p=0.027$).
There was no significant difference observed between patients with and without LM restenosis (or other artery restenosis) in analysis of achieved maximal heart rate during exercise test 1-3 and 3-6 months after PCI, also between patients groups with and without diagnosed new artery stenosis on coronary angiography (Table 6.).

	Maximal heart rate (mean ± SD)				
Exercise test control (months after PCI)	'Restenosis' group	Number of the patients	'Non-restenosis' group	Number of the patients	p (between groups)
1-3 months	114.70 ± 8.87	10	118.49 ± 19.96	49	0.49
3-6 months	120.93 ± 17.43	15	122.07 ± 16.92	58	0.82
6-12 months	119.06 ± 14.63	16	120.69 ± 15.39	55	0.71
12-24 months	112.79 ± 10.03	14	120.58 ± 15.71	38	0.09
> 24 months	112.4 6± 13.48	13	120.74 ± 15.90	38	0.10

Table 6. Maximal heart rate analysis in different exercise test control periods.

In maximal systolic blood pressure analysis, almost statistically significant difference was observed (trend) between 'restenosis' group and 'non-restenosis' patients group on exercise test 1-3 months and 3-6 months follow-ups (Table 7.).

Maximal systolic blood pressure (mean ± SD)					
Exercise test control (months after PCI)	**'Restenosis' group**	**Number of the patients**	**'Non-restenosis' group**	**Number of the patients**	**p (between groups)**
1-3 months	161.70 ± 23.64	10	182.27 ± 32.32	49	0.06
3-6 months	170.33 ± 27.55	15	185.00 ± 28.91	58	0.08
6-12 months	176.44 ± 37.51	16	182.67 ± 26.22	54	0.45
12-24 months	177.14 ± 30.76	14	184.16 ± 30.60	38	0.47
> 24 months	186.92 ± 32.27	13	183.39 ± 32.90	38	0.74

Table 7. Maximal systolic blood pressure in different exercise test control periods.

The difference in analysis of double product (maximal rate-pressure product) or Robinson index was expected, on basis of previously obtained results. The following trend was observed - patients with coronary artery restenosis at control coronary angiography 1-3 months after performed PCI showed lower parameters of Robinson index. In turn, independently of stenosis location - LM or other coronary artery, or patients with new detected coronary artery stenosis - statistically significant difference and association with Robinson index changes between patients groups was not ascertained.
Variability of Robinson index changes on exercise test could become possible additional parameter to ST-segment changes in restenosis diagnostics (Table 8., Figure 5.).

Robinson index (mean ± SD)			
Exercise test control (months after PCI)	**'Restenosis' group**	**'Non-restenosis' group**	**p (between groups)**
1-3 months	185.70 ± 32.96	217.51 ± 54.09	0.08
3-6 months	208.12 ± 56.00	226.73 ± 53.81	0.24
6-12 months	210.41 ± 51.57	223.22 ± 45.16	0.34
12-24 months	197.89 ± 27.17	223.41 ± 50.73	0.08
> 24 months	210.23 ± 46.75	221.48 ± 50.63	0.49

Table 8. Robinson index analysis in different exercise test control periods.

Patients with angiographically detected coronary artery stenosis have achieved lower physical load (in Watts), not achieving submaximal pulse, because of termination the veloergometry, if ischemic changes or typical chest pain is appearing. This explains the curve difference of Robinson index in patients with and without coronary artery restenosis, also, statistically significant difference between mentioned groups is not present in analysis of maximal achieved heart rate and maximal systolic blood pressure. However, oscillations of Robinson index parameters are obviously seen in patiens of 'restenosis' group in relative

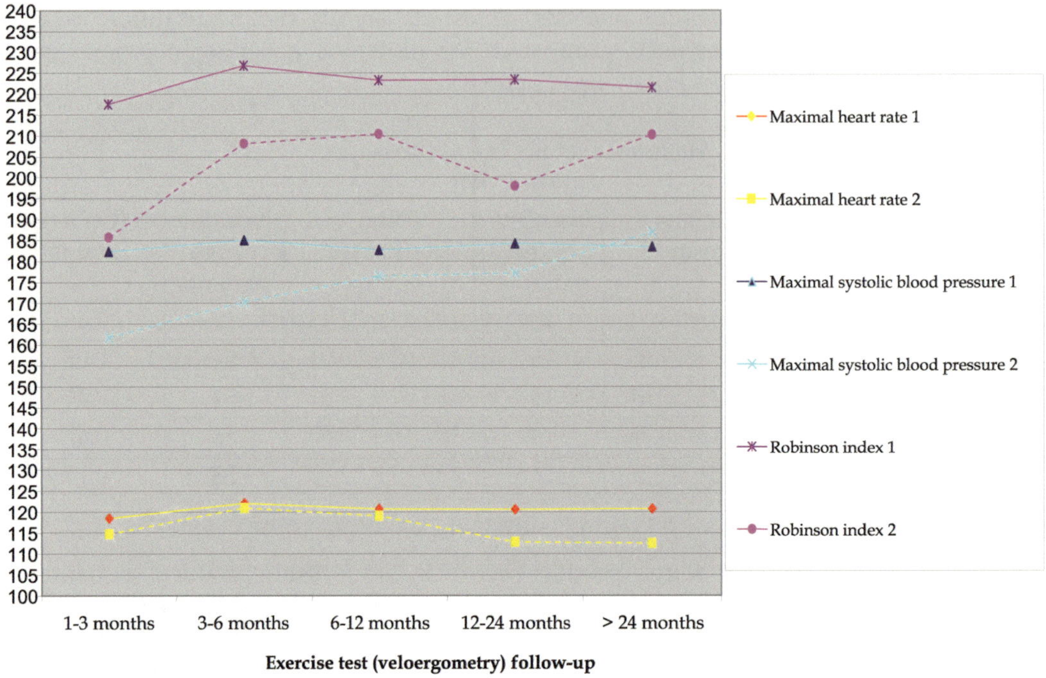

1 - without restenosis on control coronary angiography
2 - with restenosis on control coronary angiography

Fig. 5. Analysis of different exercise test parameters (Robinson index, maximal heart rate and maximal systolic blood pressure) during follow-ups in patients with and without coronary artery restsenosis (on control angiography).

risk period - 6-12 months follow-up. These curves repeatedly are establishing the role of targeted follow-up programme after performed PCI for more precise evaluation of risk of restenosis, taking into account not only patient's complaints and ischemic changes on ECG, but also the changes of Robinson index parameters in dynamics.

It is supposed, that the number of analyzed patients was not sufficient for statistical significance between groups in ST/p index analysis, in order to definitely conclude the role of this parameter in restenosis diagnostics (Table 9.)

ST/pulse index (mean ± SD)					
Exercise test control	**'Restenosis' group**	**Number of the patients**	**'Non-restenosis' group**	**Number of the patients**	**p (between groups)**
1-3 months after PCI	0.76 ± 0.55	10	0.59 ± 0.44	49	0.28
3-6 months after PCI	0.72 ± 0.35	15	0.61 ± 0.45	58	0.36
6-12 months after PCI	0.76 ± 0.47	16	0.59 ± 0.41	55	0.16

ST/pulse index (mean ± SD)					
Exercise test control	**'New stenosis' group**	**Number of the patients**	**'Without new stenosis' group**	**Number of the patients**	**p (between groups)**
1-3 months after PCI	1.07 ± 0.98	6	0.57 ± 0.34	53	0.01
3-6 months after PCI	0.80 ± 0.67	7	0.61 ± 0.40	66	0.27
6-12 months after PCI	0.76 ± 0.54	11	0.61 ± 0.40	60	0.28

Table 9. ST/pulse (ST/p) index in LM patients' group according to angiographic finding (restenosis, new stenosis of coronary artery or without detected restenosis or new stenosis of coronary artery).

In LM patients' group analysis - 50% of cases of coronary artery restenosis are detected in early period (3-6 months after PCI), left 43% and 7% - 6-12 and 12-24 months after PCI, respectively. Angiographic results in early coronary angiography follow-up period (3-6 months after performed PCI) correlate with ECG changes on 1-3 months control of physical test: there is statistically significant difference between patients groups - ST-segment depression on exercise ECG is obvious in all patients with restenosis established at control coronary angiography (Table 10.).

	3-6 months	6-12 months	12-24 months
Restenosis	50%	43%	7%
ST-segment changes	ST-segment depression	ST-segment depression	ST-segment depression

Table 10. Restenosis and ST-segment changes on exercise ECG prior the control coronary angiography.

The sensitivity of veloergometry test in 1-3 months - 29%, specificity - 100 %. Lower parameters of Robinson index also were registered in this patients' group.
Correlation of ST-segment changes with restenosis development is obvious also in later control of veloergometry (3-6 months after PCI). The sensitivity of veloergometry test - 50%, specificity - 86 %. All the patients with diagnosed new coronary artery stenosis (in other coronary artery) at control coronary angiography (3-6 months after PCI) showed ST-segment depression on exercise ECG in early stress test control (1-3 months), but in patients group without restenosis ECG without any dynamical changes is observed in 92.9% of cases. The sensitivity of the test - 33%, specificity - 93 %.

4.4 Algorithms

Basing on the previously obtained data and on the significance of exercise test in patients' follow-up after performed PCI, several algorithms were developed for evaluation of patients' functional status after PCI, also for evaluation of possible treatment strategy of coronary artery stenosis.

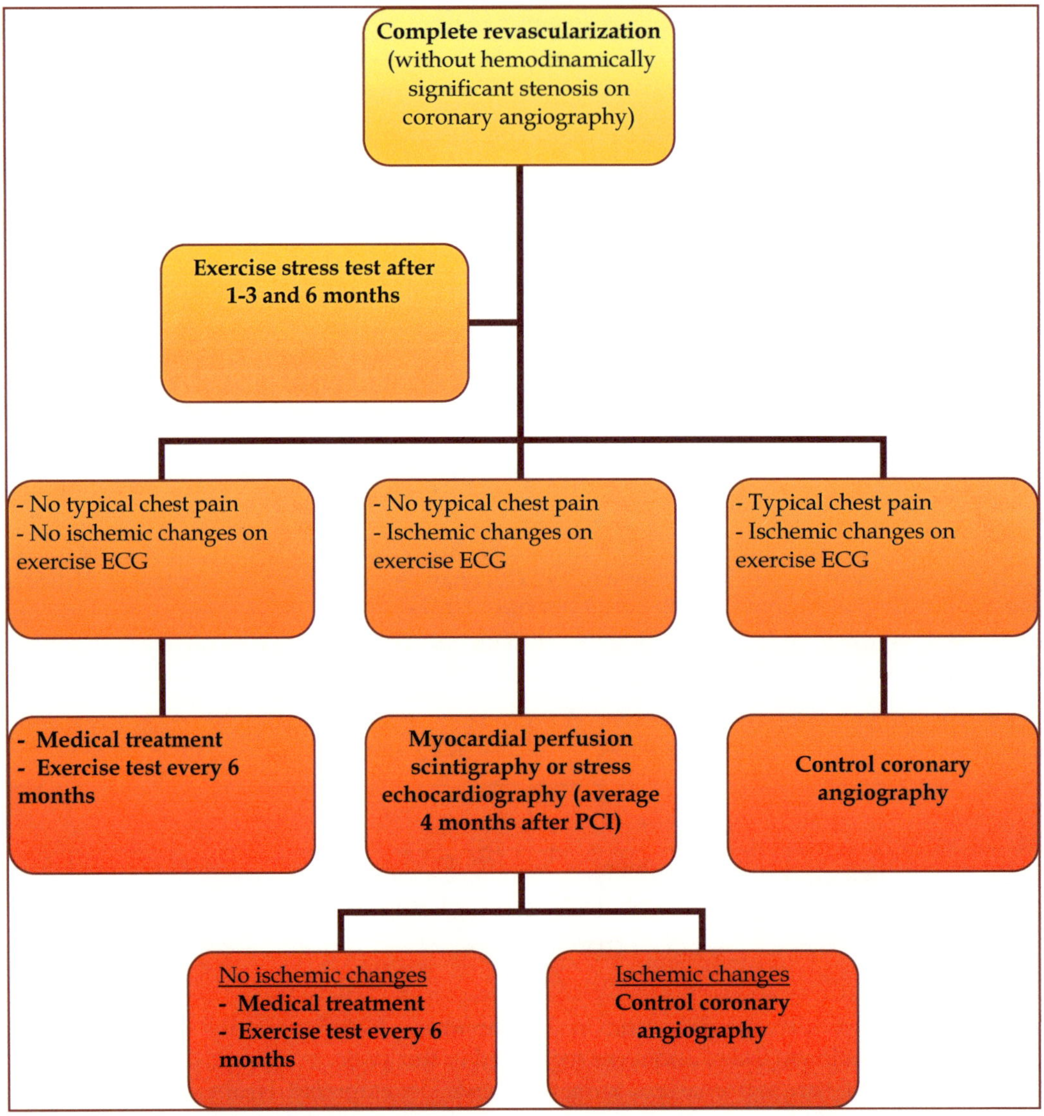

Fig. 6. Exercise test algorithm in patients after PCI (complete revascularization).

Patients with complete revascularization (Figure 6):

- Exercise test should be performed in 1-3 months after PCI in patients with complete revscularization (performed with PCI method);
- Patients should continue medical treatment and exercise test control every 6 months, if angina or ischemic changes on exercise ECG are not present;
- Patients should undergo myocardial perfusion scintigraphy investigation or stress echocardiography in case of no angina, but with presentation of ischemic changes on exercise ECG. If ischemic changes are not present on additional examination tests, medical treatment shoul be continued and control of exercise test every 6 months;

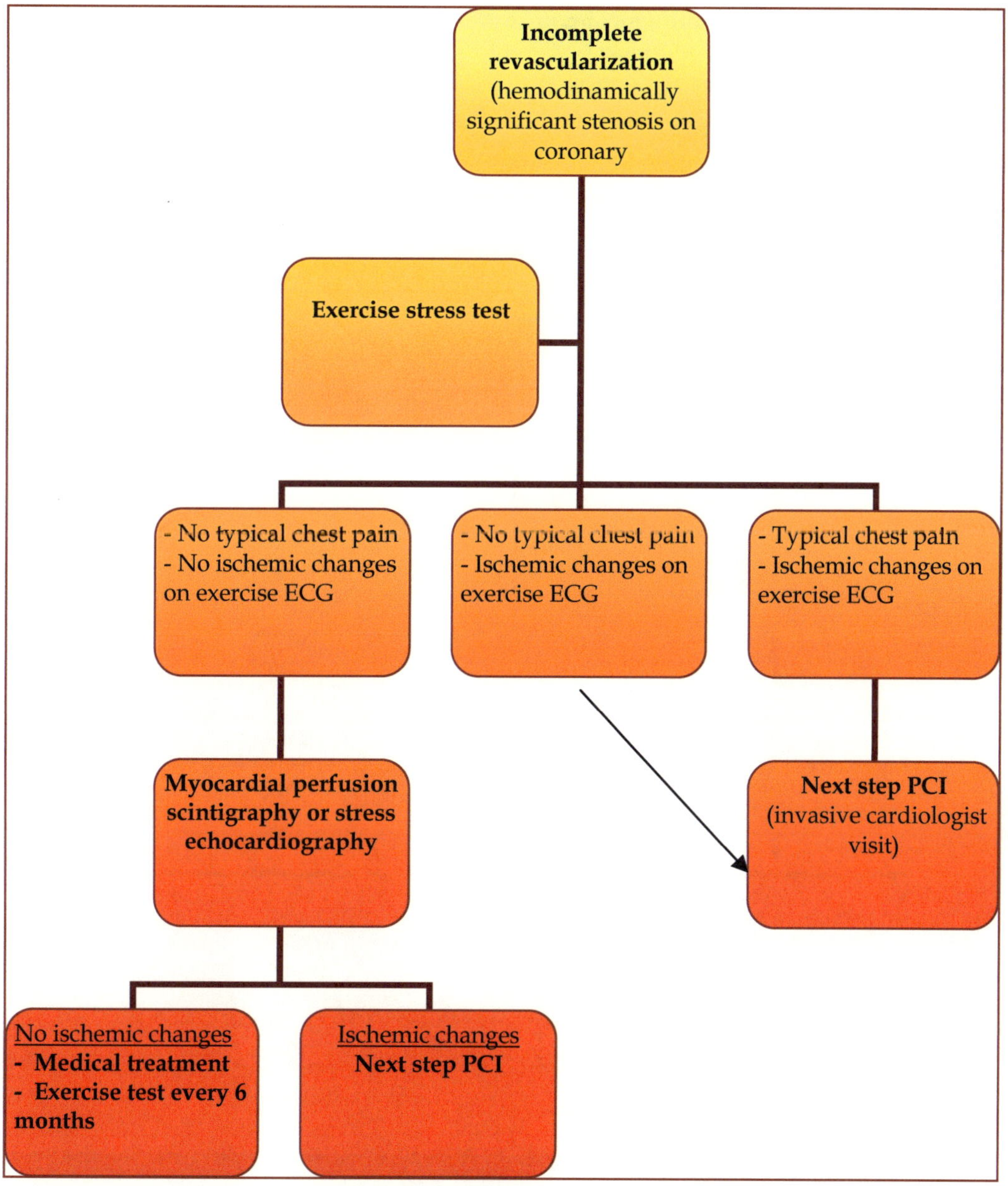

Fig. 7. Exercise test algorithm in patients after PCI (incomplete revascularization).

- In case of angina and ischemic changes on exercise ECG patients should undergo control coronary angiography.

Patients with incomplete revascularization (Figure 7.):

- Exercise test should be performed in 1-3 months after PCI in patients with incomplete revascularization (and hemodinamically sigfnificant stenosis, left on angiography);
- Myocardial perfusion scintigraphy investigation or stress echocardiography should be performed in case of no angina and no ischemic changes on exercise ECG. If ischemic

changes are present (in additional investigations), next step PCI should be performed. If ischemic changes are not present, patients should continue medical treatment and perform exercise test every 6 months;

- In case of ischemic changes on exercise ECG, independently of patient's complaints, next step PCI should be performed.

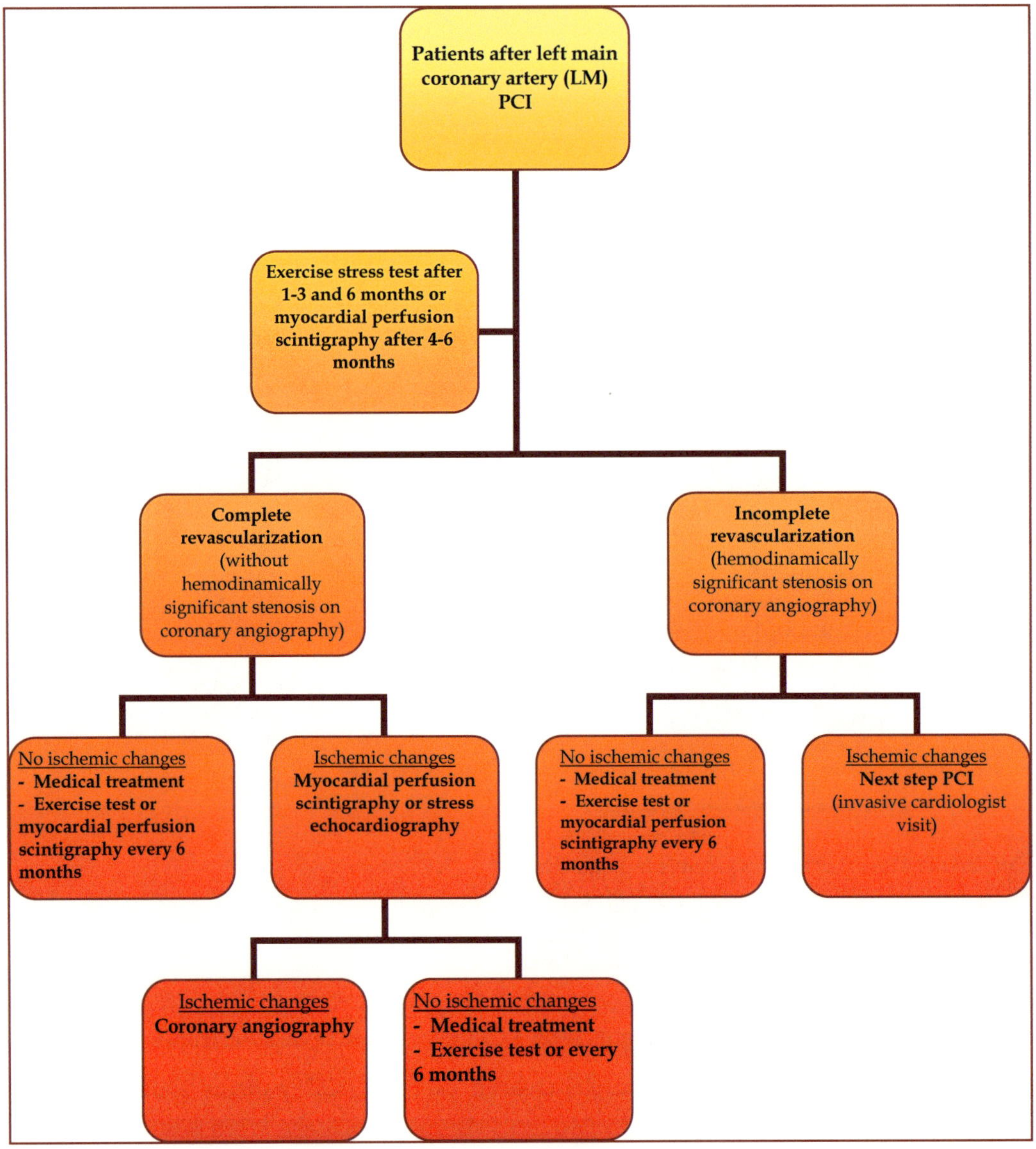

Fig. 8. Exercise test algorithm in patients after LM PCI.

Patients after left main coronary artery (LM) revascularization (Figure 8.):

- Exercise test should be performed in 1-3 months after LM PCI. Myocardial perfusion scintigraphy could be performed in 4-6 months in case of inconclusive ECG;

- Patients should continue medical treatment and should perform exercise test every 6 months in case of no hemodinamically significant stenosis on coronary angiography;
- Myocardial perfusion scintigraphy investigation or stress echocardiography should be performed in case of ischemic changes on exercise ECG. If If ischemic changes are present (in additional investigations), coronary angiography should be performed. If ischemic changes are not present, patients should continue medical treatment and perform exercise test every 6 months;
- Patients with incomplete revascularization and angiographycally with hemodynamically significant stenosis are left, exercise test should be performed in 1-3 months after PCI. If ischemic changes are not present, patients continue medical treatment and perform exercise test every 6 months. In case of ischemic changes on exercise test, patient should visit invasive cardiologist in order to make decision of next step PCI.

5. Discussion

In this study we raised the question whether physical exercise test alone beside accurate diagnosis of obstructive lesions provides an opportunity to prognose cardiovascular risk. We claim that this is possible, which is demonstrated in our study by a significant number of patients with silent ischemia. The potential gain from reducing the risk of reverse cardiac events is actually greatest in those with silent ischemia at the time of follow-up presentation, because those patients are at especially high risk (Pepine and Deedwania, 1994). Nowadays it is clear that chest pain in history does not correlate tightly with ischemic ST-segment deviation following physical loading and with haemodynamically significant stenosis on angiography either.

Published data as well as national and international guidelines state that physical exercise test following PCI is a useful method in diagnosis of restenosis in high risk or symptomatic patients and should be conducted six months after intervention (Gibbons et al., 2002). Our results showed that the exercise test should be done not later than three to six months after intervention. The highest rate of restenosis was observed in patients after interventional treatment of LM disease in 1-3 months after procedure. The importance of the physical test does not decrease later; more than third part of all documented restenosis was registered at six months after intervention (including the patients with newly diagnosed stenosis on coronary angiography). One year after PCI the specific weight of restenosis was 16.7% of all diagnosed restenosis.

The clinical value of exercise electrocardiograms following interventional therapy in the early period is high in evaluation of early post-interventional results (Roffi et al., 2003). This is supported with our results, which demonstrated high specificity of exercise test performed in the first six months after PCI. Exercise electrocardiograms 1–3 months after PCI did not show a shift of the ST-segment for all patients without restenosis. However, angiography depression of the ST-segment was registered on exercise electrocardiogram only for patients with restenosis. This demonstrates a clear correlation between ST-segment depression and restenosis.

Adequate implementation of drug therapies depending on patient clinical and functional status allow to reach goals set by national and international guidelines. Based on epidemiological studies, even small decreases in low density lipoprotein cholesterol and blood pressure levels translate into significant reductions in cardiovascular morbidity and mortality (LaRosa et al., 2005). Moreover, especially important is the patient compliance, which can be achieved through frequently scheduled visits.

The clinical course and prognosis of patients with coronary artery disease can be modified favourably by successful translation of recommendations for secondary coronary prevention into effective clinical care. Crucial to the outcome of any preventive strategy is patient attitude to lifestyle modification and compliance with drug therapies over the long term. We tend to claim that an aggressive follow-up programme could help us to reach the goals in secondary prevention of coronary artery disease set by European Societies and Latvian Society of Cardiology.

The physical exercise test is a safe method with high specificity, but is limited by poor test sensitivity for the evaluation of efficacy of interventional and medical treatment for patients with coronary artery disease. A focussed exercise test performed on a regular basis indirectly influences clinical results and prognosis. Timely set diagnosis of restenosis provides necessary treatment measures, therefore, alienating adverse cardiac events such as unstable angina and myocardial infarction. Moreover, an exercise test performed on a regular basis provides essential corrections in drug therapy. After comparison of drug therapies recommended three months and one year after PCI, we can conclude that regular follow-ups provide the opportunity to sustain acceptable patient compliance and use of medications even twelve months after an intervention.

A focussed follow-up programme with an exercise test allows to evaluate clinical status of patients as well as to determine timely possible risk of restenosis, to adapt medication doses, to reduce risk factors and to influence positively patient compliance. The exercise test provides accurate estimation of possible restenosis in patients with complete revascularization. In patients with incomplete revascularization the exercise test specificity is reduced. Taking into account the results of the current study, we are sure, that focussed physical exercise test should be advised for all patients after interventional treatment. It is of high importance to achieve submaximal heart rate during the exercise test. In all cases when this is not possible for any reason, myocardial perfusion scintigraphy is indicated.

Advantages of the study (benefits)

The results of this study can be used with a goal to determine possible risk of restenosis in a time, to prescribe medications according to patient's functional status, to correct possible risk factors, which can have negative influence on development of disease.

Regular patients' follow-ups increase the compliance of the patients and 'participation' in treatment process, thus increasing accuracy of data and foundation of the results.

Possible disadvantages (limits) of the study

Irregular patients' follow-ups, thus exclusion from statistycal analysis.

Insufficient information about patient recurrent hospitalization at district hospital. Also the variability in medical treatment (general practitioner like „middle stage" between patient and cardiologist).

The lack of patients compliance in medication use, the lack of motivation in modification of their possible risk factors.

Low availability of myocardial perfusion scintigraphy, thus, not possibility to perform necessary investigation in position of diagnosis making and more detailed evaluation of clinical situation.

6. Conclusions

1. Exercise test (veloergometry) is established as a safe method with high specificity, but lower sensitivity in evaluation of invasive and medical treatment efficiacy in patients

with CAD, evolving different invasive treatment methods (with drug-eluting stents, balloon angioplasty, etc.)
2. The database of the patients with left main coronary artery stenosis was analyzed, evaluating the efficacy of invasive treatment of left main stenosis, analyzing possible progression of restenosis and evaluating following treatment steps.
3. New specific criteria were extracted for risk evaluation and detection with exercise stress test.
4. Algorithms were developed for CAD patients' clinical status evaluation after percutaneous coronary intervention.
5. Follow-up programme with targeted exercise test allows to personalize exact treatment strategy and risk factor correction for each patient individually.

7. References

Arab D,Valeti V, Schunemann H, Lopez-Candales A (2000) Usefulness of the QTc Interval in Predicting Myocardial Ischemia in Patients undergoing Exercise Stress Testing. Am J Cardiol 85:764-766.

Babapulle M, Diodati J, Blankenship J, Huynh T, Cugno S, Puri R, Nguyen P, Eisenberg M (2007) Utility of Routine Exercise Treadmill Testing early after Percutaneous Coronary Intervention. BMC Cardiovascular Disorders 7.

Bengtson J, Mark D, Honan M, et al (1990) Detection of Restenosis after Elective Percutaneous Transluminal Coronary Angioplasty using the Exercise Treadmill Test. Am J Cardiol 65:28-34.

Berntsen R, Gjestvang F, Rasmussen K (1995) QRS Prolongation as an Indicator of Risk of Ischemia-Related Ventricular Tachycardia and Fibrillation Induced by Exercise. Am Heart J 129:542-548.

Califf R, Mark D, Harrell F (1988) Importance of Clinical Measures of Ischemia in the Prognosis of Patients with Documented Coronary Artery Disease J Am Coll Cardiol 11:20-26.

Cecchi F, Olivotto I, Gistri R, Lorenzoni R, Chiriatti G, Camici P (2003) Coronary Microvascular Dysfunction and Prognosis in Hypertrophic Cardiomyopathy. N Engl J Med 349:1027-1035.

Chalela W, Kreling J, Falcao A, Hueb W, Moffa P, Pereyra P, Ramires J (2006) Exercise Stress Testing before and after successsful Multivessel Percutaneous Transluminal Coronary Angioplasty. Brazilian Journal of Medical and Biological Research 39:475-482.

Cerqueira M D, Weissman N J, Dilsizian V, Jacobs A K, Kaul S, Lasney W K, Pennel D J, Rumberger J A, Ryan T, Verani M S (2002) Standardized Myocardial Segmentation and Nomenclature for Tomographic Imaging of the Heart. A Statement for Healthcare Professionals From the Cardiac Imaging Committee of the Council on Clinical Cardiology of the American Heart Association. Circulation 105:539-542.

Eisenberg M, Schechter D, Lefkovits J, Goudreau E, Deligonul U, Mak K, Del Core M, Duerr R, Garzon P, Huynh T, Smilovitch M, Sedlis S, Brown D, Brieger D, Pilote L (2001) ROSETTA Investigators: Use of Routine Functional Testing after Percutaneous Transluminal Coronary Angioplasty: Results from the ROSETTA Registry. Am Heart J 141:837-846

Erglis A et al. The guidelines of the Latvian Society of Cardiology on prevention and management of stable coronary heart disease, Riga, 2007.Fletcher G, Balady G, Froelicher V, Hartley L, Haskell W, Pollock M (1995) Exercise Standards. A

Statement for Healthcare Professionals from the American Heart Association. Writing Group. Circulation 91:580-615.

Foult J, Hoffman O, Ducardonnet A, Attal B, Uzan L, Weinmann P, Verdier J (2009) Exercise Testing in Cardiology.

Fox K, Garsia M, Ardissino D, Buszman P, Camici P, Crea F, Daly C, De Backer G, Hjemdahl P, Lopez-Sendon H, Marco J, Morais J, Pepper J, Sechtem U, Simoons M, Thygesen T (2006) Stable angina pectoris (Management of). ESC Practice guidelines.

Gianrossi R, Detrano R, Mulvihill D, Lehmann K, Dubach P, Colombo A, McArthur D, Froelicher V (1989) Exercise Induced ST Depression in the Diagnosis of Coronary Artery Disease: a Meta -Analysis. Circulation 80:87-98.

Gibbons R, Balady G, Bricker J, Chaitman B, Fletcher G, Froelicher V, Mark D, McCallister B, Mooss A, O'Reilly M, Winters W (2002) ACC/AHA 2002 Guideline Update for Exercise Testing. A Report of the American College of Cardiology/ American Heart Association Task Force on Practice Guidelines (Committee on Exercise Testing). ACC/AHA Practice Guidelines.

Hamasaki S, Arima S, Tahara M, Kihara K, Shono H, Nakao S, Tanaka H (1996) Increase in the delta ST/ delta Heart Rate (HR) Index: a new Predictor of Restenosis after successful Percutaneous Transluminal Coronary Angioplasty. Am J Cardiol 78:990-995.

Hamasaki S, Abematsu H, Arima S, Tahara M, Kihara K, Shono H, Nakao S, Tanaka H. A new predictor of restenosis after successful percutaneous transluminal coronary angioplasty in patients with multivessel coronary artery disease. *Am J Cardiol.* 1997; 80: 411–415.

Hesse B, Morise A, Pothier C, Blackstone E, Lauer M (2005) Can we Reliably Predict Long-Term Mortality After Exercise Testing? An External Validation Am Heart J 150:307-314.

Hjalmarson A, Goldstein S, Fagerberg B, Wedel H, Waagstein F, Kjekshus J, Wikstrand J, AlAllaf D, Vitovec J, Aldershvile J (2000) Effects of controlled-release Metoprolol on total Mortality, Hospitalizations, and well-being in Patients with Heart Failure: the Metoprolol CR/XL Randomized Intervention Trial in Congestive Heart Failure (MERIT-HF), MERIT-HF Study Group. JAMA 283:1295-1302.

Holmes DR, Vlietstra RE, Smith HC, Vetrovec GW, Kent KM, Cowley MJ, Faxon DP, Gruentzig AR, Kelsey SF, Detre KM (1984) Restenosis after Percutaneous Transluminal Coronary Angioplasty (PTCA): A Report from the PTCA Registry of the National Heart, Lung, and Blood Institute Am J Cardiol 53:C77-C81.

Imai K, Sato H, Hori M, Kusuoka H, Ozaki H, Yokoyama H, Takeda H, Inoue M, Kamada T (1994) Vagally mediated Heart Rate Recovery after Exercise is accelerated in Athletes but blunted in Patients with Chronic Heart Failure. J Am Coll Cardiol 1994:1529-1535.

Jawad E, Arora R (2008) Chronic Stable Angina Pectoris. Dis Mon 54:671-689.

Kligfield P, Lauer M (2006) Exercise Electrocardiogram Testing. Beyond the ST Segment. Circulation 114:2070-2082.

Kligfield P, Okin P (1994) Evolution of the Exercise Electrocardiogram. Am J Cardiol 73:1209-1210.

Kwok J, Miller T, Christian T, Hodge D, Gibbons R (1999) Prognostic Value of a Treadmill Exercise Score in Symptomatic Patients with Nonspecific ST-T Abnormalities on Resting ECG JAMA 282:1047-1053.

LaRosa J, Grundy S, Waters D, Shear C, Barter P, Fruchart J, Gotto A, Greten H, Kastelein J, Shepherd J, Wenger N (2005) Intensive Lipid lowering with Atorvastatin in Patients with Stable Coronary Disease. N Engl J Med 352:1425-1435.

Lauer M, Francis G, Okin P, Pashkow F, Snader C, Marwick T (1999) Impaired chronotropic Response to Exercise Stress Testing as a Predictor of Mortality. JAMA 281:524-529.

Libby P, Theroux P (2005) Pathophysiology of Coronary Artery Disease. Circulation 111:3481-3488.

Lombard A, Loperfido F, Pennestri F, Rossi e, Patrizi R, Cristinziani G, Catapano G, Maseri A (1996) Significance of Transient ST-T Segment Changes during Dobutamine Testing in Q Wave Myocardial Infarction. J Am Coll Cardiol 27:599-605.

Mackay J, Mensah G (2004) Atlas of Heart Disease and Stroke. World Health Organization, Geneva.

Margonato A, Chierchia S, Xuereb R, Xuereb M, Fragasso G, Cappelletti A, Landoni C, Lucignani G, Fazio F (1995) Specificity and Sensitivity of Exercise-Induced ST Segment Elevation for Detection of Residual Viability: Comparison with Fluorodeoxyglucose and Positron Emission Tomography. J Am Coll Cardiol 25:1032-1038.

Mark D, Shaw L, Harrell F, Hlatky M, Lee K, Bengtson J, McCants C, Califf R, Pryor D (1991) Prognostic Value of a Treadmill Exercise Score in Outpatients with Suspected Coronary Artery Disease. N Engl J Med 325:849-853.

Mastouri R, Sawada SG, Mahenthiran J (2010) Current Noninvasive Imaging Technique for Detection of Coronary Artery Disease. Expert Review of Cardiovascular Therapy 8:77-91.

Mehta S, Yusuf S, Peters R, Bertrand M, Lewis B, Natarjan M, Malmberg K, Rupprecht H, Zhao F, Chrolavicius S (2001) Effects of Pretreatment with Clopidogrel and Aspirin followed by long-term Therapy in Patients undergoing Percutaneous Coronary Intervention: the PCI-CURE Study. Lancet 358:524-533.

Mercado N, Boersma E, Wijns W, Gersh B, Morillo C, de Valk V, van Es G, Grobbee D, Serruys P (2001) Clinical and Quantitative Coronary Angiographic Predictors of Coronary Restenosis: a comparative Analysis from the Baloon-to-Stent Era. J Am Coll Cardiol 38.

Michaelides A, Ryan J, Bacon J, Pozderac R, Toutouzas P, Boudoulas H (1995) Exercise-induced QRS Changes (Athens QRS Score) in Patients with Coronary Artery Disease: a Marker of Myocardial Ischemia. J Cardiol 26:263-272.

Michaelides A, Ryan J, VanFoseen D, Pozderac R, Boudoulas H (1993) Exercise-Induced QRS Prolongation in Patients with Coronary Artery Disease: a Marker of Myocardial Ischemia. Am Heart J 126:1320-1325.

Michaelides A, Triposkiadis F, Boudoulas H, Spanos A, Papadopoulos P, Kourouklis K, Toutouzas P (1990) New Coronary Artery Disease Index based on Exercise-Induced QRS Changes. Am Heart J 120:292-302.

Mintāle I, Erglis A. Recommendations of Latvian Society of Cardiology on Physical Exercise Tests, Riga, 2008.

Miranda C, Lehmann K, Froelicher V (1991) Correlation between Resting ST Segment Depression, Exercise Testing, Coronary Angiography, and Long-Term Prognosis. Am Heart J 122:1617-1628.

Miranda C, Lehmann K, Lachterman B, Coodley E, Froelicher V (1991) Comparison of Silent and Symptomatic Ischemia during Exercise Testing in Men. Ann Intern Med 114:649-656.

Myers J, Prakash M, Froelicher V, Do D, Partington S, Atwood J (2002) Exercise Capacity and Mortality among Men referred for Exercise Testing. N Engl J Med 346:793-801.

Okin P, Kligfield P (1995) Heart Rate Adjustment of ST Segment Depression and Performance of the Exercise Electrocardiogram: a Critical Evaluation. J Am Coll Cardiol 25:1726-1735
Okin P, Kligfield P (1995) Heart Rate Adjustment of ST Segment Depression and Performance of the Exercise Electrocardiogram: a Critical Evaluation. J Am Coll Cardiol 25:1726-1735.
Pepine C, Cohnm P, Deedwania P (1994) Effects of Treatment on Outcome in Mildly Symptomatic Patients with Ischemia during Daily Life: the Atenolol Silent Ischemia Study (ASIST). Circulation 90:762-768.
Renkin J, Melin J, Robert A (1990) Detection of Restenosis after Successful Coronary Angioplasty: improved Clinical Decision Making with Use of a logistic Model Combining Procedural and Follow-Up Variables. J Am Coll Cardiol 16:1333-1340.
Roffi M, Wenaweser P, Windecker S, Mehta H, Eberli F, Seiler C, Fleisch M, Garachemani A, Pedrazzini G, Hess O, Meier B (2003) Early Exercise Test after Coronary Stenting is safe. J Am Coll Cardiol 42:1569-1573.
Ruygrok P, Webster M, De Valk V, van Es G, Ormiston J (2001) Clinical and Angiographic Factors associated with Asymptomatic Restenosis after Percutaneous Coronary Intervention. Circulation 104:2289-2294.
Serruys PW, Luijten HE, Beatt KJ, Gauskens R, de Feyter PJ, van den Brand M, Reiber JH, ten Katen HJ, van Es GA, Hugenholtz PG (1988) Incidence of Restenosis after Successful Coronary Angioplasty: a time-related Phenomenon. A quantitative angiographic Study in 342 consecutive patients at 1, 2, 3, and 4 months. Circulation 77:361-371.
Shaw L, Peterson E, Shaw L, Kesler K, DeLong E, Harrell F, Muhlbaier L, Mark D (1998) Use of a Prognostic Treadmill Score in Identifying Diagnostic Coronary Disease Subgroups Circulation 98:1622-1630.
Sheffield L (1991) Upsloping ST Segments. Circulation 84:426-428.
Sketch M, Mooss A, Butler M, Nair C, Mohiuddin S (1981) Digoxin-induced Positive Exercise Tests: their Clinical and Prognostic Significance. Am J Cardiol 48:655-659.
Strauss HW, Miller D, Wittry M, Cerqueira MD, Garcia EV, Iskandrian AS, Schelbert HR, Wackers FJ (2002) Procedure Guideline for Myocardial Perfusion Imaging The Journal of Nuclear Medicine 39:918-923.
Stuart RJ, Ellestad M (1980) National Survey of Exercise Stress Testing Facilities. Chest 77:94-97.
Viik J (2000) Diagnostic Properties of Exercise Electrocardiographic Leads and Variables in the Detection of Coronary Artery Disease. Tampere University of Technology Publications.
Weinsaft J, Wong F, Walden J, Szulc M, Okin P, Kligfield P (2005) Anatomic Distribution of Myocardial Ischemia as a Determinant of Exercise-Induced ST-segment Depression Am J Cardiol 96:1356-1360.
Wenaweser P, Surmely J-F, Windecker S, Roffi M, Togni M, Billinger M, Cook S, Vogel R, Seiler C, Hess O, Meier B (2008) Prognostic value of Early Exercise Testing After Coronary Stent Implantation. Am J Cardiol 101:807-811.
Whinnery J, Froelicher V, Stuart A (1997) The Electrocardiographic Response to Maximal Treadmill Exercise in Asymptomatic Men with Left Bundle Branch Block. Am Heart J 94:316-324.
Yusuf S, Sleght P, Pogue J, Bosch J, Davies R, Dagenais G (2000) Effects of an Angiotensin-converting-Enzyme Inhibitor, Ramipril, on Cardiovascular Events in high-risk Patients. The Heart Outcomes Prevention Evaluation Study Investigators. N Engl J Med 342:145-153.

Part 4

Cardiotoxicology

15

Toxic and Drug-Induced Changes of the Electrocardiogram

Catalina Lionte, Cristina Bologa and Laurentiu Sorodoc
"Gr.T.Popa" University of Medicine and Pharmacy, Iasi, Romania

1. Introduction

There are numerous toxins and drugs that can cause, in overdose, electrocardiogram (ECG) changes, even in patients without history of cardiac pathology. The diagnosis and management of patients with an abnormal ECG encountered in a specific toxicity can challenge experienced physicians. One must have serious knowledge of basic cardiac physiology, in order to understand the ECG changes associated with various drugs and toxins.

The main mechanisms involved include membrane - depressant action (sodium channel blockers, slow calcium channel blockers, outward potassium (K^+) channel blockers, and sodium-potassium adenosine-triphosphatase blockers), and action on autonomic nervous system and its sites of cardiovascular action (beta-adrenergic blockers and other sympathetic-inhibitors, sympathomimetic, anticholinergic and cholinomimetic substances). Many toxins and medications have actions that involve more than one of these mechanisms, including hypoxia, electrolyte and metabolic imbalances, and thus may result in a combination of electrocardiographic changes.

In resting state, the myocardial cell membrane is impermeable to positively charged sodium ions (Na^+). The Na^+/K^+ ATPase maintains a negative electric potential of approximately 90 mV in the myocyte. The rapid opening of Na^+ channels and massive Na^+ influx (phase 0 of action potential) explains depolarization of the cardiac cell membrane (fig.1), causing the rapid upstroke of the cardiac action potential, which is conducted through the ventricles and is expressed as the QRS complex of the ECG. The closure of Na^+ channels and the transient opening of I_{to} K^+ efflux channels (phase 1) mark the peak of the action potential. Then, phase 2 of the action potential occurs when the opening of slow calcium (Ca^{2+}) channels produces an influx of positive ions with a steady maintenance of the membrane potential and myocardial contraction continues. The end of the cardiac cycle is marked by the closure of the Ca^{2+} channels and the activation of the K^+ efflux channels, which allow the action potential to return to its resting potential of - 90 mV (phase 3). This K^+ efflux from the myocardial cell is directly responsible for the QT interval on the ECG (Holstege et al., 2006). During phase 4 of the cardiac cell action potential, some cardiac fibers allow sodium ions to enter the cell, increasing the resting membrane potential, known as spontaneous diastolic depolarization. When the threshold in membrane potential is reached, the Na^+ channels open and another action potential is generated.

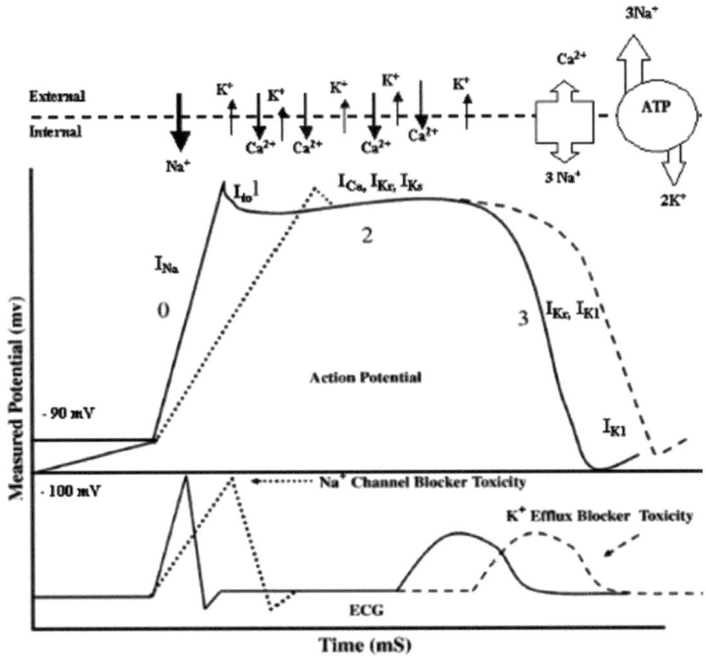

Fig. 1. Cardiac cycle action potential with corresponding ion changes across the membrane and electrocardiographic tracing. Dotted line indicates the changes associated with Na^+ channel blocker toxicity. Dashed line indicates the changes associated with K^+ efflux blocker toxicity. I_{to}= transient outward K^+ current; I_{Ca}= L-type Ca^{2+} current; I_{Na}= late sodium channel current; I_{Kr}= rapidly activating delayed-rectifier K^+ current; I_{Ks}= slowly activating delayed rectifier K^+ current; I_{K1}= inward rectifier K^+ current (adapted from Holstege et al., 2005).

The atrial and ventricular myocardium contraction, and the conduction in the His-Purkinje system depend on sodium entry via the fast sodium channels in phase 0 of the action potential, while the conduction in sinoatrial node and atrioventricular (AV) node depend on Ca^{2+} entry during phase 0 via the slow Ca^{2+} channels (Patel & Benowitz, 2005).

Cardiac activity is controlled, among other mechanisms, by the autonomic nervous system. Sympathetic fibers increase the heart rate, the rate of AV nodal conduction and the contracility of the myocardium. The norepinephrine released by postganglionic fibers leads to an interaction with beta 1-adrenergic cardiac receptors, and increasing cells' permeability to Na^+ and Ca^{2+}, with an increase of contractility, excitability, and conduction. The parasympathetic postganglionic fibers innervate the sinus node and AV node. Stimulation of muscarinic receptors via releasing of acetylcholine decreases atrial excitability and slows the conduction of impulses to the ventricles (Patel & Benowitz, 2005).

In the setting of drug overdose or of a toxic exposure, ECG abnormalities, especially arrhythmias, are produced by direct or indirect sympathomimetic effects, anticholinergic effects, the effects of altered central nervous system (CNS) regulation of peripheral autonomic system, and myocardial membrane depression. Genesis of arrhythmias in the poisoned patient is based on the same three mechanisms as in an ischemic patient: abnormal impulse formation, abnormal impulse conduction, and triggered activity. Contributing factors to ECG changes are hypotension, hypoxia, acid-base and electrolyte imbalances.

2. Membrane – depressant drugs and toxins

Cardiotoxins are responsible of ECG changes through a combination of membrane depressant effects, autonomic disturbances and metabolic changes. The severity of a toxic-induced conduction block varies depending on the toxin involved and its site of action.

2.1 Sodium channel blockers

Inhibition of the fast Na^+ channels, in the phase 0 of the action potential (AP), decreases the rate of rise and amplitude of the AP in Purkinje fibers, and in atrial and ventricular myocardial cells. As a result, the upslope of depolarization is slowed and the QRS complex becomes wide. In a toxicological situation, QRS complex widening likely results directly from Na^+ channel blockage or indirectly from toxin-induced hyperkalemia (Holstege et al.,

Inhibitors of fast Na^+ channels	1. Cardiovascular drugs: - Type Ia antiarrhythmics (Quinidine, Disopyramide, Procainamide) - Type Ic antiarrhythmics (Flecainide, Encainide, Propafenone, Moricizine) - Propranolol and other membrane depressant beta-blockers* - Verapamil, Diltiazem 2. Psychiatric drugs: - Carbamazepine - Cyclic antidepressants (Amitriptyline, Amoxapine, Desipramine, Doxepin, Imipramine, Nortriptyline, Maprotiline) - Neuroleptics (Thioridazine, Mesoridazine) - Other antidepressants (Citalopram) - Antipsychotics (Loxapine) 3. Other drugs: - Amantadine - Antihistamines (Diphenhydramine) - Chloroquine, Hydroxychloroquine - Orphenadrine - Narcotic pain relievers (Propoxyphene) 4. Illicit drugs: Cocaine 5. Toxins: Quinine, Saxitoxin, Tetrodotoxin
ECG changes	QRS widening Right bundle branch pattern R wave elevation in aVR lead Rightward deviation of QRS axis Ventricular tachycardia (VT) and ventricular fibrillation (VF) Bradycardia with wide QRS complex Asystole ST/T changes consistent with ischemia (cocaine toxicity)

*mechanism not involving the beta-receptor.

Table 1. Na^+ channel blockers and the resulting ECG changes.

2005). Direct toxin-induced blockade of cardiac Na^+ channels will cause QRS complex widening, and it has been described as a membrane stabilizing effect, a local anesthetic effect, or a quinidine-like effect. Some drugs in this category (Table 1) may also affect other myocardial ion transfers, such as the Ca^{2+} influx and K^+ efflux (Holstege et al., 2006). Other abnormal QRS complex configurations are also possible. In the most severe cases, the QRS complex widening becomes so profound that the ultimate origin of the rhythm disturbance is impossible (fig. 2).

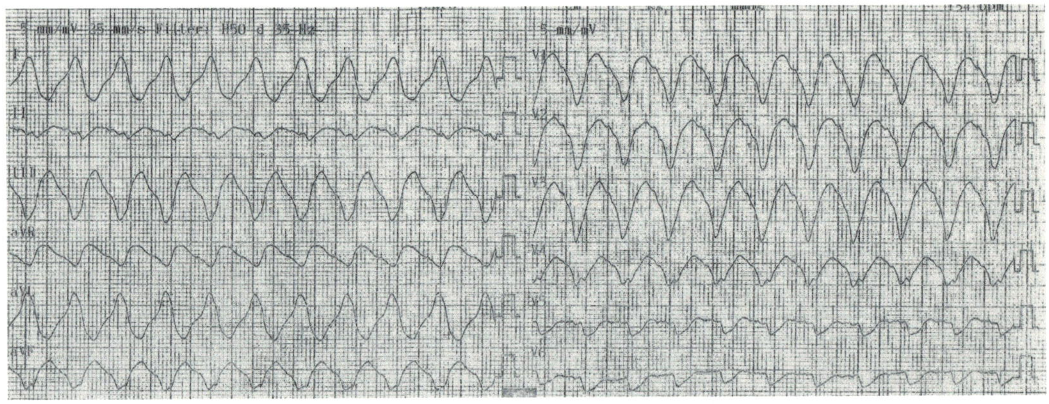

Fig. 2. Na^+ channel blocker toxicity (patient with acute Propafenone overdose). Note the wide QRS complex, at a rate of 134/min, which suggests, at a first view, monomorphic VT.

R wave elevation in aVR ≥ 3 mm (fig.3) is the only ECG variable that significantly indicates the risk of seizures and arrhythmias in acute tricyclic antidepressant poisoning (Liebelt et al., 1995). In addition, QT interval prolongation can occur with tricyclic antidepressant poisoning, as well as rightward axis deviation of the terminal 40 msec of the frontal plane QRS axis, which is unknown in other Na^+ channel blocking agents (Wolfe et al. 1989; Berkovitch et al, 1995). Continued prolongation of the QRS complex may result in a sine wave pattern and eventual asystole.

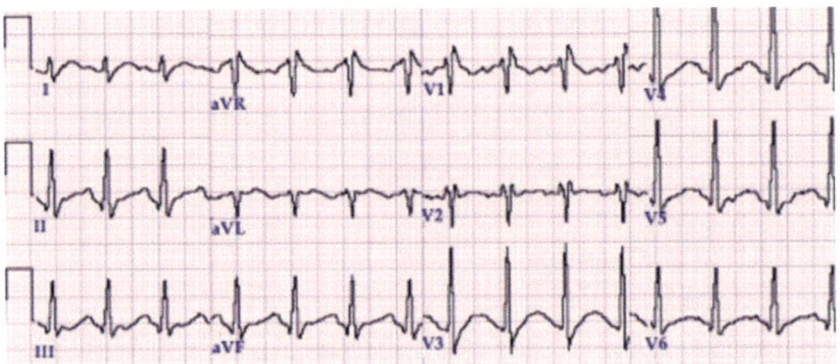

Fig. 3. Acute poisoning with Amitriptyline. ECG reveals sinus tachycardia 148/min, RBBB pattern, QRS complex ≥ 120 ms, as well as R wave elevation in aVR ≥ 3 mm.

Na^+ channel blockers may determine slowed intraventricular conduction, unidirectional block, the development of a reentrant circuit, and a resulting VT as well as VF. Because many of the Na^+ channel blocking agents have also anticholinergic or sympathomimetic effects, bradydisrrhythmias are rare. In Na^+ channel blocker poisoning by anticholinergic and sympathomimetic drugs, the combination of a wide QRS complex and bradycardia is a sign of severe poisoning, indicating that the Na^+ channel blockade is so profound that tachycardia does not occur, despite the clinical muscarinic antagonism or adrenergic agonism (Holstege et al., 2006). Nevertheless, bradycardia may occur because of slowed depolarization of pacemaker cells that depend on entry of Na^+ ions.

2.2 Slow Calcium Channel Blockers (CCB)

All CCBs (Table 2) inhibit the voltage sensitive L-type Ca^{2+} channel within the cell membrane. In the pacemaker cells of the sinoatrial node and AV node, the primary ion channel, which controls depolarization, is the slow Ca^{2+} channel. When inhibited, there is a slowing or an inhibition of the specialized tissue to conduct a cardiac impulse (Patel & Benowitz, 2005).

Inhibitors of slow Ca^{2+} channels	1. Dihydropyridines: - 1st generation: Nicardipine, Nifedipine - 2nd generation: Felodipine, Isradipine, Nimodipine - 3rd generation: Amlodipine, Nitrendipine - 4th generation: Lercanidipine, Lacidipine 2. Phenylalkylamine: - Verapamil - Gallopamil 3. Benzothiazepine: - Diltiazem 4. Non-selective: - Bepridil - Mibefradil - Fluspirilene
ECG changes	Sinus bradycardia Reflex tachycardia (ex. Nifedipine) Varying degrees of AV block Sinus arrest with AV junctional rhythm Asystole Wide QRS complex ST/T changes

Table 2. Calcium channel blockers and the resulting ECG changes.

In CCB toxicity initially occurs a sinus bradycardia, followed by various degrees of AV block (fig.4), and junctional and ventricular bradydysrhythmias on ECG. Depending on the agent involved, other dysrhythmias may be seen (Gordon, 2006): sinus tachycardia (specifically Nifedipine), atrial arrhythmias, and junctional rhythms (fig. 5, 6,7). A wide QRS complex may appear, caused by ventricular escape rhythms or by CCB-induced Na^+ channel blockade which delays of phase 0 of depolarization. Sudden shifts from bradydysrhythmias to cardiac arrest have been reported.

In addition, ECG changes associated with cardiac ischemia (fig.8) may occur as a result of the hypotension and changes in the cardiovascular status, especially in patients with pre-existing cardiac disease (Patel & Benowitz, 2005; Holstege et al., 2006).

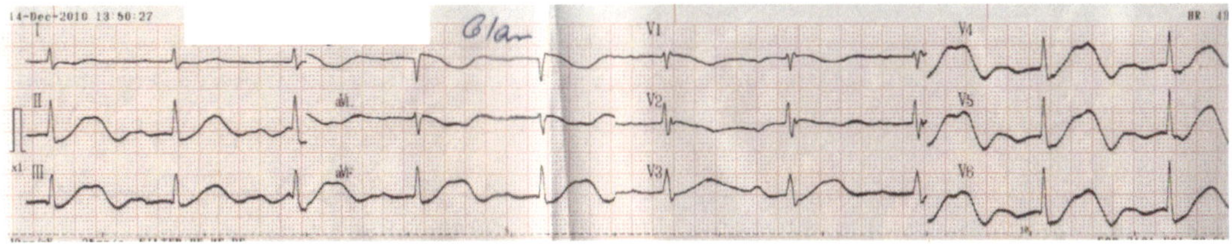

Fig. 4. Acute poisoning with Verapamil in a 61-years old female. ECG reveals sinus bradycardia 41/min, minor right bundle ranch block (RBBB), first-degree AV block (PR 0.32 sec) and long QT interval (0.64 sec).

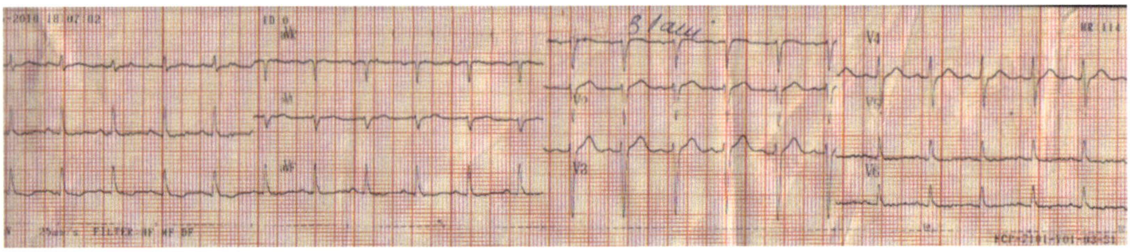

Fig. 5. Acute poisoning with Norvasc 300 mg in a 31-years old female. ECG reveals sinus tachycardia 114/min, signs of ischemia in infero-lateral leads, 14 hours after ingestion (systolic blood pressure 70 mmHg).

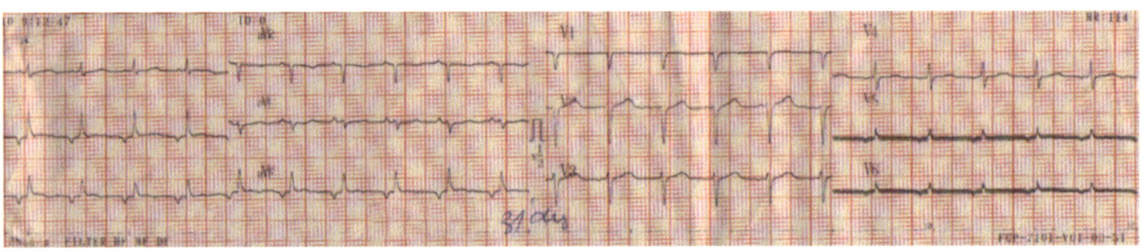

Fig. 6. Same patient, two days after ingestion. ECG reveals accelerated junctional rhythm (sinus coronary rhythm, or Zahn rhythm) 114/min, with negative P waves in leads DII, DIII, aVF, and disappearance of ischemic changes present at admission.

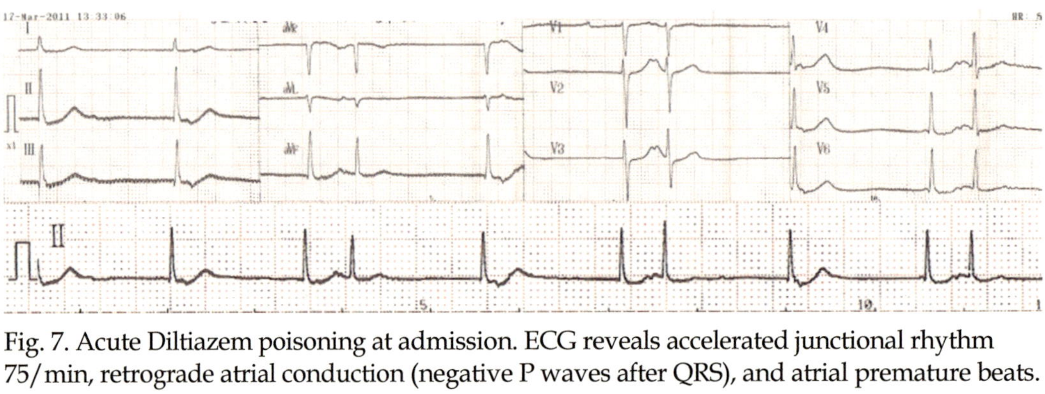

Fig. 7. Acute Diltiazem poisoning at admission. ECG reveals accelerated junctional rhythm 75/min, retrograde atrial conduction (negative P waves after QRS), and atrial premature beats.

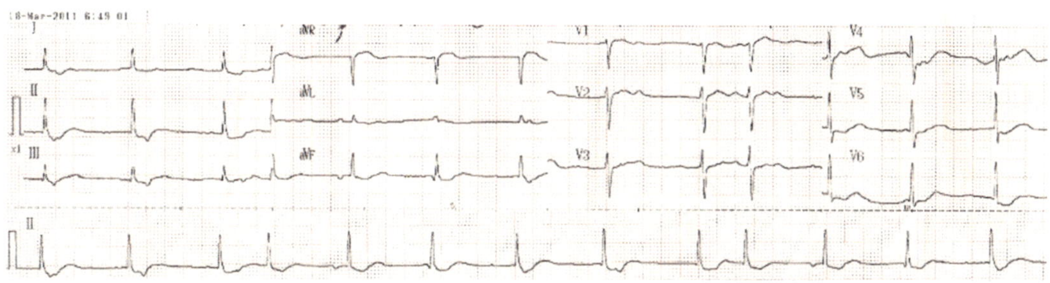

Fig. 8. Same patient (Diltiazem poisoning), second day of evolution. ECG reveals atrio-ventricular dissociation, with escape junctional rhythm and some ventricular captures, and signs of ischemia (in inferior and lateral leads).

2.3 Outward potassium channel blockers

Medications in the K^+ efflux blocker category block the outward flow of K^+ from intracellular to extracellular spaces. Blockade of the outward K^+ currents may prolong the cardiac cycle action potential (Fig. 1). The primary electrocardiographic manifestation is QT interval prolongation (QTc interval greater than 0.45 seconds in men and 0.47 seconds in women). Delay of repolarization causes the myocardial cell to have less charge difference across its membrane, and result in the activation of the inward depolarization current (early after-depolarization), which is seen on ECG as prominent U waves (Murphy et al., 2007). This may promote triggered activity, which potentially can progress to re-entry and subsequent polymorphic VT. Toxin-induced blockade of K^+ efflux channels during phase 3 of the action potential corresponding with repolarization and QT interval prolongation may place the patient at risk for polymorphic VT or torsades de pointes (Holstege et al., 2005; Holstege et al., 2006). The drugs and toxins reported to have this effect are listed in table 3.

Risk factors for torsades de pointes (TdP) among patients treated with medications that prolong QT interval include, among others, female gender, hypokalemia, hypomagnesemia, bradycardia, overdose, drug interactions (fig.9), digitalis therapy, and background of the patient (preexisting cardiac disease, long QT interval or family history of long QT). (Murphy et al., 2007; Roden, 2004)

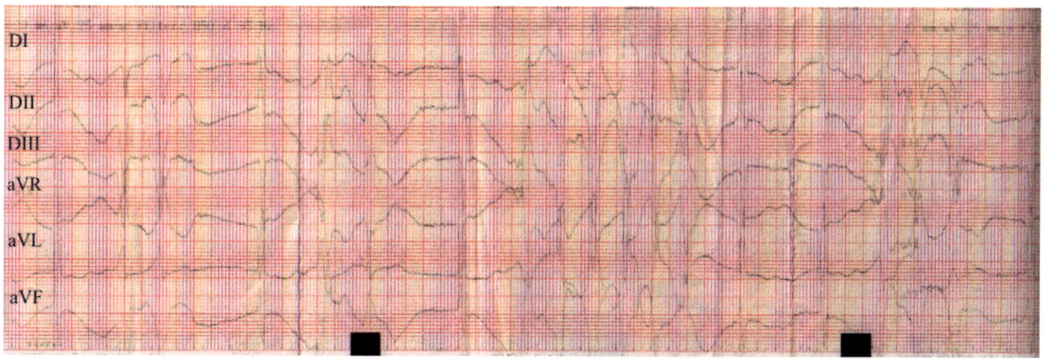

Fig. 9. Drug-induced long QT interval, following interaction between Bisoprolol and Amiodarone. ECG shows long QT interval (0.80 sec), couples of PVB with R/T phenomenon preceding a short episode of polymorphic VT.

Inhibitors of outward K^+ channel	1. Cardiovascular drugs: - Class IA antidysrhythmics**(Disopyramide, Quinidine, Procainamide) - Class IC antidysrhythmics (Encainide, Flecainide, Moricizine, Propafenone) - Class III antidysrhythmics** (e.g. Amiodarone, Dronedarone, Dofetilide, Ibutilide, Sotalol, Vernakalant) - Anti-anginal/vasodilators*,** (Bepridil, Prenylamine, Terodiline) - Antihypertensives (Ketanserin*) 2. Psychiatric drugs: - Antipsychotics (Chlorpromazine, Droperidol, Haloperidol, Mesoridazine, Pimozide, Quetiapine, Risperidone, Thioridazine, Ziprasidone) - Cyclic antidepressants (Amitriptyline, Amoxapine, Desipramine, Doxepin, Imipramine, Nortriptyline, Maprotiline) - Other antidepressants (Citalopram, Venlafaxine) - Phenothiazines 3. Other drugs: - Antihistamines (Astemizole, Diphenhydramine, Loratidine, Terfenadine*, Hydroxyzine) - Serotonin $5\text{-}HT_4$ receptor agonist (Cisaprid*,**) - Antimicrobials and antimalarics (Ciprofloxacin, Gatifloxacin, Levofloxacin, Moxifloxacin, Sparfloxacin, Clarithromycin**, Erythromycin**, Pentamidine**, Chloroquine**, Halofantrine, Hydroxychloroquine, etc.) - Arsenic trioxide - Probucol* 4. Synthetic opioids: Levomethadyl 5. Opium alkaloids: Papaverine** 6. Toxins: Quinine, Organophosphates (fig.10)
ECG changes	QT interval prolongation T- or U-wave abnormalities Premature ventricular beats (PVB) followed by TdP Sinus tachycardia

*removed from the market; ** TdP reported.

Table 3. K^+ efflux channel blockers, and the resulting ECG changes.

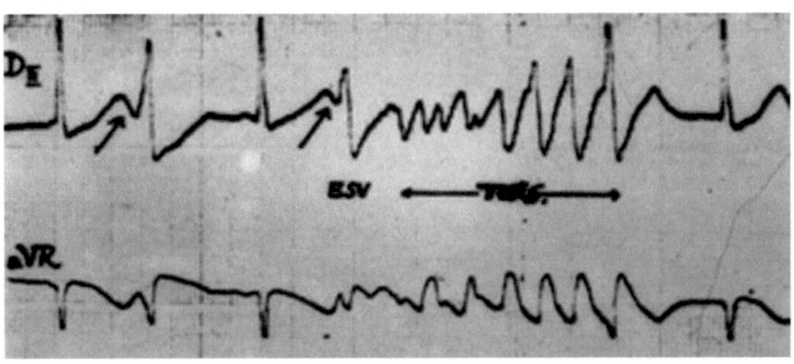

Fig. 10. Acute organophosphate poisoning, five days after ingestion. ECG shows long QT interval (0.60 sec), PVB with R/T phenomenon (arrows) preceding a short episode of TdP (TORS).

Many of these drugs have other effects that can result in significant electrocardiographic changes, such as antipsychotics, that can cause muscarinic acetylcholine receptor and alpha-adrenergic receptor blockade and cardiac cell K^+, Na^+, and Ca^{2+} channel blockade (Holstege et al., 2006). These effects lead to sinus tachycardia (secondary to anticholinergic effect) or reflex tachycardia (secondary to alpha-adrenergic blockade).

2.4 Sodium–potassium ATPase blockers

Cardiac glycosides (table 4) inhibit the Na^+/K^+ adenosine triphosphatase (Na^+/K^+ATPase) pump. As a result, there is an inhibition of the active transport of Na^+ and K^+ across cell membrane, intracellular Na^+ increases and the Na^+/Ca^{2+}exchanger is secondary activated. The intracellular Ca^{2+} level increases, and augments myofibril activity in cardiac myocytes, which results in a positive inotropic effect, and increased automaticity. The cardiac glycosides also increase vagal tone that may lead to a direct atrioventricular (AV) nodal depression (Holstege et al., 2006). Digitalis derivatives in therapeutic doses are used to increase myocardial contractility or slow AV conduction. They modify ECG, changes known as "digitalis effect", expressed by abnormal inverted or flattened T waves coupled with ST segment depression (most pronounced in leads with tall R waves), QT interval shortening (as a result of decreased ventricular repolarization time), PR interval lengthening (increased vagal activity), and prominent U-waves. Sagging ST segments, inverted T waves, and normal or shortened QT intervals are sometimes identified by their similar appearance to "Salvador Dali's mustache" (Clancy, 2007). These ECG changes are seen with therapeutic Digoxin levels and do not represent toxicity (Chung, 1981).

Na^+/K^+ ATPase blockers	1.	Drugs:
	-	Digoxin (Lanoxin)
	-	Digitoxin
	2.	Plants producing cardiac glycosides:
	-	Cardenolide type: *Strophanthus* - ouabain g/k/e-strophanthin, *Digitalis lanata* and *Digitalis purpurea* (foxglove) - digoxin, digitoxin, *Nerium oleander* (oleander) - oleandrin, *Convallaria majalis* (Lily of the valley), *Apocynum cannabinum* (Dogbane), *Asclepias species.*
	-	Bufadienolide type: *Urginea maritima* (Red squill)
	3.	Animals producing cardiac glycosides:
	-	Bufadienolide type: *Bufo marinus* toads
ECG changes	-	Excitant activity: atrial and junctional premature beats, atrial tachycardia, atrial flutter (rare), AF (rare), accelerated junctional rhythms, PVB, bigeminy and multifocal, VT, bi-directional VT, VF.
	-	Suppressant activity: sinus bradycardia, sinoatrial block, type I second degree AV block (Wenckebach), bundle branch blocks, complete AV block, type II second degree AV block (rare).
	-	Combination of these: atrial tachycardia with AV block, sinus bradycardia with junctional tachycardia, Wenckebach with junctional premature beats, regularization of ventricular rhythm with AF.

Table 4. Na+/K+ ATPase blocking agents and ECG changes in intoxication (adapted from Gordon, 2006; Lapostolle & Borron, 2007).

Electrocardiographic abnormalities with cardiac glycoside toxicity are the result of increased automaticity (from increased intracellular Ca^{2+}) accompanied by slowed conduction through the AV node. In 10% to 15% of cases, ectopic rhythms will be the first sign of intoxication. AV block or an increase in ventricular automaticity are the most common manifestations of Digoxin toxicity and have been shown to occur in 30%to 40%of verified cases of toxicity. The nonspecific dysrhythmias consist of premature ventricular contractions (especially bigeminal and multiform), first-, second-, and third degree AV block, sinus bradycardia (fig.11), sinus tachycardia, sino-atrial block or arrest, atrial fibrillation (AF) with slow ventricular response (fig.12), atrial tachycardia, junctional escape rhythm, AV dissociation, ventricular bigeminy and trigeminy, VT (fig.13), TdP, and VF. The more specific dysrhythmias are AF with slow, regular ventricular rate (AV dissociation), nonparoxysmal junctional tachycardia (rate 70-130), atrial tachycardia with block (atrial rate is usually 150-200), and bi-directional VT. Bi-directional VT is particularly characteristic of severe toxicity and is the result of alterations of intraventricular conduction, junctional tachycardia with aberrant intraventricular conduction, or, on rare occasions, alternating ventricular pacemakers. Typically, in the young, slow rhythms and conduction defects predominate over ventricular ectopy, which is more prominent in older Digoxin-toxic patients. (Litonjua et al., 2005)

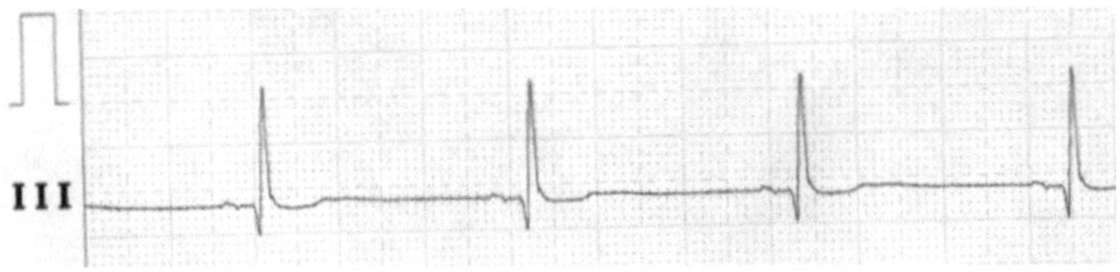

Fig. 11. Sinus bradicardia 47/min, with ST/T changes, 20 hours after attempted suicide with 10 mg Digoxin, in an 18 years old man.

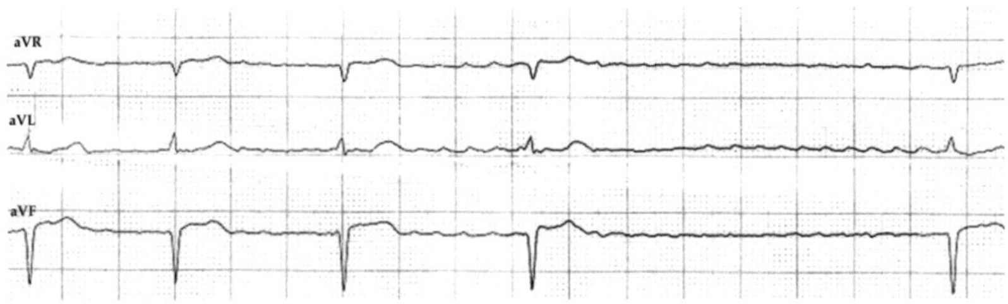

Fig. 12. AF 56/min, with a pause of 2.96 sec, 15 hours after attempted suicide with Digoxin, in a 68 years old woman.

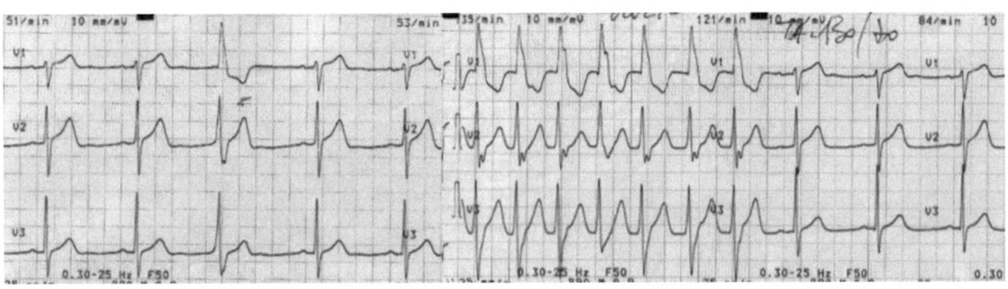

Fig. 13. PVB and a short episode of non-sustained VT 135/min, in a 56 years old male with Digoxin overdose in attempted suicide.

3. Drugs and toxins acting on autonomic nervous system

In an acute poisoning, ECG changes, especially arrhythmias, can be explained by direct or indirect sympathomimetic effects, anticholinergic effects, and the effects of altered central nervous system (CNS) regulation of peripheral autonomic activity. Sympathetic fibers innervate most parts of the heart. Postganglionic fibers release norepinephrine, which interacts with the beta 1- adrenergic cardiac receptors, to increase permeability to Na^+ and Ca^{2+}, thus leading to increased excitability, conduction and contractility. The vagal postganglionic parasympathetic fibers locally release acetylcholine. Vagal stimulation of the muscarinic receptors primarily decreases excitability of the atria, and slows the conduction of impulse into the ventricles, to a complete blockade of transmission in the AV node, with modest direct effects on contractility (Patel & Benowitz, 2005).

Beta-adrenergic blockers	1st generation - Oxprenolol (membrane stabilizing effect, intrinsic sympathomimetic activity) - Propranolol (membrane stabilizing effect) - Alprenolol, Nadolol - Pindolol (intrinsic sympathomimetic activity) - Sotalol (K^+ channel blockade) - Timolol 2nd generation - Acebutolol (membrane stabilizing effect, intrinsic sympathomimetic activity) - Practolol, Atenolol, Metoprolol - Betaxolol (membrane stabilizing effect, vasodilation secondary to calcium channel blocking properties) - Bisoprolol - Esmolol 3rd generation - Labetalol (vasodilation, alpha-adrenergic antagonist activity) - Carvedilol (vasodilation, alpha-adrenergic antagonist activity) - Nebivolol (vasodilation by release of nitric oxide) - Carteolol (vasodilation by release of nitric oxide) - Celiprolol (vasodilation, alpha 2-adrenergic antagonism activity)
ECG changes	Sinus or nodal bradycardia AV blocks (first-degree AV block is common) Prolonged PR, and QTc intervals Prolonged QRS complex (membrane stabilizing agents) Ventricular tachydysrhythmias (membrane stabilizing agents) - fig.14 Multifocal ventricular extrasystoles, VT, VF (Sotalol) Asystole (in severe poisoning) Mild tachycardia (Pindolol overdose)

Table 5. Beta-blockers and ECG changes in intoxication (adapted from Gordon, 2006; Holstege et al., 2006; Brubacher, 2007)

3.1 Beta-adrenergic blockers (BB)

BBs competitively inhibit various β-adrenergic receptors, and are listed in table 5.
They cause in most cases sinus bradycardia. Serious arrhythmias result from purely anticholinergic compound poisoning, especially in patients with underlying ischemic heart disease (e.g. atrial tachycardia and PVB). In acute BB overdose, the most pronounced effects are bradycardia (from decreased sinoatrial node function), varying degrees of AV block, and hypotension. Beta-adrenergic antagonists competitively antagonize the effects of catecholamines at the beta-adrenergic receptor and blunt the chronotropic and inotropic response to catecholamines (Bird, 2007).
Inhibition of the conducting system most commonly causes first-degree AV block, but higher levels of toxicity can promote second- and third-degree AV block (fig.15), junctional rhythms, and intraventricular conduction delays (Anderson, 2008).
Three beta-blockers are known to prolong QTc intervals: Sotalol (fig.16), Propranolol, and Acebutolol. Sotalol blocks K^+ channels, thereby prolonging the action potential and the repolarization duration. The prolongation of the QTc interval predisposes the patient to ventricular tachyarrhythmias and TdP, which have been described after both Sotalol overdose and therapeutic administration. Propranolol overdose has caused QTc prolongation and torsades on rare occasion (Delk et al., 2006).

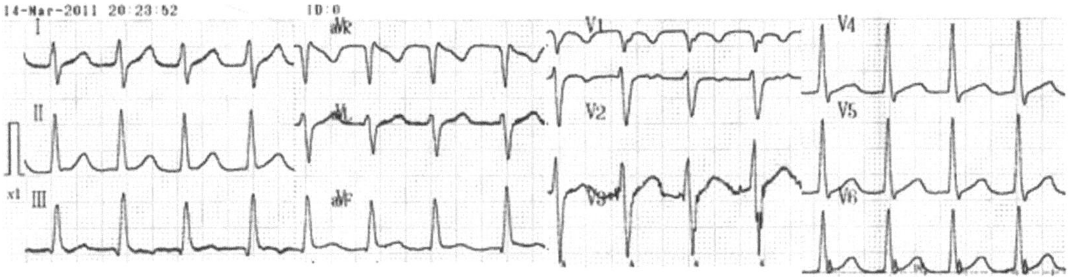

Fig. 14. Acute poisoning 3 hours after ingestion of 2 grams of Propranolol, presenting with accelerated idioventricular rhythm 115/min, in a young female. Note the absence of P waves, wide QRS complex (0.12 msec).

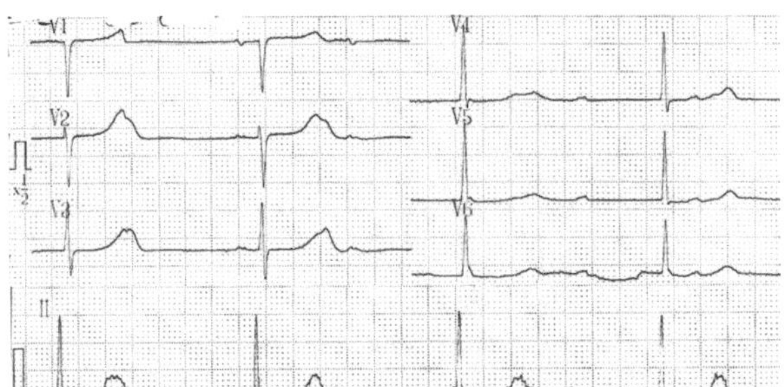

Fig. 15. Acute Metoprolol poisoning presenting with third degree AV block, with narrow QRS complex at a rate of 35/min. Atrial activity is represented by P waves, 80/min.

Beta-adrenergic antagonists also cause myocardial depression, at least in part, by an action independent of either catecholamine antagonism or membrane-depressant activity (Brubacher, 2007).

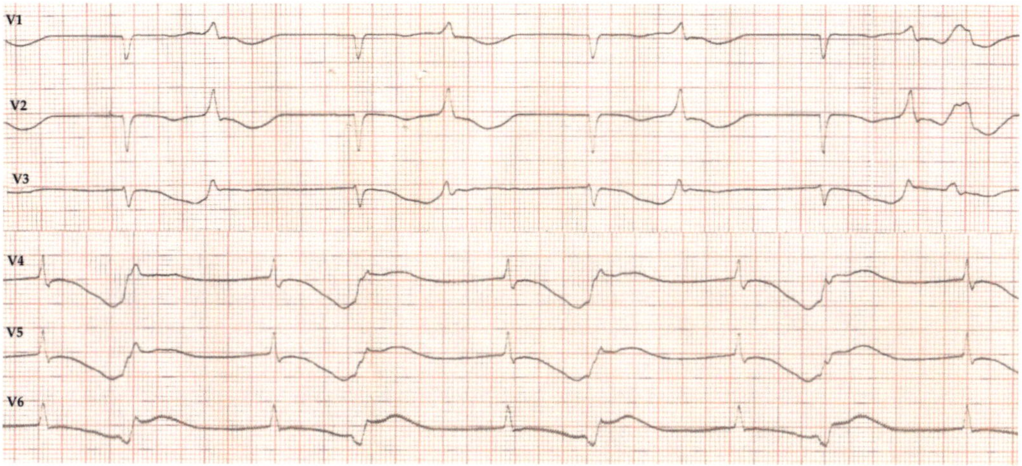

Fig. 16. Acute Sotalol poisoning presenting with bradyarrhythmias, with severe QT prolongation, and monomorphic PVB, R/T phenomenon, and a couple of polymorphic PVB (leads V1-V3).

3.2 Other sympathetic – inhibitors (other than BB)

Cardiac disturbances caused by sympathetic-inhibiting drugs are listed in table 6.

Sympathetic-inhibiting agents	Methyldopa Clonidine and other imidazoline derivatives Reserpine, Guanethidine Prazosin and other alpha-blockers
ECG changes	Sinus, atrial, junctional and ventricular bradyarrhythmias First degree AV block Ventricular tachyarrhythmias

Table 6. Sympathetic-inhibitors and the resulting ECG changes.

These drugs are used for their antihypertensive action, explained by central and peripheral alpha 2-adrenergic agonist effects. In acute overdose they cause ECG changes, along with hypotension, and cardiac failure. Cardiac arrests have been described in adults with Clonidine poisoning. Over-the-counter topical decongestants commonly contain imidazoline derivatives (naphzoline, tetrahydrozoline, oxymetazoline, and xylometazoline), and can cause systemic toxicity after topical exposure, or ingestion, with sympatholytic effects, such as bradyarrhythmias and hypotension, related to central alpha 2-adrenergic and imidazoline receptor stimulation (Murphy et al., 2007; Wiley II, 2007).

3.3 Sympathomimetic toxicity

Sympathetic overactivity can be caused by a number of drugs and toxins (table 7), such as illicit drugs, and hydrocarbon solvents, but also by sedative drug withdrawal syndromes. The typical ECG changes are sinus and atrial tachycardia, and occasionally ventricular dysrrhythmias (in massive exposures). Sinus tachycardia may be the first manifestation of exposure to a sympathomimetic.

Sympathomimetic drugs and toxins	1. Drugs: - Monoamine oxidase inhibitors - Phenylpropanolamine and other over-the-counter sympathomimetics (decongestants containing phenylephrine, pseudoephedrine, ephedrine) - Theophylline - Ergot alkaloids - Beta-adrenoreceptor agonists (Albuterol, Dobutamine, Epinephrine, Isoproterenol, Norepinephrine, Ritodrine, Terbutaline) - Caffeine - Chloral hydrate (sedative and hypnotic drug) 2. Illicit drugs: - Amphetamines - Cocaine - Phencyclidine - Delta-tetrahydrocannabinol (cannabis) - fig.17 - Lysergic acid diethylamide - Psilocybin and other hallucinogens 3. Toxins: - Ethanol - Hydrocarbon solvents (e.g. toluene, benzene, chloroform, etc.) - Freon (and other fluorocarbon aerosols)
ECG abnormalities	Sinus tachycardia Sinoatrial slowing with escape junctional or ventricular rhythms (solvent inhalation) Atrial tachycardia - fig. 18 Ventricular premature beats VT, VF Myocardial ischemia or infarction (cocaine, amphetamines, or hydrocarbons ingestion)

Table 7. Sympathomimetic drugs and toxins and the resulting ECG changes.

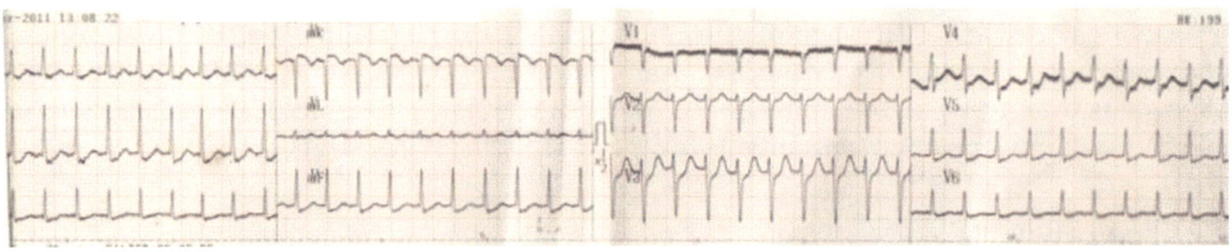

Fig. 17. Paroxysmal supraventricular tachycardia 169/min, in a young female with acute cannabis and ethanol poisoning.

However, other supraventricular or ventricular dysrhythmias may develop if an abnormal rhythm is generated in another part of the heart.

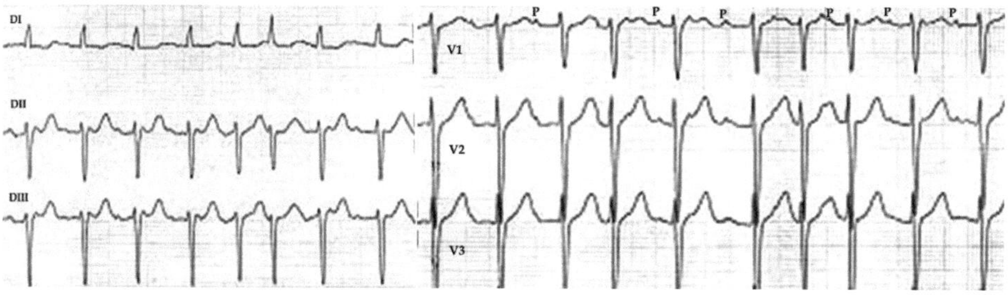

Fig. 18. Atrial tachycardia 150/min, with variable AV block, in a female with a chronic respiratory disease and Theophylline overdosage.

Either as a result of excessive circulating catecholamines observed with cocaine and sympathomimetics, or myocardial sensitization secondary to halogenated hydrocarbons or thyroid hormone, or increased second-messenger activity secondary to theophylline, the extreme inotropic and chronotropic effects cause dysrhythmias. Altered repolarization, increased intracellular Ca^{2+} concentrations, or myocardial ischemia may cause the dysrhythmia. Additionally, cocaine that produce focal myocardial ischemia, can lead to malignant ventricular dysrhythmias (Clancy, 2007). In high dose, along with its potent sympathomimetic action, cocaine blocks fast Na^{+} channels in the myocardium, with a depression of depolarization, and slowing of conduction velocity, manifested on ECG with prolonged PR, QRS, and QT intervals (Murphy et al., 2007).

3.4 Anticholinergic toxicity

There are numerous and various anticholinergic drugs and toxins that may be ingested (table 8) and produce ECG abnormalities.

Anticholinergic drugs and toxins	1. Drugs: - Antihistamines - Atropine, scopolamine - Tricyclic antidepressants - Antipsychotics (e.g. Phenothiazines, Clozapine, Olanzapine) 2. Toxins: - Toxic plants from Solanaceae family containing belladonna alkaloids: Belladonna (Atropa belladonna), Henbane (Hyoscyamus niger), Jimson Weed (Datura stramonium), Mandrake (Mandragora officinarum) - Toxic mushrooms: Amanita muscaria
ECG changes	Sinus and atrial tachycardia Premature ventricular beats

Table 8. Drugs and toxins with anticholinergic effect, with induced ECG abnormalities.

They cause in most cases sinus tachycardia. Serious arrhythmias result from purely anticholinergic compound poisoning, especially in patients with underlying ischemic heart disease (e.g. atrial tachycardia and ventricular premature beats). Atropine, for example, increases myocardial oxygen demand secondary to tachycardia, and can lead to VT and fibrillation in patients after myocardial infarction. Patients presenting with anticholinergic toxidrome (mydriasis, diminished bowel sounds, urinary retention, dry mouth, flushed skin, tachycardia, and agitation) may have ingested antihistamine-sympathomimetic combinations, or tricyclic antidepressants and neuroleptics, having both anticholinergic and membrane-depressant effects, which can explain the presence of serious cardiovascular disturbances (such as widening of the QRS complex, and a rightward deflection of the terminal 40 msec of the QRS complex, with prolongation of the QTc, which creates a substrate for the development of TdP). (Murphy et al., 2007; Juurlink, 2007)

3.5 Cholinomimetic toxicity

Poisoning by cholinomimetic drugs and toxins (table 9) lead to different ECG aspects. The most common type of cholinomimetic toxicity is poisoning with organophosphate and carbamate pesticides, resulting in the excessive inhibition of the cholinesterase. The ECG changes are unpredictable and often change over the time course of the poisoning.

Cholinomimetic drugs and toxins	1. Drugs: - Causing acetylcholine release (Alpha 2-adrenergic antagonists, Aminopyridines, Carbachol, Guanidine) - Direct muscarinic agonists (Pilocarpine, Bethanechol, Methacholine) - Direct nicotinic agonists (Carbachol, Succinylcholine) - Indirect neuronal nicotinic agonists (Chlorpromazine, local and volatile anesthetics, Ketamine) - Anticholinesterases (Pyridostigmine, Neostigmine, Physostigmine) - Central cholinesterase inhibitors (Rivastigmine, Galantamine, Donepezil) 2. Toxins: - Organophosphate and carbamate pesticides - Nicotine - Muscarine - Black widow spider venom - Coniine (alkaloid found in poison hemlock and the yellow pitcher plant)
ECG abnormalities	Sinus bradycardia Atrial, junctional, or ventricular bradycardia AV block Sinus tachycardia (seen in early stages of cholinesterase inhibition and nicotine poisoning due to ganglionic stimulation) VT associated with QT interval prolongation Asystole

Table 9. Cholinomimetic drugs and toxins, and ECG changes induced in acute exposure.

Early in the course, tachycardia is present, due to acetylcholine stimulation of nicotinic receptors, followed by bradycardia, secondary to muscarinic receptor stimulation. In severe poisonings, advanced AV block, bradydysrhythmias and asystole may occur (Murphy et al., 2007). Up to 5 days after exposure, QTc interval prolongation is followed by ventricular tachyarrhythmias (fig.19), including TdP (fig.10), due to persistent imbalance between sympathetic and parasympathetic influences on the heart, as well as dyselectrolytemias. A rare feature is acute myocardial infarction (fig.20), with a complex mechanism (fig.21) explaining its presence (coronary spasm induced by parasympathetic hyperactivity, direct toxic effect of pesticide on myocardium).

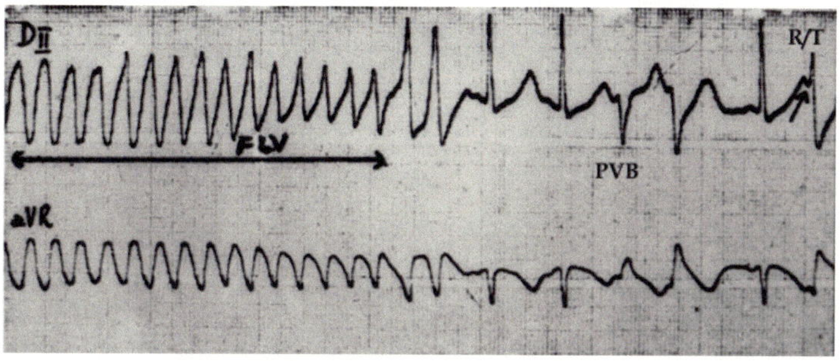

Fig. 19. Acute organophosphate poisoning, five days after exposure. ECG shows QT interval prolongation (0.60 sec), short episode of ventricular flutter (FLV), a couple of PVB, and one PVB with R on T phenomenon (R/T).

Patients with clinical signs of cholinesterase inhibition and abnormal ECG (including long QT interval) should be monitored continuously, because of the risk of developing ventricular arrhythmias (Lionte et al., 2007). Reversible acetylcholinesterase inhibitors, such as Donepezil, have a high selectivity for neuronal acetylcholinesterase, and in accidental overdose were reported to produce sinus bradycardia (Murphy et al., 2007).

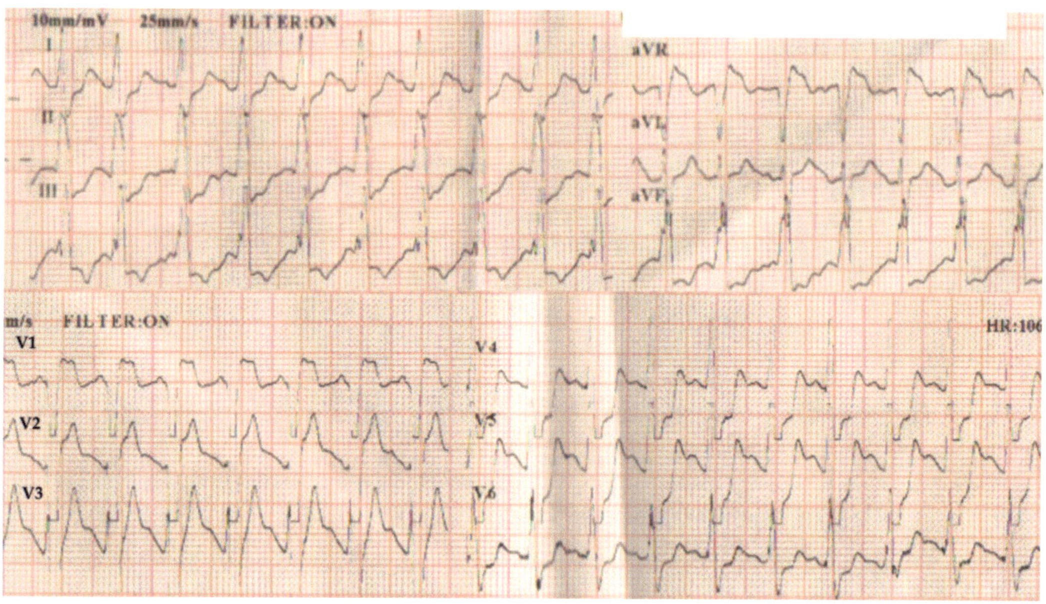

Fig. 20. Acute organophosphate poisoning, four days after exposure, serum cholinesterase normalized with antidote. ECG shows acute ST segment elevation anterior myocardial infarction (with increased cardiac enzymes), sinus tachycardia 106/min, QT interval 0.32 sec.

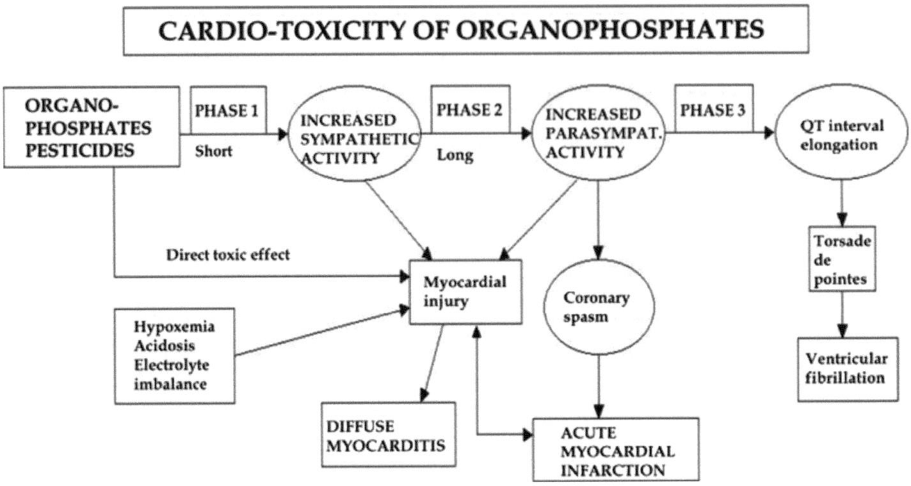

Fig. 21. Cardiac manifestations of organophosphate poisoning and mechanisms involved.

4. Other substances inducing ECG changes

4.1 Chemical asphyxiants

Chemical asphyxiants act in one of two ways. Some prevent the uptake of oxygen in the blood. Carbon monoxide interferes with the transport of oxygen to the tissues by strongly binding with hemoglobin to form carboxyhemoglobin, which leaves inadequate hemoglobin available for oxygen transport. Hydrogen cyanide does not permit the normal oxygen transfer either from the blood to the tissues or within the cell itself, resulting in tissue hypoxia. Acute exposure to these agents leads to coma and metabolic acidosis, the last explaining in part ECG abnormalities (table 10) recorded in such poisoning.

Chemical asphyxiants	ECG changes
Carbon monoxide (CO)	T wave flattening or inversion ST segment depression or elevation Conduction disturbance Myocardial infarction (fig.22, 23, 24) Arrhythmias occasionally (PVB, atrial fibrillation)
Hydrogen cyanide	Tachycardia (early) Bradicardia, heart block (late) Shortening of the ST segment with eventual fusion of the T wave into the QRS complex. Erratic supraventricular and vntricular arrhythmias Ischemic changes Asystole
Zinc phosphide	Atrial extrasystoles Ventricular arrhythmias ST/T changes (fig.25)

Table 10. Major chemical asphyxiants and their effect on ECG in acute poisoning (adapted from Hall, 2007; Murphy et al., 2007; **Schraga** et al., 2008)

Myocardial injury from CO poisoning results from tissue hypoxia, and as damage at the cellular level. The affinity of hemoglobin for CO is 200 to 250 times greater than its affinity for oxygen. This results in competitive inhibition of oxygen release due to a shift in the oxygen-hemoglobin dissociation curve, reduced oxygen delivery, and subsequent tissue hypoxia. In CO poisoning, magnitude of ST/T changes doesn't correlate with the severity of the myocardial impairment, other tests, such as echocardiography, being necessary. All cardiovascular changes are more prominent in patients with underlying cardiac pathology (Murphy et al., 2007; Satran et al., 2005).

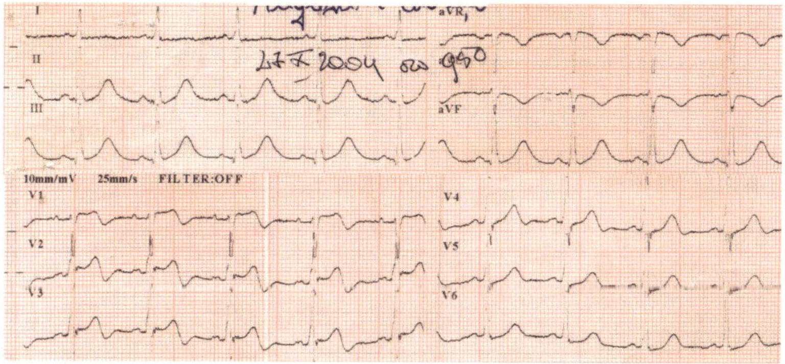

Fig. 22. ECG in acute CO poisoning, 24 hours after exposure (flattened T wave in DI, negative T wave in aVL, ST segment elevation and T wave changes in V1-V3).

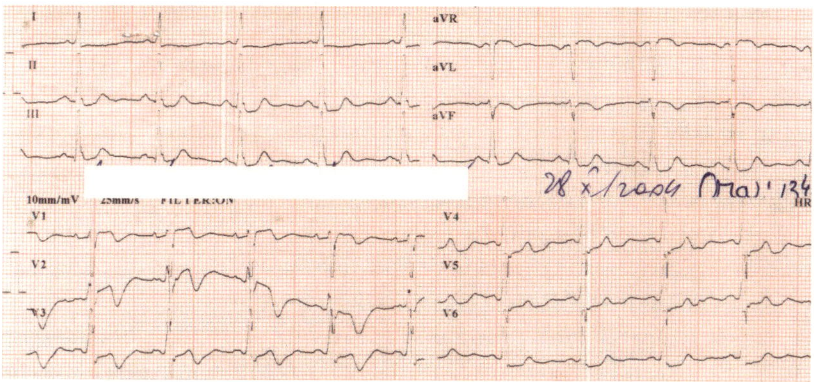

Fig. 23. ECG in acute CO poisoning, same patient, 52 hours after exposure. Note the evolution of ST/T changes in precordial leads.

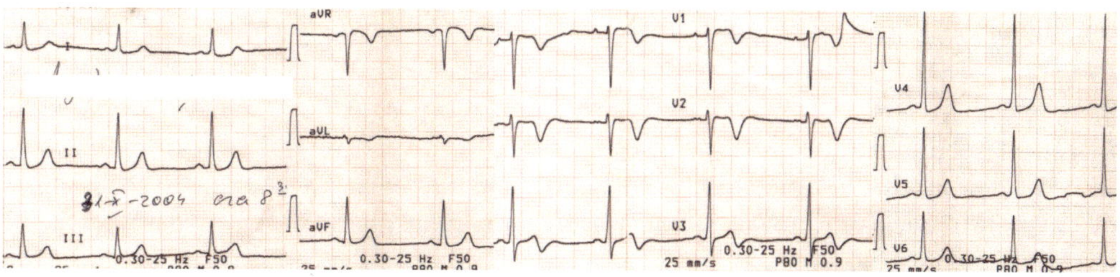

Fig. 24. Same patient, 4 days after exposure. Note the evolution of ST/T changes in precordial and lateral leads.

In humans, cyanide produces histotoxic hypoxia by combining with the ferric ion in mitochondrial cytochrome oxidase, preventing electron transport in the cytochrome system and bringing oxidative phosphorylation and ATP production to a halt. The inhibition of oxidative metabolism puts increased demands on anaerobic glycolysis, which results in lactic acid production and may produce severe acid-base imbalance. Myocardial depression with decreased cardiac output produces stagnation hypoxia. Abnormal heartbeat can occur in cases of severe poisoning. Bradycardia, intractable low blood pressure, and death may result (Hall, 2007).

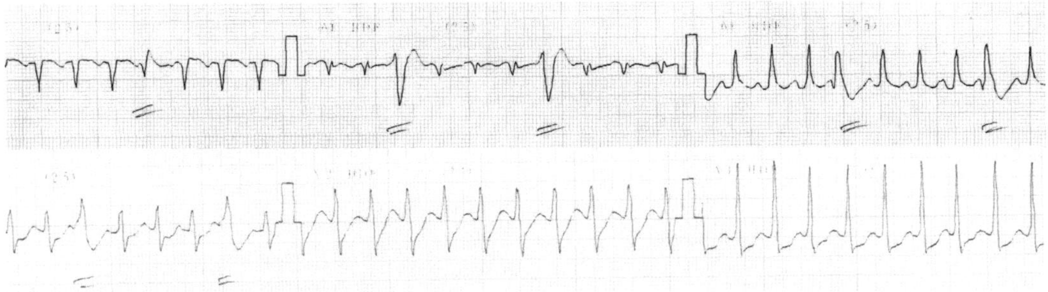

Fig. 25. Attempted suicide with zinc phosphide ingestion in a 19 years old female, presenting circulatory collapse and dyspnea. ECG (leads aVR, aVL, aVF, V1-V3) reveals tachycardia 160 /min with wide QRS complex, multiple PVC (trigeminy), some with R/T phenomenon, and ST/T changes.

Zinc phosphide is a highly effective insecticide and rodenticide. It is mediated by phosphine, which inhibits cytochrome C oxidase. It has been shown recently in nematodes that phosphine rapidly perturbs mitochondrial morphology, inhibits oxidative respiration by 70%, and causes a severe drop in mitochondrial membrane potential. This failure of cellular respiration is likely to be due to a mechanism other than inhibition of cytochrome C oxidase. In addition, phosphine and hydrogen peroxide can interact to form the highly reactive hydroxyl radical and phosphine also inhibits catalase and peroxidase; both mechanisms result in hydroxyl radical associated damage such as lipid peroxidation. The major lethal consequence of zinc phosphide ingestion, profound circulatory collapse, is secondary to factors including direct effects on cardiac myocytes, fluid loss, and adrenal gland damage. There is usually only a short interval between ingestion and the appearance of systemic toxicity. Phosphine-induced impairment of myocardial contractility and fluid loss leads to circulatory failure, and pulmonary edema. Metabolic acidosis, or mixed metabolic acidosis and respiratory alkalosis, are frequent, and contribute to ECG changes (Lionte et al., 2004; Proudfoot, 2009).

4.2 Natural products

Many natural products and toxins have cardiovascular effects, leading to ECG changes (table 11). The clinical and myocardial histological manifestations of scorpion sting resemble those of catecholamine infusion. Myocardial infarction has been documented in scorpion envenomation with a pathophysiological mechanism involving transient myocardial "stunning" (Thomas et al., 2007).

Poisonous animals and plants	ECG abnormalities
Poisonous scorpion stings (venom)	Sinus tachycardia, conduction abnormalities, ST/T changes with peaked T waves, QT prolongation, atrial and ventricular arrhythmias, myocardial infarction
Black widow spider bites (venom)	Tachycardia Atrial arrhythmias
Hymenoptera (bees and wasps) stings (venom)	Tachycardia, dysrhythmias, myocardial infarction
Ciguatera fish (ciguatoxin)	Bradycardia, arrhythmias
Puffer fish (tetrodotoxin)	Bradycardia, arrhythmias
Scombroid fish (scombrotoxin)	Bradycardia, sinus tachycardia, ventricular arrhythmias, acute myocardial infarction (fig.26)
Aconite poisoning (Chinese herbs or teas that contain *Aconitum carmichaelii* or *A. kusnezoffii*)	Bradycardia VT (monomorphic or polymorphic) VF

Table 11. ECG changes induced by natural products poisoning (adapted from Hahn, 2007; Lionte, 2010; Murphy et al., 2007; Wandersee, 2006).

In the pathogenesis of clinical syndrome produced by black widow spider bites was suggested to be also involved an excess of catecholamines, while in patients affected by *Hymenoptera* stings, histamine plays a role in pathogenesis.

Fish-borne poisoning has multiple pathogenic mechanisms, depending on the toxin involved. Some of these toxins are heat stable, therefore unaffected by cooking, and gastric acid, while others produce the poisoning because of improper fish handling.

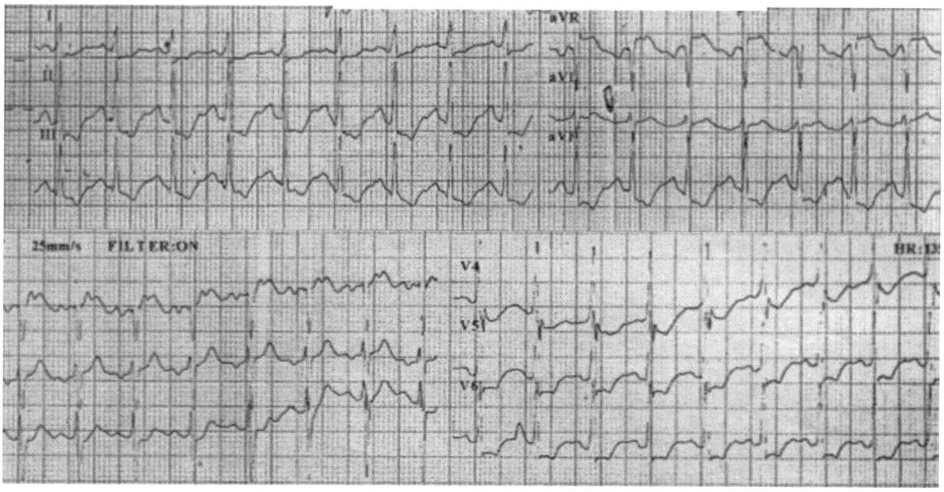

Fig. 26. Scombroid fish poisoning, 1 hour after ingestion, in a young female, presenting chest pain and hypotension (BP 70/45 mmHg). ECG reveals signs of subendocardial myocardial infarction (sustained by enzymatic evidence), and sinus tachycardia 139/min.

Aconite poisoning results from alkaloids contained in teas and herbs, which are not boiled enough before ingestion, such as aconitine and mesaconitine (Murphy et al., 2007).

Aconitine has Na^+ channel-binding properties (maintaining them in an open position), which explain, in part, its neurological and cardiovascular toxicity (cardiodepressant effects). Vagal stimulation is also involved in pathogenesis of aconitine poisoning. Aconitine has a propensity to cause early and delayed after-depolarizations in ventricular myocytes that may be due to increased intracellular Ca^{2+} and Na^+. This explains the presence of biventricular tachycardia and TdP on ECG (Smolinske et al., 2007).

4.3 Drugs of abuse

Some of the most commonly abused drugs are alcohol, nicotine, marijuana, amphetamines, cocaine, opium alkaloids and synthetic opioids, gamma-hydroxybutyrate, 3,4-methylenedioxymethamphetamine (MDMA, ecstasy), and phencyclidine. Drug abuse may lead to organ damage, addiction, and disturbed patterns of behavior. Some illicit drugs, such as heroin, lysergic acid diethylamide, and phencyclidine hydrochloride, have no recognized therapeutic effect in humans. Cardiovascular toxicity of illicit drugs relies on multiple pathophysiological mechanisms. Table 12 presents major categories of drugs, and the ECG abnormalities reported in acute setting.

Illicit drug	ECG
Amphetamines and derivatives (including "ecstasy")	Sinus tachycardia and supraventricular tachyarrhythmias Myocardial ischemia, and infarction PVB and ventricular tachydysrhythmias
Cannabis (marijuana)	Tachycardia (fig. 17) Non-specific ST/T changes PVC (occasional) and AF
Cocaine	Sinus bradycardia, complete heart block, bundle branch block Prolonged QTc, and QRS Supraventricular tachyarrhythmias VT or fibrillation Myocardial infarction
Gamma-hydroxybutyrate (GHB)	Bradycardia Transient P wave inversion in DII, right bundle branch block, ST-segment elevation (pediatric) U waves (in adults) First degree AV block, transient AF (rare)
Hallucinogens	Tachycardia
Opiates and opioids	Bradycardia (opioids) Cardiac conduction abnormalities and dysrhythmias (heroin) Prolonged QT interval and TdP (methadone) QRS prolongation, dysrhythmias (Propoxyphene) Tachycardia (Tramadol)

Table 12. Drugs of abuse and consequent ECG changes in acute poisoning (adapted from Albertson, 2004; Albertson et al., 2007, a; Delgado, 2007; Quang, 2007; Traub, 2007; Yip et al., 2007).

Amphetamine and related drugs activate the sympathetic nervous system via central nervous system stimulation, peripheral release of catecholamines, inhibition of neuronal reuptake of catecholamines, and inhibition of monoamine oxidase. Fenfluramine and dexfenfluramine cause serotonin release and block neuronal serotonin uptake. Methamphetamine (crank, speed), 3,4-methylenedioxymethamphetamine (MDMA, ecstasy), and several other amphetamine derivatives (Lysergic Acid Diethylamide), as well as a number of prescription drugs, are used orally and intravenously as illicit stimulants. "Ice" is a smokable form of methamphetamine (Albertson, 2004). Direct catecholamine effects, and ischemic effects, after coronary vasospasm explain arrhythmias, in amphetamine use. The last is involved in the pathogenesis of myocardial infarction after amphetamine use, together with direct cardiac toxicity (myocarditis), and thrombus formation (Albertson et al., 2007, b).

Most of the hallucinogens are indoleamine or phenylethylamine derivatives, structurally similar to the neurotransmitter serotonin. Commonly used hallucinogens include lysergic acid diethylamide (LSD), mescaline, 5-methoxy-N,N-diisopropyltriptamine, and psilocybin ("magic mushrooms"). They produce a variety of autonomic effects, both parasympathetic and sympathetic (Traub, 2007).

Cocaine is one of the most popular drugs of abuse. Rapidly after smoking or intravenous injection (mediated by sympathetic overactivity) appear cardiovascular signs of toxicity. Coronary artery spasm and/or thrombosis may result in myocardial infarction, even in patients with no coronary disease. Chest pain with electrocardiographic evidence of ischemia or infarction in a young, otherwise healthy person suggests cocaine use (Benowitz, 2004). At low doses, occur sinus bradycardia and ectopic rhythms, based on cocaine's local anesthetic properties and its effects on catecholamines. At high doses, cocaine produces direct Na^+ and K^+ channel blockade (see section 3.3). Enhanced sympathetic stimulation will increase intracellular Ca^{2+} within myocardial cells, and will enhance automaticity, leading to afterdepolarizations, and ectopic rhythms (Albertson et al., 2007, a).

The cannabinoid delta 9-tetrahidrocannabinol (THC) is the principal psychoactive constituent of *Cannabis sativa* (marijuana consists of the leaves and flowering parts of the plant). Cardiovascular toxicity is dose-related, and is explained by stimulation of the autonomic nervous system, involving both parasympathetic and sympathetic pathways. The effects tend to be more serious in patients with preexisting cardiovascular pathology (for example, an increased risk of myocardial infarction was reported in the hour following marijuana use), but in young, healthy patients, these effects have no serious consequences (Delgado, 2007).

Opiates are a group of naturally occurring compounds derived from the juice of the poppy *Papaver somniferum*. The term opioid refers to these and other derivatives of naturally occurring opium (e.g., morphine, heroin, codeine, and hydrocodone) as well as new, totally synthetic opiate analogs (e.g., fentanyl, butorphanol, meperidine, methadone, and propoxyphene). In general, opioids share the ability to stimulate a number of specific opiate receptors in the CNS. With mild or moderate overdose, pulse rate is decreased. Cardiotoxicity similar to that seen with tricyclic antidepressants and quinidine can occur in patients with severe propoxyphene intoxication. Heroin and propoxyphene toxicity is associated with ECG changes, such as non-specific ST/T wave abnormalities, first-degree AV block, AF, prolonged QTc intervals, and ventricular dysrhythmias. In the pathogenesis of these cardiovascular findings contribute electrolyte, and metabolic derangements, hypoxia, or adulterants (e.g. quinine) found in street drugs (Yip et al., 2007).

5. Conclusions

ECG is a valuable source of information in poisoned patients and has the potential to enhance and direct their care. Although it seems obvious that an ECG is required following exposure to a drug used for cardiovascular indications, many drugs with no overt cardiovascular effects from therapeutic dosing become cardiotoxic in overdose. An ECG should be examined extremely early in the initial evaluation of most poisoned patients.

6. References

Albertson, T.E. (2004). Amphetamines, In: *Poisoning & Drug Overdose, 4th Ed.*, Olson, K.R. et al. (Eds.), pp. 72-74, Lange Medical Books/McGraw-Hill, ISBN 0-8385-8172-2, New York, USA.

Albertson, T.E.; Chan, A. & Tharratt, R.S. (2007). Cocaine, In: *Haddad and Winchester's Clinical Management of Poisoning and Drug Overdose* (4th Ed.), Shannon, M.W. et al. (Eds.), pp. 755-772, Saunders Elsevier, ISBN 978-0-7216-0693-4, Philadelphia, USA.

Albertson, T.E.; Kenyon, N.J. & Morrissey, B. (2007). Amphetamines and derivatives, In: *Haddad and Winchester's Clinical Management of Poisoning and Drug Overdose* (4th Ed.), Shannon, M.W. et al. (Eds.), pp. 781-792, Saunders Elsevier, ISBN 978-0-7216-0693-4, Philadelphia, USA.

Anderson, A.C. (2008). Management of Beta-Adrenergic Blocker Poisoning. *Clinical Pediatric Emergency Medicine,* Vol. 9, No. 1, (March, 2008), pp.4-16, ISSN 1522-8401.

Benowitz, N.L. (2004). Cocaine, In: In: *Poisoning & Drug Overdose, 4th Ed.*, Olson, K.R. et al. (Eds.), pp. 171-173, Lange Medical Books/McGraw-Hill, ISBN 0-8385-8172-2, New York, USA.

Berkovitch, M., et al. (1995). Assessment of the terminal 40-millisecond QRS vector in children with a history of tricyclic antidepressant ingestion. *Pediatric Emergency Care,* Vol.11, No.2, (Apr 1995), pp.75–77, ISSN 0749-5161.

Bird, S.B.(2007). Beta-Adrenergic anatagonists, In: *Haddad and Winchester's Clinical Management of Poisoning and Drug Overdose* (4th Ed.), Shannon, M.W. et al. (Eds.), pp. 975-982, Saunders Elsevier, ISBN 978-0-7216-0693-4, Philadelphia, USA.

Brubacher, J.R. (2007). Beta-adrenergic antagonists, In: *Goldfrank's Manual of Toxicologic Emergencies,* Hoffman R.S. et al. (Eds.), pp. 518-529, The McGraw-Hill Companies, Inc., http://www.mhprofessional.com/product.php?cat=116&isbn=007144310X.

Chung, D.C. (1981). Anaesthetic problems associated with the treatment of cardiovascular disease: I. Digitalis toxicity. *Can Anaesth Soc J.,* Vol. 28, No.1, (Jan 1981), pp.6-16, ISSN 0008-2856.

Clancy, C. (2007). Electrocardiographic principles, In: *Goldfrank's Manual of Toxicologic Emergencies,* Hoffman R.S. et al. (Eds.), pp. 29-40, The McGraw-Hill Companies, Inc., http://www.mhprofessional.com/product.php?cat=116&isbn=007144310X.

Delgado, J. (2007). Marijuana, In: *Haddad and Winchester's Clinical Management of Poisoning and Drug Overdose* (4th Ed.), Shannon, M.W. et al. (Eds.), pp. 747-754, Saunders Elsevier, ISBN 978-0-7216-0693-4, Philadelphia, USA.

Delk, C.; Holstege, C.P. & Brady, W.J. (2007). Electrocardiographic abnormalities associated with poisoning. *American Journal of Emergency Medicine,* Vol.25, No. 6, (July 2007), pp. 672-687, ISSN 0735-6757.

Gordon, B. (2006). Cardiovascular drugs, In: *The Toxicology Handbook for Clinicians*, Harris, C.R. (Ed.), pp. 61-75, Mosby Elsevier, ISBN 1-56053-711-6, Philadelphia, USA.

Hahn, I-H. (2007). Arthropods, In: *Goldfrank's Manual of Toxicologic Emergencies*, Hoffman R.S. et al. (Eds.), pp. 901-911, The McGraw-Hill Companies, Inc., http://www.mhprofessional.com/product.php?cat=116&isbn=007144310X.

Hall, A.H. (2007). Cyanide and related compounds - sodium azide, In: *Haddad and Winchester's Clinical Management of Poisoning and Drug Overdose* (4th Ed.), Shannon, M.W. et al. (Eds.), pp. 1309-1316, Saunders Elsevier, ISBN 978-0-7216-0693-4, Philadelphia, USA.

Holstege, C.; Baer, A. & Brady, W.J. (2005). The electrocardiographic toxidrome: the ECG presentation of hydrofluoric acid ingestion. *American Journal of Emergency Medicine*, Vol. 23, No.2, (March 2005), pp.171-176. ISSN 0735-6757.

Holstege, C.P.; Eldridge, D.L. & Rowden, A.K. (2006). ECG manifestations: the poisoned patient. *Emergency Medicine Clinics of North America,* Vol.24, No.1, (Feb 2006), pp.159-177, ISSN 0733-8627.

Juurlink, D.N. (2007). Antipsychotics, In: *Goldfrank's Manual of Toxicologic Emergencies*, Hoffman R.S. et al. (Eds.), pp. 583-590, The McGraw-Hill Companies, Inc., http://www.mhprofessional.com/product.php?cat=116&isbn=007144310X.

Lapostolle, F. & Borron, S.W. (2007). Digitalis, In: *Haddad and Winchester's Clinical Management of Poisoning and Drug Overdose* (4th Ed.), Shannon, M.W. et al. (Eds.), pp. 949-962, Saunders Elsevier, ISBN 978-0-7216-0693-4, Philadelphia, USA.

Liebelt, E.L.; Francis, P.D & Woolf, A.D. (1995). ECG Lead aVR versus QRS interval in predicting seizures and arrhythmias in acute tricyclic antidepressant toxicity. *Annals of Emergency Medicine*, Vol. 26, No.2, (Aug 1995), pp. 195-201, ISSN 0196-0644.

Lionte, C. (2010). An unusual cause of hypotension and abnormal electrocardiogram (ECG) — scombroid poisoning. *Central European Journal of Medicine*, Vol. 5, No. 3, (June 2010), pp. 292-297, ISSN 1895-1058.

Lionte, C., et al. (2007). Electrocardiographic changes in acute organophosphate poisoning. *Revista Medico-Chirugicala a Societatii de Medici si Naturalisti Iasi*, Vol.111, No.4, (Oct-Dec, 2007), pp. 906-911, ISSN 0048-7848.

Lionte, C.; Sorodoc, L. & Laba, V. (2004). Zinc phosphide poisoning - diagnosis, complications, management. *Terapeutica, Farmacologie si Toxicologie Clinica,* Vol. VIII, No. 4, (Dec 2004), pp. 87-91, ISSN 1583-0012.

Litonjua, R.M., et al. (2005). Digoxin: The Monarch of Cardiac Toxicities. *Journal of Pharmacy Practice,* Vol. 18, No. 3, (June 2005), pp.157–168, ISSN 0897-1900.

Murphy, N.G; Benowitz, N.L. & Goldschlager, N. (2007). Cardiovascular toxicology, In: *Haddad and Winchester's Clinical Management of Poisoning and Drug Overdose* (4th Ed.), Shannon, M.W. et al. (Eds.), pp. 133-165, Saunders Elsevier, ISBN 978-0-7216-0693-4, Philadelphia, USA.

Patel, M.M. & Benowitz, N. (2005). Cardiac conduction and rate disturbances, In: *Critical care toxicology: diagnosis and management of the critically poisoned patient*, Brent, J. et al. (Eds.), pp. 241-260, Elsevier Mosby, ISBN 0-8151-4387-7, Philadelphia, USA.

Proudfoot, A.T. (2009). Aluminium and zinc phosphide poisoning. *Clin Toxicol (Phila).* Vol. 47, No.2, (Feb 2009), pp. 89-100, ISSN 1556-3650.

Quang, L.S. (2007). GHB and related compounds, In: *Haddad and Winchester's Clinical Management of Poisoning and Drug Overdose* (4th Ed.), Shannon, M.W. et al. (Eds.), pp. 803-823, Saunders Elsevier, ISBN 978-0-7216-0693-4, Philadelphia, USA.

Roden, D.M. (2004). Drug-induced prolongation of the QT interval. *New England Journal of Medicine*, Vol. 350, No.10, (March, 2004), pp.1013-1022, ISSN 0028-4793.

Satran, D. et al. (2005). Cardiovascular Manifestations of Moderate to Severe Carbon Monoxide Poisoning. *Journal of the American College of Cardiology*, Vol. 45, No. 9, (June 2005), pp. 1513–1516, ISSN 0735-1097.

Schraga, E.D. et al. (Updated: Mar 11, 2008). Hydrogen Cyanide Poisoning, In: *Medscape Reference*, accessed 16 April, 2011, http://emedicine.medscape.com/article/832840-overview.

Smolinske, S.C.; Daubert, G.P. & Spoerke, D.G. (2007). Poisonous plants, In: *Haddad and Winchester's Clinical Management of Poisoning and Drug Overdose* (4th Ed.), Shannon, M.W. et al. (Eds.), pp. 473-506, Saunders Elsevier, ISBN 978-0-7216-0693-4, Philadelphia, USA.

Thomas, J.D.; Thomas, K.E. & Kazzi, Z.N. (2007). Scorpion and stinging insects, In: *Haddad and Winchester's Clinical Management of Poisoning and Drug Overdose* (4th Ed.), Shannon, M.W. et al. (Eds.), pp. 440-454, Saunders Elsevier, ISBN 978-0-7216-0693-4, Philadelphia, USA.

Traub, S.J. (2007). Hallucinogens, In: *Haddad and Winchester's Clinical Management of Poisoning and Drug Overdose* (4th Ed.), Shannon, M.W. et al. (Eds.), pp. 793-802, Saunders Elsevier, ISBN 978-0-7216-0693-4, Philadelphia, USA.

Wandersee, S. (2006). Toxic foods, In: *The Toxicology Handbook for Clinicians*, Harris, C.R. (Ed.), pp. 194-204, Mosby Elsevier, ISBN 1-56053-711-6, Philadelphia, USA.

Wiley II, J.F. (2007). Clonidine and related imidazoline derivatives, In: *Haddad and Winchester's Clinical Management of Poisoning and Drug Overdose* (4th Ed.), Shannon, M.W. et al. (Eds.), pp. 1001-1008, Saunders Elsevier, ISBN 978-0-7216-0693-4, Philadelphia, USA.

Wolfe, T.R.; Caravati, E.M. & Rollins, D.E. (1989). Terminal 40-ms frontal plane QRS axis as a marker for tricyclic antidepressant overdose. *Annals of Emergency Medicine*, Vol.18, No.4, (Apr 1989), pp.348–351, ISSN 0196-0644.

Yip, L.; Mégarbane, B. & Borron, S.W. (2007). Opioids, In: *Haddad and Winchester's Clinical Management of Poisoning and Drug Overdose* (4th Ed.), Shannon, M.W. et al. (Eds.), pp. 635-658, Saunders Elsevier, ISBN 978-0-7216-0693-4, Philadelphia, USA.

16

Electrocardiogram (ECG) Abnormality Among Residents in Arseniasis-Endemic and Non-Endemic Areas of Southwestern Taiwan – A Study of Gene-Gene and Gene-Environment Interactions

Ya-Tang Liao, Wan-Fen Li, Chien-Jen Chen,
Wei J. Chen, Hsiao-Yen Chen and Shu-Li Wang
National Health Research Institutes and National Taiwan University
Taiwan

1. Introduction

Natural occurrence of arsenic in groundwater is found in the Americas, European, Western Africa, and Asia including Taiwan, Japan, southern Thailand and China where in some areas, drinking water supplies are primarily based on groundwater resources [2]. For general population in southwestern coast Taiwan, the major arsenic exposure resource is the ingestion of arsenic contaminated groundwater. The residents have used high-arsenic contaminated well water for drinking and cooking for many decades since early 1910s. The tap water supply system was implemented in the early 1960s, however artesian well water has not been used for drinking or cooking until mid-1970s [3].

Because arsenic toxicity operates in a highly nonlinear manner and different levels of exposure measurements applied result in large discrepancy across studies and made it difficult to come up a reliable dose-response relationship for arsenic hazard. There is a long-standing observation of individual variability in susceptibility to arsenic toxicity [4] and this variation may be partly due to differences in age and sex distribution across areas, and also individual arsenic metabolism capabilities [5,6]. Inter-individual differences in the speciation and amounts of arsenic metabolites have been reported among subjects chronically exposed to arsenic [7] and significant genetic determinants of arsenic metabolism was supported by epidemiological study [8]. Toenail and hair arsenic has been reported to provided an integrated measure of internal arsenic exposure [9]. However epidemiologic studies showed that external contamination lead to overestimation of internal dose and urinary arsenic concentration seems to be a better marker than concentrations in drinking water[10]. Growing epidemiological evidence also suggests that some factors such as age, sex and genetic susceptibility are related to its metabolism and can be important predictors for arsenic-related health hazard [11,12].

1.1 Nature history of cardiovascular disease (CVD)

Heart disease or cardiovascular disease is defined as the class of disease that involved the cardiac or blood vessels including arteries and veins. Although the term technically refers to

any disease that affects the cardiovascular system, it is usually to refer to those related to atherosclerosis and arterial disease since they shared similar conditions of causes, mechanisms and treatments[13]. The primary underlying disease process that leads to atherosclerosis is the deposition of lipid on the arterial surface progress to form plaques that reduced blood flow and induced blood clots that blocked flow entirely [14].
Most countries face high and increasing rates of cardiovascular disease. In United States, mortality from heart and hypertensive diseases was greater than mortality from neoplasm. In recent years, cardiovascular risk in women has been increasing and has killed more women than breast cancer [15]. The estimated age-adjusted mortalities of cardiovascular disease in US is 152.1 per 100,000 in year 2002 and is 48.3 in Taiwan 2005 [16]. By the time that heart problems are detected, the underlying causes, atherosclerosis, is usually quite advanced, have progressed for decades [17]. Therefore increased emphasis on preventing atherosclerosis by modifying risk factors is remained important.

1.2 Arsenic-related CVD

Chronic arsenic exposure can lead to hyperkeratosis and loss of skin pigmentation as well as cancers of the skin, bladder, and lung. The international Agency for Research on Cancer [18] and the U.S. EPA [19] have classified arsenic as a group 1 and group A carcinogen based on human evidence. However, the mechanism of action for iAs-induced carcinogenicity is not known [20]. Cardiovascular death is the major cause of mortality worldwide, and a small increased risk may imply a large quantity of excess mortality [21]. Arsenic has also been shown to be a major risk factor of an unique form of peripheral vascular disease, Blackfoot disease (BFD) [22,23], especially in southwest Taiwan. Although the etiology of BFD development is still unclear, the dose-response relationships between arsenic and the prevalence of cardiovascular diseases have been documented including atherosclerosis, peripheral vascular disease (PVD), ischemic heart disease (IHD), hypertension, and cerebrovascular disease [21]. IHD is a disease characterized by reduced blood supply to heart muscle, usually due to atherosclerosis of the coronary arteries. Its risk increases with age, smoking, hypercholesterolemia, diabetes, hypertension, and is more common in men and those who have close relatives with ischemic heart disease. Standard diagnosis of IHD including electrocardiogram, blood tests with cardiac enzymes, history and physical examinations.
Although both population-based and occupational studies had shown that long-term exposure to inorganic arsenic has significant toxic effects on the cardiovascular system and the maximum arsenic contamination level in drinking water has been lowered from 0.05 to 0.01 ppm by US Environmental Protection Agency in 2006. The allowable limit for arsenic in drinking water is 0.025 for Canada [24] and 0.05 ppm for Bengal, India, and Bangladesh [25]. , the long-term association with chronic exposure to arsenic remains unclear and there is still epidemiological evidence needed for developing regulatory guidelines [26,27].

1.3 Genetic factors associated with arsenic metabolism and CVD

Although the mechanism of action for iAs-induced CVD hazards is not known [20]. Proposed mechanisms include arsenic metabolism, pathogenesis of atherosclerosis and oxidative stress [28-30]. More than one of these mechanisms may occur, and some may work together.

1.4 Arsenic metabolism genes

In general, the distribution of arsenic in human urine is 10-30% iAs, 10-20% MMA(V), and 60-70% DMA(V) [6]. However, some populations showed significant variation of arsenic methylation levels in urine [31] which suggests that there are genetic factors in the regulation of the enzymes that metabolize arsenic, which may lead to difference in toxicity related to arsenic exposure. Not until recently have genes encoding enzymes that are responsible for arsenic metabolism been cloned and characterized. These genes include AS3MT and GSTO. The AS3MT gene directly encodes a cytosolic enzyme, arsenic methyltransferase, which catalyzes the multi-step process to convert inorganic arsenic to monomethyl arsenical (MMA) and dimethyl arsenical (DMA) [32]. Glutathione S-transferases (GSTs) are Phase II detoxification enzymes that catalyze the conjugation of reduced glutathione (GSH) to a wide variety of endogenous and exogenous electrophilic compounds [33]. A subfamily of GSTs, GST omega class,was shown to be identical with human monomethylarsonic acid (MMAV) reductase that is the rate-limiting enzyme for biotransformation of inorganic arsenic. Polymorphisms of GSTO genes were shown associated with the intracellular thiol status and arsenic biotransformation efficiency of the cell [34].

1.5 Atherosclerosis- and CVD-related genes

High-density lipoprotein (HDL) is postulated to prevent the development of atherosclerosis by inhibiting the oxidation of low-density lipoprotein (LDL). Human paraoxonase (PON1) is a serum esterase/lactonase transported on HDL particles which is considered the major determinant of the antioxidant action of HDL [35]. Both in vitro studies and animal studies using PON1-knockout mice have shown that PON1 can prevent both HDL and LDL oxidation and therefore a protective enzyme against the development of atherosclerosis [36-38]. Our previous data also showed significant synergistic effects of genetic variations in the PON gene cluster and chronic arsenic exposure on electrocardiogram abnormality [39].

1.6 Other genes may linked to arsenic-related CVD

A recent review article also pointed out that some other genes that associated with arsenic toxicity and altered gene expression in humans including genes involved in stress response, DNA damage response and apoptosis related genes, cell cycle regulatory genes and cell signaling and altered growth factor [40]. Evidence from experimental studies had also suggested that arsenic increases the production of reactive oxygen species (ROS) [41-43]. The induction of oxidative stress by arsenic may influence gene expression, inflammatory responses, and endothelial nitric oxide homeostasis [44], which play an important role in maintaining vascular tone. Genes involved in endogenous defenses against ROS thus may modify arsenic's effect. Genetic material is constantly being subjected to insult from a wide range of DNA damage agents and this damage is controlled by the action of DNA repair enzymes.

1.7 Arsenic-related early effect-biomarkers for CVD

Preclinical or subclinical disease was defined as the pathological changes in the heart and arteries that develop early in the course of cardiovascular disease before symptoms or morbid events occur. They were developed before the evaluation of any of the risk factors or the determination of the subsequent incidence and mortality and thus are unbiased. Persons with subclinical disease, regardless of whether other risk factors are present, are at greater risk of future cardiovascular events than are those without subclinical disease [45]. Although standard methods of cardiac risk assessment from the physical examination, laboratory tests, and treadmill exercise testing are often used clinically in cardiovascular disease stratification [46], evaluation of subclinical disease often not taken into account.

Epidemiology studies have showed that the population attributable fractions to CHD of subclinical disease was 36.8% and 42.5% for men and women respectively, which is much higher than for most of the known risk factors or combination of risk factors and further documents the importance of subclinical disease as a contributor to subsequent incident clinical disease [45]. Among coronary artery disease (CAD) patients, the preoperative electrocardiogram (ECG) is shown to be predictive of long-term outcome independent of clinical findings and perioperative ischemia [47]. Moreover, unrecognized silent myocardial infarction as diagnosed by electrographic changes is a major risk factor for subsequent myocardial infarction and coronary disease deaths [48], and it is also a useful additional tool for differentiating the x-lined form of hereditary cardiac myopathies [49]. Subclinical disease and clinical disease shared similar risk factors and thus aggressive interventions to prevent clinical disease should be oriented to individuals with subclinical disease [50].

Various ECG abnormalities have been observed among cases of acute arsenic poisoning and in acute promyelocytic leukemia patients treated with arsenic trioxide. Individuals exposed to excess arsenic through drinking water showed some of the ECG abnormalities [51]. QT prolongation and dispersion have been implicated in the genesis of ventricular arrhythmia and directly predictors of cardiovascular and all-cause mortality [52,53]. The gradient relationship of chronic arsenic poisoning and prolonged QT interval and increased QT dispersion has been reported recently [54,55] and arsenic-induced QT dispersion was associated with atherosclerosis disease and predicted cardiovascular mortality. However, evidence was based on risk assessment on subjects with previous exposure to high arsenic level and biomarkers for methylation metabolism were not considered. Besides, the accuracy and reproducibility of ECG reading including QT dispersion measurement have been restricted by difficulties with reliable determination of T-waves offset. Further study with a standardize measurement of ECG reading is warranted for a reliable assessment of ECG abnormality.

Although an association between chronic arsenic exposure and CVD has been found in many studies, nearly all of these studies were limited by use of cross-sectional data, and longitudinal evidence by follow-up study was still limited. Besides, majority of previous studies were focus on the clinical arsenic-related cardiovascular disease, instead of the manifest of preclinical or subclinical detections. Morbidity and mortality from peripheral vascular disease, ischemic heart disease, and cerebral infarction are relative late clinical manifestations of chronic arsenic damage. These health effects may be the consequence of the interactions between predisposing and precipitating factors for cardiovascular diseases. The risk assessment based on these late cardiovascular events may be underestimated due to competing causes of death and the correctness in the diagnosis of the sudden death from cardiovascular diseases. Studies based on subclinical finding including ECG abnormality are needed to detect the early sign of chronic poisoning.

Furthermore, the variation in distribution of arsenic in human urine across areas [31] suggested that there are genetic factors in the regulation of the enzymes that metabolize arsenic, which may lead to difference in toxicity related to arsenic exposure. Association studies based on genetic polymorphisms have not provided consensus data that could generate a viable hypothesis on the molecular mechanism that determines the genetic basis of arsenic toxicity. The major objective of this study is to investigate the joint contribution of genetic factors including PON1, AS3MT, and GSTO gene families and the long-term arsenic impacts on cardiovascular disease through measuring ECG abnormality as subclinical phenotypes and to evaluate whether the arsenic methylation patterns modifies the association between cumulative arsenic exposure and the risk of CVD.

2. Materials and methods

2.1 Study area and population

The study included a community-based cohort from previous arseniasis-endemic area in southwestern Taiwan and a non-exposed population recruited from documented non-endemic area in the same county with similar age, gender contribution and ecological status in 2002. The arseniasis-endemic area included Homei, Fusin and Hsinming villages in Putai Township on the southwestern coast of Taiwan which had been described previously [56-58]. In short, residents in the study area consumed high-arsenic contaminated well water for decades since the 1910s because of the high salinity in shallow village wells [23]. The arsenic concentration of artesian well water measured in the early 1960s was from 0.035 to 1.14 ppm, with a median of 0.78 ppm [59,60]. An estimated total daily amount of arsenic ingested by local residents was as high as 1 mg, mainly from drinking water [61]. A tap water supply system was implemented in the area in the early 1960s and the entire arseniasis-endemic area has been supplied with municipal water since the early 1970s. The arsenic concentration of tap water supplied in the study area was less than 0.01 ppm [62]. The original cohort established in 1989 including 1571 residents and 1081 subjects provided informed consents and enrolled in the study cohort. In 1993, 732 residents from the villages had a 12-lead baseline Electrocardiogram (ECG) recorded. In 2002, after an average follow up period of eight years, 216 out of 380 subjects recruited provided a second ECG recording; 141 of them provided blood and urine specimens without an ECG recording; 229 were dead and their mortality determined through linkage with the national database; and the remaining 146 were lost to follow-up. Among the 121 residents with normal baseline ECGs, 42 developed an ECG abnormality at follow up. The non-exposed area was Chiali Township where the arsenic concentration of well water was very low according to the results of surveys conducted in 1960s and 1970s[60,63]. Climate, ethnic background (Han Chinese), urbanization degree and socioeconomic status were similar between Putai and Chiali. Frequency matching by age strata and gender were conducted for recruitment of resident and a total of 303 subjects were recruited.

2.2 Measurement of arsenic exposure

Arsenic level of well water for this study area was measured by the National Taiwan University group[60]. The water-contained arsenic recovery efficiencies were 95 percent or greater and were obtained using a PerkinElmer UV-VIS Spectrophotometer incorporating with Klett-Summerson Colorimeter. Detail validations of the water arsenic levels have been presented previously[57,64]. For villages which used more than one artesian well as a source of potable water, the medial levels of water arsenic contamination across those wells were assigned. The arsenic levels in artesian well water in this study area have been reported to be stable[65]. An index of cumulative arsenic exposure (micrograms per liter-years) were defined as the summation of products derived by multiplying the arsenic concentration (in micrograms per liter) in well water by duration of water consumption (in years) during consecutive periods of living in the defacement villages. Both cumulative arsenic exposure and average arsenic concentrations in drinking water were calculated only for subjects who had complete information on arsenic exposure from drinking water throughout his or her lifetime.

2.3 Questionnaire interview

At both baseline and follow-up, well trained public health nurses carried out the standardized personal interview based on a structured questionnaire to acquire information regarding demographic and socioeconomic characteristics, artesian well water usage, residential history, lifestyle variables, personal and family disease history of hypertension, diabetes, and cardiovascular diseases. Cumulative arsenic exposure (in ppm-years) was derived from the median arsenic concentration in artesian well water (ppm) in the village where the subject lived and the duration of consuming the artesian well water (years)while residing in the village. The human Ethical Committee of the National Health Research Institutes in Taiwan approved the study protocol which based on the ethical standards formulated from the Helsinki Declarations of 1964 and revised in 2000 [66]. Informed consent was provided to each subject before participation.

2.4 Biochemical measurements

Fasting plasma was used for quantitative determination of blood glucose, cholesterol, triglycerides, high- and low-density lipoproteins, and urine acid were analyzed using the same instrument.

Urinary samples were collected from each subject for arsenic species analyses. Subjects were asked not to consume seafood three days before urine collection. Arsenic species in urine including arsenite (AsIII), arsenate (AsV), monomethyl arsenical (MMA) and dimethyl arsenical (DMA) were quantified using high-performance liquid chromatography (HPLC) coupled with flow injection atomic absorption spectrometry. The HPLC system consisted of a solvent delivery pump (PU-1580, Jasco, Tokyo, Japan) and a silica-based anion-exchange column (Nucleosil 10 SB, 250 mm×4.6 mm; Phenomenex, CA, USA) with a guard column packed with the same material. A flow injection analysis system (FIAS-400, PerkinElmer, CT, USA) was designed as the on-line interface to the continuous hydride generation system (Analyst 100, PerkinElmer, CT, USA) used in this study. With this method, the within-say and between-day precision (coefficient of variance, CV%) for AsIII, AsV, MMA, and DMA determinations ranged from 1.0 to 3.7% were observed. Furthermore, the recoveries for AsIII, AsV, MMA, and DMA were 99.0, 98.9, 99.0, and 99.0% while the detection limits were 0.75, 1.47, 1.19, and 0.76 μg/L, respectively. The primary methylation index (PMI) was defined as the ratio between MMA and iAs levels, and the secondary methylation index (SMI) was defined as the ratio between DMA and MMA.

2.5 Genotyping

Eight functional polymorphisms: C-108T (promoter), L55M (exon 3) and Q192R (exon 6) of PON1, A148G (exon 5) and C311S (exon 9) of PON2, M287T (exon 9) of AS3MT, A140D (exon 4) of GSTO1, and N142D (exon 5) of GSTO2. SNPs were selected from NCBI's SNP database based on prior implication in disease and minor allele frequency. Genomic DNA was extracted from whole blood using standard techniques. The AS3MT M287T polymorphism was determined using a commercially designed TaqMan SNP Genotyping Assay (Applied Biosystems, USA). All other genotypes will be conducted by PCR amplification followed by polymorphism-specific restriction enzyme digestion and gel analysis.

2.6 Physical examination

Resting twelve-lead conventional ECG recording was performed at the Beimen Branch, Shinyin Hospital. Minnesota standardized code classification [1] was evaluated for both baseline and follow-up ECG readings at Epidemiological Cardiology Research Center (EPICARE), Department of Public Health Sciences, Wake Forest University School of Medicine, Winston-Salem, North Carolina, USA (blinded to all other study data). ECG readings were classified into normal and abnormal (including minor and major abnormality) according to the definition of cardiac function by myocardial infarction or ischemia (Q wave and STT change) (MC_1, MC_4, MC_5, MC_92), conduction defect (MC_7), arrhythmias (MC_6, MC_81~MC_88), atrial enlargement or ventricular hypertrophy (LVH_MC3/LVH_CV), and prolonged ventricular repolarization. Fasting plasma was analyzed for blood glucose, cholesterol, triglycerides, high- and low-density lipoproteins, and urine acid by Beckmen SYNCHRON LX20 System (Beckman Coulter, Fullerton, CA).

2.7 Statistical analysis

Differences in demographic characteristics and cardiovascular risk factors between ECG normal and abnormal subjects were assessed. Continuous variables were expressed as mean ± standard deviation (SD) and evaluated by student's t or Wilcoxon rank-sum test. Categorical variables were expressed as proportions and compared using chi-square test or Fisher's exact test. Allele frequencies, genotype frequencies, and Hardy-Weinberg equilibrium were assessed separately in ECG abnormal and normal groups using SAS-genetics package. Relative distribution of polymorphisms in the ECG abnormal and ECG normal groups was assessed by chi-square analyses. Linkage disequilibrium (LD) as measured by D′ was assessed using Haploview 4.0 (http://www.broad.mit.edu/mpg/haploview/). Haplotypes and tag SNPs were inferred using SAS. Logistic regression analysis was used to assess the effect of cardiovascular risk factors and genetic polymorphisms in relation to ECG abnormality. Arsenic exposure and ECG abnormality in between study subjects in Putai and Chiali areas were also compared. Arsenic exposure in Putai area were stratified into two categories by median levels and subjects in Chiali area were used as reference group, and a trend test was conducted to evaluate the dose-relationship. ANOVA was conducted to evaluate urinary arsenic species between subjects with normal and abnormal ECG reading. A p value <0.05 was considered statistically significant. Permutation test, a significance test used to obtain the unknown reference distribution by calculating all possible values of the test statistic under random rearrangements of the disease status on the observed study subjects , was used to control for type 1 error for multiple testing due to the limited sample size, and the empirical p-values were reported [67]. Statistical analyses were conducted using SAS version 9.1 (SAS, Inc., Cary, NC).

3. Results

Baseline characteristics of arsenic exposure and cardiovascular risk factors among study subjects are summarized in Table 1. A total of 42 incident cases among the 121 baseline-normal study subjects showed ECG deterioration at follow-up. Compared to ECG normal subjects, those with an ECG abnormality had significantly higher arsenic exposure as shown by both years of drinking artesian water and cumulative arsenic exposure index. Age and proportion of cigarette smoking in the ECG abnormal group tended to be higher but did not reach statistical significance. No differences were observed in other cardiovascular risk factors including gender, alcohol consumption, BMI, serum lipids, blood pressure, and plasma glucose.

Variable	ECG normal (n=79)	ECG abnormal (n=42)
Age (years)	62.0 ± 7.3	64.9 ± 8.7
Male (%)	29 (36.7)	18 (42.9)
Cigarette Smoking (%)	14 (17.7)	13 (31.0)
Alcohol consumption (%)	10 (12.7)	6 (14.3)
Residency (years)	41.5 ± 12.4	43.3 ± 14.3
Drinking Artesian Water (years)	19.2 ± 9.3	25.1 ± 9.7
Cumulative As exposure (ppm-years)	13.6 ± 8.4	18.0 ± 8.4
BMI (kg/m^2)	24.9 ± 3.13	24.5 ± 3.4
Triglycerides (mg/dl)	113.1 ± 64.7	132.3 ± 106.9
Total Cholesterol (mg/dl)	220.2 ± 45.0	211.7 ± 42.5
HDL (mg/dl)	60.3 ± 18.1	59.2 ± 14.3
LDL (mg/dl)	121.9 ± 48.1	124.6 ± 76.3
Cholesterol /HDL ratio	4.0 ± 1.6	3.8 ± 1.2
Uric acid (mg/dl)	6.1 ± 1.9	5.7 ± 1.8
SBP (mmHg)	124.8 ± 19.3	128.2 ± 17.3
DBP (mmHg)	82.2 ± 11.1	84.2 ± 8.6
AC glucose (mg/dl)	98.6 ± 23.1	104.4 ± 37.3
PC glucose (mg/dl)	127.3 ± 52.2	129.1 ± 78.1

Data are reported as mean ± SD or counts (%)
HDL: high density lipoprotein; LDL: low density lipoprotein; CHOL: total cholesterol levels; SBP: systolic blood pressure; DBP: diastolic blood pressure, AC: ante cibum, PC: post cibum

Table 1. Baseline characteristics of arsenic and CVD risk factors among baseline-normal study participants classified by ECG status at follow-up

3.1 Univariate SNPs association analysis

Eight functional polymorphisms: C-108T, L55M and Q192R of PON1, A148G and C311S of PON2, M287T of AS3MT, A140D of GSTO1, and N142D of GSTO2 were screened for association with ECG abnormality and Hardy-Weinberg equilibrium (HWE). None reached statistical significance, suggesting no univariate SNP association in the analysis. Genotypic frequencies of M287T showed a significant departure from HWE but because of the limited number of participants carrying the T alleles in this study population, they were excluded from subsequent analysis.

Gene	SNP	ECG status		OR (95% CI)
		Normal	Abnormal	
PON1	Q192R			
	RR	18	14	1.00 (reference)
	QR	27	9	0.43 (0.15-1.20)
	QQ	11	3	0.35 (0.08-1.50)
	L55M			
	LL	48	21	1.00 (reference)
	LM	14	4	0.65 (0.19-2.22)
	MM	0	0	-
	C-108T			
	CC	17	7	1.00 (reference)
	CT	30	15	1.21 (0.41-3.56)
	TT	15	6	0.97 (0.27-3.54)
PON2	C311S			
	SS	31	18	1.00 (reference)
	CS	24	7	0.50 (0.18-1.40)
	CC	2	2	1.72 (0.22-13.30)
	A148G			
	AA	30	15	1.00 (reference)
	AG	28	10	0.71 (0.28-1.85)
	GG	3	2	1.33 (0.20-8.86)
AS3MT	M287T			
	MM	67	30	1.00 (reference)
	MT	2	1	1.12 (0.10-12.80)
	TT	0	0	-
GSTO1	A140D			
	AA	41	21	1.00 (reference)
	AD	22	9	0.80 (0.31-2.04)
	DD	5	2	0.78 (0.14-4.37)
GSTO2	N142D			
	NN	35	16	1.00 (reference)
	ND	30	14	1.02 (0.43-2.43)
	DD	4	2	1.09 (0.18-6.60)

Hardy-Weinberg Equilibrium (HWE) test was conducted among all study subjects

Table 2. Association of SNPs and Hardy-Weinberg equilibrium test

Figure 1 shows the related position and linkage disequilibrium (LD) between SNPs in the PON and GSTO gene clusters. Two SNPs within PON2 (C311S and A148G) and GSTO1-A140D and GSTO2-N142 were in high LD but SNPs within PON1 or adjacent SNPs between PON1 and PON2 (C-108T and C311s) had low LD measurements, implying they were not in the same LD block. Q192R, C-108T, C311S and A140D were identified as tag-SNPs.

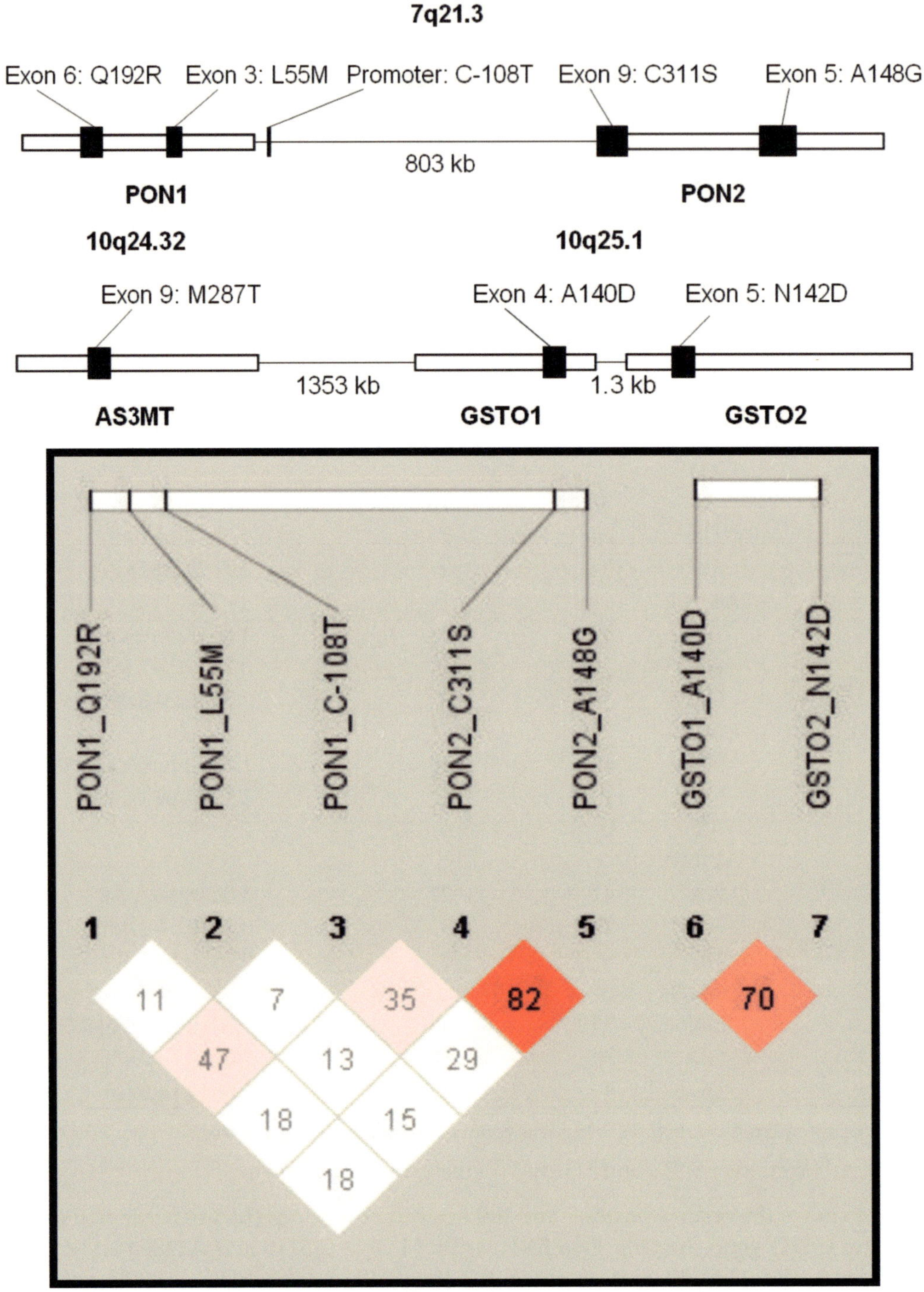

Fig. 1. Linkage disequilibrium (LD) plot of PON1 and GSTO gene clusters in 121 study subjects. The measure of LD (D′) among all possible pairs of SNPs is shown graphically. Dark red represents high D′ while white represents low D′

3.2 Haplotype analysis and association with ECG abnormality

Haplotypes of PON1, PON2, GSTO1, GSTO2 and tag-SNPs of the PON gene cluster were constructed, and those whose frequencies were <5% were excluded from association analysis (Table 3). Overall, the effects of these haplotypes on ECG abnormality were not statistically significant after 10,000 permutations; however, the haplotype R-C-S constructed by Q192R, C-108T and C311S had the highest odds, 1.92 (95% CI: 0.76-4.85) times increased risk toward ECG abnormality.

Haplotypes			ECG normal	ECG abnormal	OR
Q192R	L55M	C-108T			
R	L	T	46 (37.1%)	24 (42.9%)	1.00 (reference)
Q	L	C	38 (30.7%)	10 (17.9%)	0.50 (0.22-1.18)
R	L	C	18 (14.5%)	15 (26.8%)	1.60 (0.69-372)
Q	M	C	8 (6.5%)	4 (7.1%)	0.96 (0.26-3.51)
Q	L	T	8 (6.5%)	3 (5.4%)	0.72 (0.17-2.96)
Q192R	C-108T				
R	T		52 (41.9%)	24 (42.9%)	1.00 (reference)
Q	C		46 (37.1%)	14 (25.0%)	0.66 (0.31-1.42)
R	C		18 (14.5%)	15 (26.8%)	1.81 (0.78-4.18)
Q	T		8 (6.5%)	3 (5.4%)	0.81 (0.20-3.33)
C311S	A148G				
S	A		89 (71.8%)	40 (70.4%)	1.00 (reference)
C	G		32 (25.8%)	10 (17.9%)	0.70 (0.31-1.56)
A140D	N142D				
A	N		96 (69.5%)	43 (67.2%)	1.00 (reference)
D	D		28 (20.3%)	10 (15.6%)	0.80 (0.36-1.77)
A	D		10 (7.3%)	8 (12.5%)	1.79 (0.66-4.84)
Q192R	C-108T	C311S			
R	T	S	47 (37.9%)	21 (37.5%)	1.00 (reference)
Q	C	S	27 (21.7%)	9 (16.1%)	0.75 (0.30-1.86)
R	C	S	14 (11.3%)	12 (21.4)	1.92 (0.76-4.85)
Q	C	C	19 (15.3%)	5 (8.9%)	0.59 (0.19-1.79)
Q	T	S	8 (6.5%)	3 (5.4%)	0.84 (0.20-3.48)

Haplotypes with a frequency less than 5% were removed.
Empirical P-value: [a] Haplotype-specific test, [b] Haplotype-global test

Table 3. Estimated haplotype frequencies and haplotypes association analysis with ECG abnormality

The relative odds of lipid profiles for PON-haplotype R-C-S carrier compared with non-carriers are shown in Figure 2. The R-C-S haplotype was positively correlated with higher serum HDL-cholesterol, LDL-cholesterol, and triglyceride levels without statistical significance, but was significantly associated with increased total cholesterol levels (OR=2.91, 95% CI: 1.13-7.70).

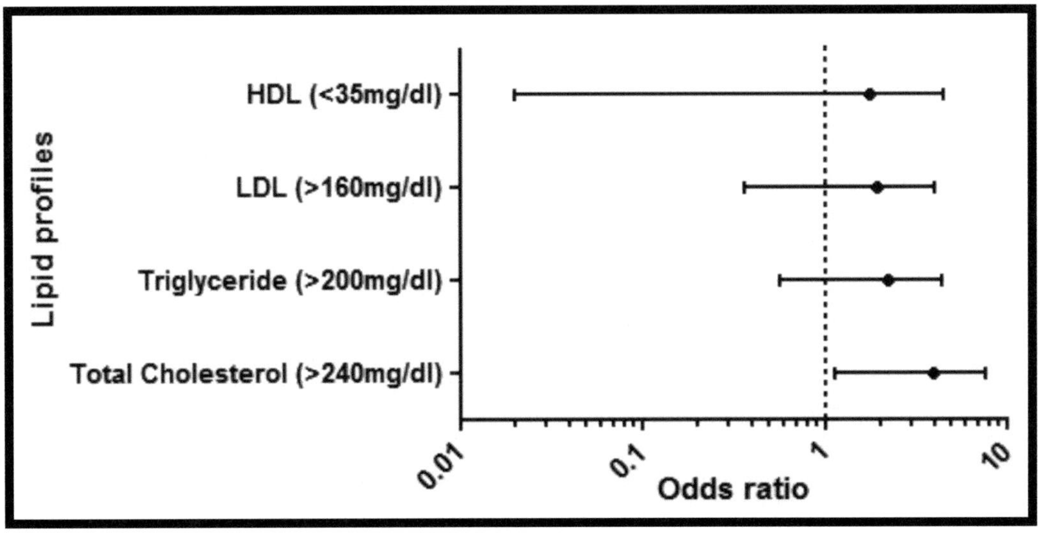

Fig. 2. Odds ratios of lipid profiles for Q192R, C-108T and C311S R-C-S haplotype carrier among study subjects (N=121)

3.3 Synergistic association of PON haplotype and arsenic on ECG abnormality

The synergistic associations between PON haplotype and arsenic exposure are summarized in Table 4. The PON R-C-S haplotype carrier with higher cumulative arsenic exposure (greater than the median value of 14.7 ppm-years) showed a >14.66 (95% CI: 1.83-117.64) increased risk for ECG abnormality compared to non-RCS haplotype carriers with low cumulative arsenic exposure (<14.7 ppm-years) (Table 4a). The PON R-C-S haplotype carrier with more years of drinking artesian water (greater than the median of 21 years) had a 10.83-fold (95% CI: 1.83-64.03) increased risk (Table 4b). These associations were even stronger after adjusting for age, gender, and cigarette smoking, when the odds increased to 19.19 (95% CI: 1.86-197.76) and 21.09 (95% CI: 2.77-160.35) for cumulative exposure index and drinking years, respectively.

Table 5 showed the correlation between cumulative arsenic exposure and urinary arsenic species from arsenic endemic and non-endemic areas in southwestern Taiwan. Subjects with higher cumulative arsenic exposure had significantly higher levels of As (III), iAs, MMA, Summation of iAs and MMA. However, DMA levels and SMI were significantly lower among subjects with high arsenic exposure. Similar pattern was observed when urinary arsenic was analyzed in percentage. Subjects with higher cumulative arsenic exposure had higher percentages of As(III), iAs and MMA in urinary and lower DMA percentage.

R-C-S	CAE	ECG Normal	ECG Abnormal	OR (95% CI)	OR (95% CI)[a]	Empirical P-value [a]
-	-	22	3	1.00 (reference)	1.00 (reference)	-
+	-	8	2	1.83 (0.26-13.06)	1.57 (0.19-13.00)	0.319
-	+	17	11	4.74 (1.14-19.72)	4.27 (0.83-22.08)	0.632
+	+	2	4	14.66 (1.83-117.64)	19.19 (1.86-197.76)	0.014

[a] Permutation analysis adjusted by age, gender and cigarette smoking
CAE: Cumulative arsenic exposure (ppm-years)
R-C-S: Q192R, C-108T and C311S R-C-S haplotype

Table 4a. Synergistic effects of Q192R, C-108T, and C311S R-C-S haplotypes carrier and high cumulative arsenic exposure (CAE) (> median of 14.7 ppm-years) on ECG abnormality

R-C-S	DAW	ECG Normal	ECG Abnormal	OR (95% CI)	OR (95% CI)[a]	Empirical P-value [a]
-	-	26	3	1.00 (reference)	1.00 (reference)	-
+	-	8	2	2.17 (0.31 15.33)	1.90 (0.24-14.94)	0.190
-	+	19	15	6.84 (1.73-27.02)	10.66 (2.12-53.55)	0.055
+	+	4	5	10.83 (1.83-64.03)	21.09 (2.77-160.35)	0.010

[a] Permutation analysis adjusted by age, gender and cigarette smoking
DAW: Drinking artesian water (years)
RCS: Q192R, C-108T & C311S R-C-S haplotype

Table 4b. Synergistic effects of Q192R, C-108T, and C311S R-C-S haplotypes carrier and more years of drinking artesian water (DAW) (> mean of 21 years) on ECG abnormality

Variable	Non-exposed (Chiali) (N=302)	≤ 14.7 (Putai) (N=191)	> 14.7 (Putai) (N=103)
Urinary arsenic level			
As (III) (μg/g creatinine)**	2.07 (2.98)	4.61 (9.46)	4.73 (6.24)
As (V) (μg/g creatinine)	2.78 (3.16)	3.13 (3.66)	2.21 (1.92)
iAs (μg/g creatinine)**	4.85 (4.66)	7.73 (11.54)	6.95 (6.74)
MMA (μg/g creatinine)**	3.13 (3.79)	4.48 (6.30)	4.21 (3.25)
Σ(iAs +MMA) (μg/g creatinine)**	7.98 (6.84)	12.21 (14.66)	11.15 (7.84)
DMA (μg/g creatinine)*	42.87 (34.48)	33.64 (27.34)	37.37 (24.32)
Σ(iAs + MMA + DMA) (μg/g creatinine)	50.85 (37.86)	45.87 (33.60)	48.58 (28.53)
PMI (MMA/iAs)	0.87 (1.02)	0.84 (0.75)	0.85 (0.60)
SMI (DMA/MMA)**	23.68 (22.80)	15.44 (28.38)	15.94 (20.86)
Urinary arsenic percentage			
As (III) %**	4.59 (5.18)	10.08 (13.22)	9.18 (9.08)
As (V) %**	6.23 (5.62)	8.27 (7.76)	5.81 (7.58)
iAs %**	10.82 (8.37)	18.35 (16.50)	14.99 (10.73)
MMA %**	7.45 (8.59)	10.90 (9.05)	10.12 (7.57)
DMA %**	81.73 (13.84)	70.75 (20.23)	74.89 (13.99)

[a] P-value for ANOVA
*P-value < 0.05, ** P-value < 0.01

Table 5. Correlation of cumulative arsenic exposure and urinary metabolism capacity

Distribution between levels of cumulative arsenic exposure and ECG abnormality was summarized in Table 6. Significant dose-response relationships were observed between higher levels of cumulative arsenic exposure and ECG reading regarding abnormalities, myocardial infarction or ischemia disease, and also atrial enlargement and ventricular hypertrophy. Increased cumulative arsenic exposure was also correlated with a higher proportion of abnormality in prolonged ventricular repolarization however not reach statistical significance.

Variable	Non-exposed (Chiali) (N=302)	≤ 14.7 (Putai) (N=191)	> 14.7 (Putai) (N=103)
ECG reading (ECG group)**			
0: Normal	155 (51.3)	96 (50.3)	40 (38.8)
1: Minor abnormal	122 (40.3)	70 (36.7)	40 (38.8)
2: Major abnormal	25 (8.3)	25 (13.0)	23 (22.4)
Myocardial Infarction or Ischemia (MC_MI)*			
0: Normal	216 (71.5)	136 (71.2)	68 (66.0)
1: Minor abnormal	72 (23.8)	37 (19.4)	20 (19.4)
2: Major abnormal	14 (4.6)	18 (9.4)	15 (14.6)
Conduction defect (BBB; Bundle Branch Block)			
0: Normal	261 (86.4)	174 (91.1)	86 (83.5)
1: Abnormal	41 (13.6)	17 (8.9)	17 (16.5)
Arrhythmia (Arrhythmia)			
0: Normal	265 (87.8)	170 (89.0)	97 (94.2)
1: Abnormal	37 (12.3)	21 (11.0)	6 (5.8)
Atrial enlargement/Ventricular hypertrophy (Hypertrophy)**			
0: Normal	286 (94.7)	167 (87.4)	85 (82.5)
1: Abnormal	16 (5.3)	24 (12.6)	18 (17.5)
Prolonged ventricular repolarization (Long_QT)			
0: Normal	299 (99.0)	187 (98.0)	99 (96.1)
1: Abnormal	3 (1.0)	4 (2.0)	4 (3.9)

[a] P-value for trend test
*P-value < 0.05, ** P-value < 0.01

Table 6. Distribution of ECG reading by cumulative arsenic exposure

4. Discussion

Various ECG abnormalities have been observed among cases of acute arsenic poisoning and in acute promyelocytic leukemia patients treated with arsenic trioxide. Individuals exposed to excess arsenic through drinking water showed some of the ECG abnormalities[51]. Several epidemiologic studies showed that QT prolongation and increased CVD mortality among high levels of arsenic-exposed subjects. However, the results might not be applicable in subjects with low to moderate arsenic. Our data replicated this association in an arseniasis-endemic area and a well-matched control area which no previous history of water contamination. We highlighted the correlation between previous chronic arsenic exposure and ECG abnormalities after cessation of arsenic-contaminated water consumption for decades.

The major strength of this study was to apply a standardized Minnesota coding classification of ECG reading that ensures good quality assurance and control. Furthermore, detailed parameters regarding ECG abnormalities allowed us to evaluate the minor changes due to arsenic toxicity. In current analyses, higher duration of arsenic water consumption was associated with ECG abnormality, myocardial infarction or ischemia, atrial enlargement or ventricular hypertrophy in a dose-response relationship. Besides, it was also positively correlated to arrhythmia and prolonged ventricular repolarization without reached the statistical significance. Moreover, higher levels of cumulative arsenic exposure were also associated with ECG parameters including higher PR duration, QRS duration and QRS axis and smaller JT duration, JT index and RaVL (data not shown).

There were still some limitations for this study. First, results from this study were based on a population with history of arsenic exposure. Insignificant association between urinary methylation capabilities might due to attrition of high-level arsenic exposed subjects, competing risks for CVD mortality was not considered in current analysis. Another limitation of the present study was that the measurement of urinary metabolism species and physical evaluation were conducted at a cross-sectional design. The causal-relationship between urinary species of arsenic and ECG abnormality could not be inferred given current evidence. However, the previous exposure status was significantly correlated with current urinary arsenic species implied it was more efficient among subjects after cessation of long-term exposure to high levels of arsenic. These results may have implications for arsenic mediation strategies in areas currently exposed to potentially harmful levels of arsenic in drinking water. Furthermore, CVD usually took years for disease development. Correlation may be biased due to unmeasured factors during a relative short follow-up period. Longer duration of follow-up with serial changes for ECG abnormality would help better understand the underlying mechanism regarding arsenic-induced hazards.

The major significance by this study was the assessment of arsenic risk from subjects without exposure of inorganic arsenic to moderate and relatively high levels of cumulative arsenic exposure. Causal inference can be strengthened by the dose-response relationship by the stronger effect in a susceptible subgroup of the population. Besides, this study demonstrated significant gene-gene and gene-environment interactions by showing PON1 gene cluster including polymorphisms of PON1: Q192R, PON1: C-108T, and PON2: C311S and latent effect of arsenic exposure on incidence of ECG abnormality. Besides, PON2: C311S was independently associated with LDH elevation and further predicted future CVD mortality independent to other conventional risk factors including age, gender, cigarette smoking, hypertension and diabetes mellitus. After cessation of arsenic-contaminated water consumption for decades, biomarkers for CVD mortality and morbidity was still associated with reduced risks for arsenic and attributable to underlying genetic predisposition. Such data may also help risk assessment in the population and provide knowledge about the underlying mechanisms.

HDL has been shown to prevent atherogenesis in vivo and in vitro through anti-oxidative and anti-inflammatory activities[35]. The major part of anti-atherogenic properties associated with HDL is explained by the activity of Paraoxonase 1[68]. Both PON1 and PON2 belong to the protein family of Paraoxonase 1 that includes PON3 which has been suggested that involved in CVD[69]. PON1 directly form part of HDL particles whereas PON2 found in endothelial cells, smooth muscle cells and macrophages that possesses antioxidant properties similar to PON1 by delays cellular oxidative stress and prevents apoptosis in vascular endothelial cells[70,71]. Regarding three common polymorphisms in coding region of the human PON1 gene, the frequencies of Q192R, L55M, and C-108T for Taiwanese population were similar to those reported in the literature for the Chinese population [72,73]. Besides, we confirmed that paraoxonase, diazoxonase and arylesterase activities were directly influenced by the Q192R and C-108T polymorphisms. Previous studies had also shown that 311 C allele in PON2 was associated with increased risks of coronary artery disease, MI and also diabetic nephropathy[74-76]. Our data confirmed the significance of PON2: C311S polymorphism during pathogenesis of CVD among chronic arsenic exposed subject. This finding could help to identify subjects at higher risk of cardiovascular damage for arsenic toxicity.

However, some other factors that might have influenced the arsenic methylation profiles were not considered. Nutritional status and dietary intake may also be uncontrollable factors. Besides, we could not obtain the accurate data on allele distribution three polymorphisms: PON1: C-108T, GSTO1:A140D, and AS3MT: L55M in our samples. We still could not rule out the intra- and inter-individual variability to arsenic methylation and also their impacts on pathogenesis of CVD morbidity and mortality. Besides, the arsenic levels in rice growing in the arsenic contaminated area or inorganic arsenic from fish intake may be elevated. This might potentially increase arsenic exposure in the endemic area[77-80]. Future study of exposure assessment is needed. In addition, arsenic exposure has also been shown to alter the methylation level of both global DNA and certain genes in studies that analyzed a limited number of epigenetic endpoints[81]. Therefore, it is necessary to enlarge sample size for the evaluation of genetic association and ECG abnormality and other confounders that may be directly related to arsenic risks.

Genome-wide association studies (GWAS) have been applied in the search for suscepitibility genes to coronary artery disease, myocardial infarction and heart failure[82-84]. However, none of the candidate regions and genes showed a powerful association with CVD at genome-wide significance and the molecular and biological mechanisms remains unclear. Atherosclerosis is a multifactorial disease that may lead to myocardial infarction or heart failure. A conservative estimate would be that at least 100 genes have the potential to affect the modifying factors including atherosclerosis, myocardial infarction and congestive heart failure with each having a genetic contribution of as much as 2% to the phenotype[84]. Since CVD usually took years to develop, correlation may be biased due to unmeasured factors during a relative short follow-up period or relatively underestimated by competing risk. Our studies with longer duration of follow-up with serial changes for ECG abnormality did help better understand the underlying mechanism and duration regarding arsenic-induced hazards. These findings emphasize the importance of long term arsenic effect, along with the necessity of intensive follow-up for preclinical or subclinical phenotypes such as ECG abnormality for preventing excessive CVD mortality.

5. References

[1] Prineas RJ, Crow RS, Blackburn H. The Minnesota Code Manual of Electrocardiographic Findings. In: John Wright PSB Inc.,1st edition. Boston: MA; 1982.

[2] Kapaj S, Peterson H, Liber K, Bhattacharya P. Human health effects from chronic arsenic poisoning--a review. *J Environ Sci Health A Tox Hazard Subst Environ Eng.* 2006;41(10):2399-2428.

[3] Tseng WP. Blackfoot disease in Taiwan: a 30-year follow-up study. *Angiology.* Jun 1989;40(6):547-558.

[4] NRC. Arsenic in drinking water. Washington, DC: National Academy Press; 1999.

[5] Watanabe C, Inaoka T, Kadono T, et al. Males in rural Bangladeshi communities are more susceptible to chronic arsenic poisoning than females: analyses based on urinary arsenic. *Environ Health Perspect.* Dec 2001;109(12):1265-1270.

[6] Vahter M. Genetic polymorphism in the biotransformation of inorganic arsenic and its role in toxicity. *Toxicol Lett.* Mar 15 2000;112-113:209-217.

[7] Loffredo CA, Aposhian HV, Cebrian ME, Yamauchi H, Silbergeld EK. Variability in human metabolism of arsenic. *Environ Res.* Jun 2003;92(2):85-91.

[8] Chung JS, Kalman DA, Moore LE, et al. Family correlations of arsenic methylation patterns in children and parents exposed to high concentrations of arsenic in drinking water. *Environ Health Perspect.* Jul 2002;110(7):729-733.

[9] Karagas MR, Morris JS, Weiss JE, Spate V, Baskett C, Greenberg ER. Toenail samples as an indicator of drinking water arsenic exposure. *Cancer Epidemiol Biomarkers Prev.* Oct 1996;5(10):849-852.

[10] Cohen SM, Arnold LL, Eldan M, Lewis AS, Beck BD. Methylated arsenicals: the implications of metabolism and carcinogenicity studies in rodents to human risk assessment. *Crit Rev Toxicol.* Feb 2006;36(2):99-133.

[11] Tseng CH. Metabolism of inorganic arsenic and non-cancerous health hazards associated with chronic exposure in humans. *J Environ Biol.* Apr 2007;28(2 Suppl):349-357.

[12] Tseng CH. Arsenic methylation, urinary arsenic metabolites and human diseases: current perspective. *J Environ Sci Health C Environ Carcinog Ecotoxicol Rev.* Jan-Mar 2007;25(1):1-22.

[13] Maton A. *Human Biology and Health* Englewood Cliffs, New Jersey: Prentice Hall; 1993.

[14] McGill HC, Jr., McMahan CA, Zieske AW, et al. Associations of coronary heart disease risk factors with the intermediate lesion of atherosclerosis in youth. The Pathobiological Determinants of Atherosclerosis in Youth (PDAY) Research Group. *Arterioscler Thromb Vasc Biol.* Aug 2000;20(8):1998-2004.

[15] CDC, US. Chronic Disease Overview: Center for Disease control and Prevention 1999.

[16] Department of Health, Executive Yuan, Taiwan. *Health and Vital statistics-vital statistics*2005.

[17] Rainwater DL, McMahan CA, Malcom GT, et al. Lipid and apolipoprotein predictors of atherosclerosis in youth: apolipoprotein concentrations do not materially improve prediction of arterial lesions in PDAY subjects. The PDAY Research Group. *Arterioscler Thromb Vasc Biol.* Mar 1999;19(3):753-761.

[18] IARC. Arsenic and arsenic compounds. In: Cancer IAfRo, ed. Vol 23: IARC Monogr Eval Carcinog Risks Hum; 1987:100-103.

[19] EPA US. Inorganic Arsenic. Washington, DC, U.S.: Integrated Risk Information System; 1993.

[20] Hughes MF. Biomarkers of exposure: a case study with inorganic arsenic. *Environ Health Perspect.* Nov 2006;114(11):1790-1796.

[21] Wang CH, Hsiao CK, Chen CL, et al. A review of the epidemiologic literature on the role of environmental arsenic exposure and cardiovascular diseases. *Toxicol Appl Pharmacol.* Aug 1 2007;222(3):315-326.

[22] Ch'i IC, Blackwell RQ. A controlled retrospective study of Blackfoot disease, an endemic peripheral gangrene disease in Taiwan. *Am J Epidemiol.* Jul 1968;88(1):7-24.

[23] Wu HY, Chen KP, Tseng WP, Hsu CL. Epidemiologic studies on blackfoot disease: prevalence and incidence of the disease by age, sex, year, occupation, and geographic distribution. *Memoirs of College of Medicine (National Taiwan University).* 1961;7:1-18.

[24] Grantham DA, Jones FJ. Arsenic contamination of water wells in Nova Scotia. *Journal of the American Water Works Association.* 1977;69:653-657.

[25] Rahman MM, Chowdhury UK, Mukherjee SC, et al. Chronic arsenic toxicity in Bangladesh and West Bengal, India--a review and commentary. *J Toxicol Clin Toxicol.* 2001;39(7):683-700.

[26] Smith AH, Lopipero PA, Bates MN, Steinmaus CM. Public health. Arsenic epidemiology and drinking water standards. *Science.* Jun 21 2002;296(5576):2145-2146.

[27] Navas-Acien A, Sharrett AR, Silbergeld EK, et al. Arsenic exposure and cardiovascular disease: a systematic review of the epidemiologic evidence. *Am J Epidemiol.* Dec 1 2005;162(11):1037-1049.

[28] Hughes MF. Arsenic toxicity and potential mechanisms of action. *Toxicol Lett.* Jul 7 2002;133(1):1-16.

[29] Kitchin KT. Recent advances in arsenic carcinogenesis: modes of action, animal model systems, and methylated arsenic metabolites. *Toxicol Appl Pharmacol.* May 1 2001;172(3):249-261.

[30] Rossman TG. Mechanism of arsenic carcinogenesis: an integrated approach. *Mutat Res.* Dec 10 2003;533(1-2):37-65.

[31] Vahter M, Concha G, Nermell B, Nilsson R, Dulout F, Natarajan AT. A unique metabolism of inorganic arsenic in native Andean women. *Eur J Pharmacol.* Dec 7 1995;293(4):455-462.

[32] Lin S, Shi Q, Nix FB, et al. A novel S-adenosyl-L-methionine:arsenic(III) methyltransferase from rat liver cytosol. *J Biol Chem.* Mar 29 2002;277(13):10795-10803.

[33] Townsend D, Tew K. Cancer drugs, genetic variation and the glutathione-S-transferase gene family. *Am J Pharmacogenomics.* 2003;3(3):157-172.

[34] Tanaka-Kagawa T, Jinno H, Hasegawa T, et al. Functional characterization of two variant human GSTO 1-1s (Ala140Asp and Thr217Asn). *Biochem Biophys Res Commun.* Feb 7 2003;301(2):516-520.

[35] Aviram M, Rosenblat M, Bisgaier CL, Newton RS, Primo-Parmo SL, La Du BN. Paraoxonase inhibits high-density lipoprotein oxidation and preserves its functions. A possible peroxidative role for paraoxonase. *J Clin Invest.* Apr 15 1998;101(8):1581-1590.

[36] Mackness MI, Arrol S, Durrington PN. Paraoxonase prevents accumulation of lipoperoxides in low-density lipoprotein. *FEBS Lett.* Jul 29 1991;286(1-2):152-154.

[37] Watson AD, Berliner JA, Hama SY, et al. Protective effect of high density lipoprotein associated paraoxonase. Inhibition of the biological activity of minimally oxidized low density lipoprotein. *J Clin Invest.* Dec 1995;96(6):2882-2891.

[38] Shih DM, Gu L, Xia YR, et al. Mice lacking serum paraoxonase are susceptible to organophosphate toxicity and atherosclerosis. *Nature.* Jul 16 1998;394(6690):284-287.

[39] Liao YT, Li WF, Chen CJ, et al. Synergistic effect of polymorphisms of paraoxonase gene cluster and arsenic exposure on electrocardiogram abnormality. *Toxicol Appl Pharmacol.* Sep 1 2009;239(2):178-183.

[40] Ghosh P, Banerjee M, Giri AK, Ray K. Toxicogenomics of arsenic: classical ideas and recent advances. *Mutat Res.* Sep-Oct 2008;659(3):293-301.

[41] Barchowsky A, Klei LR, Dudek EJ, Swartz HM, James PE. Stimulation of reactive oxygen, but not reactive nitrogen species, in vascular endothelial cells exposed to low levels of arsenite. *Free Radic Biol Med.* Dec 1999;27(11-12):1405-1412.

[42] Chen YC, Lin-Shiau SY, Lin JK. Involvement of reactive oxygen species and caspase 3 activation in arsenite-induced apoptosis. *J Cell Physiol.* Nov 1998;177(2):324-333.

[43] Wang TS, Kuo CF, Jan KY, Huang H. Arsenite induces apoptosis in Chinese hamster ovary cells by generation of reactive oxygen species. *J Cell Physiol.* Nov 1996;169(2):256-268.

[44] Simeonova PP, Luster MI. Arsenic and atherosclerosis. *Toxicol Appl Pharmacol.* Aug 1 2004;198(3):444-449.

[45] Kuller LH, Shemanski L, Psaty BM, et al. Subclinical disease as an independent risk factor for cardiovascular disease. *Circulation.* Aug 15 1995;92(4):720-726.

[46] Califf RM, Armstrong PW, Carver JR, D'Agostino RB, Strauss WE. 27th Bethesda Conference: matching the intensity of risk factor management with the hazard for coronary disease events. Task Force 5. Stratification of patients into high, medium and low risk subgroups for purposes of risk factor management. *J Am Coll Cardiol.* Apr 1996;27(5):1007-1019.

[47] Jeger RV, Probst C, Arsenic R, et al. Long-term prognostic value of the preoperative 12-lead electrocardiogram before major noncardiac surgery in coronary artery disease. *Am Heart J.* Feb 2006;151(2):508-513.

[48] Kannel WB, Abbott RD. Incidence and prognosis of unrecognized myocardial infarction. An update on the Framingham study. *N Engl J Med.* Nov 1 1984;311(18):1144-1147.

[49] Emery AE. Abnormalities of the electrocardiogram in hereditary myopathies. *J Med Genet.* Mar 1972;9(1):8-12.

[50] Kuller L, Borhani N, Furberg C, et al. Prevalence of subclinical atherosclerosis and cardiovascular disease and association with risk factors in the Cardiovascular Health Study. *Am J Epidemiol.* Jun 15 1994;139(12):1164-1179.

[51] Ahmad SA, Khatun F, Sayed MH, et al. Electrocardiographic abnormalities among arsenic-exposed persons through groundwater in Bangladesh. *J Health Popul Nutr.* Jun 2006;24(2):221-227.

[52] de Bruyne MC, Hoes AW, Kors JA, Hofman A, van Bemmel JH, Grobbee DE. QTc dispersion predicts cardiac mortality in the elderly: the Rotterdam Study. *Circulation.* Feb 10 1998;97(5):467-472.

[53] Zabel M, Klingenheben T, Franz MR, Hohnloser SH. Assessment of QT dispersion for prediction of mortality or arrhythmic events after myocardial infarction: results of a prospective, long-term follow-up study. *Circulation.* Jun 30 1998;97(25):2543-2550.

[54] Wang CH, Chen CL, Hsiao CK, et al. Increased risk of QT prolongation associated with atherosclerotic diseases in arseniasis-endemic area in southwestern coast of Taiwan. *Toxicol Appl Pharmacol.* Sep 15 2009;239(3):320-324.

[55] Wang CH, Chen CL, Hsiao CK, et al. Arsenic-induced QT dispersion is associated with atherosclerotic diseases and predicts long-term cardiovascular mortality in subjects with previous exposure to arsenic: A 17-Year follow-up study. *Cardiovasc Toxicol.* Mar 2010;10(1):17-26.

[56] Chen CJ, Chuang YC, Lin TM, Wu HY. Malignant neoplasms among residents of a blackfoot disease-endemic area in Taiwan: high-arsenic artesian well water and cancers. *Cancer Res.* Nov 1985;45(11 Pt 2):5895-5899.

[57] Chen CJ, Hsueh YM, Lai MS, et al. Increased prevalence of hypertension and long-term arsenic exposure. *Hypertension.* Jan 1995;25(1):53-60.

[58] Tseng CH, Chong CK, Tseng CP, et al. Long-term arsenic exposure and ischemic heart disease in arseniasis-hyperendemic villages in Taiwan. *Toxicol Lett.* Jan 31 2003;137(1-2):15-21.

[59] Chen KP, Wu TC, Wu TC. Epidemiologic studies on blackfoot disease in Taiwan. 3. Physicochemical characteristics of drinking water in endemic blackfoot disease areas. *Memoirs of College of Medicine (National Taiwan University).* 1962;8:115-129.

[60] Kuo TL. *Arsenic Content of Artesian Well Water in Endemic Area of Chronic Arsenic Poisoning* Institute of Pathology, National Taiwan University; 1964.

[61] Blackwell RQ. Estimation total arsenic ingested by residents in the endemic blackfoot area. *J Formosan Med. Assoc.* 1961;60:1143-1144.

[62] Chen WY, Chen KP. Study on arsenic artesian well water and blackfoot disease progress. *Taichung, Taiwan: Taiwan Provincial Institute of Environmental Sanitation*: Taichung, Taiwan: Taiwan Provincial Institute of Environmental Sanitation; 1975.

[63] Lo MC, Hsen YC, Lin BK. *Arsenic content of underground water in Taiwan: Second report.* Taichung, Taiwan: Taiwan Provincial Institute of Environmental Sanitation;1977.

[64] Hsueh YM, Lin P, Chen HW, et al. Genetic polymorphisms of oxidative and antioxidant enzymes and arsenic-related hypertension. *J Toxicol Environ Health A.* Sep 2005;68(17-18):1471-1484.

[65] MC L, YC H, BK L. *Arsenic content of underground water in Taiwan: Second report.* Taichung, Taiwan1977.

[66] World Medical Association. Declaration of Helsinki: Ethical Principles for Medical Research Involving Human Subjects. *Bulletin of Medical Ethics* Vol 1622000:8-11.

[67] Potter DM. A permutation test for inference in logistic regression with small- and moderate-sized data sets. *Stat Med.* Mar 15 2005;24(5):693-708.

[68] Mackness MI, Arrol S, Abbott C, Durrington PN. Protection of low-density lipoprotein against oxidative modification by high-density lipoprotein associated paraoxonase. *Atherosclerosis.* Dec 1993;104(1-2):129-135.

[69] Wheeler JG, Keavney BD, Watkins H, Collins R, Danesh J. Four paraoxonase gene polymorphisms in 11212 cases of coronary heart disease and 12786 controls: meta-analysis of 43 studies. *Lancet.* Feb 28 2004;363(9410):689-695.

[70] Horke S, Witte I, Wilgenbus P, Kruger M, Strand D, Forstermann U. Paraoxonase-2 reduces oxidative stress in vascular cells and decreases endoplasmic reticulum stress-induced caspase activation. *Circulation.* Apr 17 2007;115(15):2055-2064.

[71] Ng CJ, Wadleigh DJ, Gangopadhyay A, et al. Paraoxonase-2 is a ubiquitously expressed protein with antioxidant properties and is capable of preventing cell-mediated oxidative modification of low density lipoprotein. *J Biol Chem.* Nov 30 2001;276(48):44444-44449.

[72] Li WF, Pan MH, Chung MC, Ho CK, Chuang HY. Lead exposure is associated with decreased serum paraoxonase 1 (PON1) activity and genotypes. *Environ Health Perspect.* Aug 2006;114(8):1233-1236.

[73] Wang X, Fan Z, Huang J, et al. Extensive association analysis between polymorphisms of PON gene cluster with coronary heart disease in Chinese Han population. *Arterioscler Thromb Vasc Biol.* Feb 1 2003;23(2):328-334.

[74] Jalilian A, Javadi E, Akrami M, et al. Association of cys 311 ser polymorphism of paraoxonase-2 gene with the risk of coronary artery disease. *Arch Iran Med.* Sep 2008;11(5):544-549.

[75] Martinelli N, Girelli D, Olivieri O, et al. Interaction between smoking and PON2 Ser311Cys polymorphism as a determinant of the risk of myocardial infarction. *Eur J Clin Invest.* Jan 2004;34(1):14-20.

[76] Pinizzotto M, Castillo E, Fiaux M, Temler E, Gaillard RC, Ruiz J. Paraoxonase2 polymorphisms are associated with nephropathy in Type II diabetes. *Diabetologia.* Jan 2001;44(1):104-107.

[77] Meharg AA, Rahman MM. Arsenic contamination of Bangladesh paddy field soils: implications for rice contribution to arsenic consumption. *Environ Sci Technol.* Jan 15 2003;37(2):229-234.

[78] Meharg AA. Arsenic in rice--understanding a new disaster for South-East Asia. *Trends Plant Sci.* Sep 2004;9(9):415-417.

[79] Ruiz-Chancho MJ, Lopez-Sanchez JF, Schmeisser E, Goessler W, Francesconi KA, Rubio R. Arsenic speciation in plants growing in arsenic-contaminated sites. *Chemosphere.* Apr 2008;71(8):1522-1530.

[80] Peshut PJ, Morrison RJ, Brooks BA. Arsenic speciation in marine fish and shellfish from American Samoa. *Chemosphere.* Mar 2008;71(3):484-492.

[81] Ren X, McHale CM, Skibola CF, Smith AH, Smith MT, Zhang L. An emerging role for epigenetic dysregulation in arsenic toxicity and carcinogenesis. *Environ Health Perspect.* Jan 2011;119(1):11-19.

[82] Larson MG, Atwood LD, Benjamin EJ, et al. Framingham Heart Study 100K project: genome-wide associations for cardiovascular disease outcomes. *BMC Med Genet.* 2007;8 Suppl 1:S5.

[83] Keating BJ, Tischfield S, Murray SS, et al. Concept, design and implementation of a cardiovascular gene-centric 50 k SNP array for large-scale genomic association studies. *PLoS One.* 2008;3(10):e3583.

[84] Dorn GW, Cresci S. Genome-wide association studies of coronary artery disease and heart failure: where are we going? *Pharmacogenomics.* Feb 2009;10(2):213-223.

17

Abnormal Electrocardiogram in Patients with Acute Aluminum Phosphide Poisoning

Amine Ali Zeggwagh and Maha Louriz
Medical Intensive Care Unit - Faculty of Medicine and Pharmacy, University Mohamed V, Rabat, Morocco

1. Introduction

Aluminum phosphide (AlP) is used throughout the world as pesticides to protect stored grains from rodents and other pests **(Cienki, 2001)**. The chemical is usually formulated in pellets, granules or as a dust. Upon contact with moisture in the environment, AlP undergoes a chemical reaction yielding phosphine gas (PH_3), which is the active pesticidal component and a very toxic system poison, makes acute AlP poisoning (AAlPP) extremely dangerous **(Sasser et al., 1998)**.

AAlPP has been reported in literature since 1985. The majority of cases of AlP poisoning involving intentional suicide acts. It is a major health problem with a high mortality rate especially in developing countries where AlP is low cost and easily accessible **(Mehpour et al., 2008; Louriz et al., 2009)**. Patients who intend to commit suicide take tablets. Once mixed with hydrochloric acid in the stomach, PH_3 is immediately released and absorbed rapidly via the lungs causing systemic poisoning **(Proudfoot, 2009)**. However, accidental exposure to AlP is a relatively common cause of poisoning from agriculture chemical exposure in many countries. The manufacture and application of AlP fumigants pose risks of inhalation exposure to PH_3 **(Sudakin, 2005)**.

During the past 35 years, high mortality rates have been reported following significant exposures to aluminum phosphide. This mortality rates vary from 40% to 80% **(Chugh et al., 1991)**.

2. Toxicology of phosphine gas

The toxicity of AlP is attributed to the liberation of PH_3 gas which is cytotoxic and causes free radical mediated injury **(Sudakin, 2005)**.

PH_3 a nucleophile, acts as a strong reducing agent capable of inhibiting cellular enzymes involved in several metabolic processes. Early studies on PH_3 demonstrated specific inhibitory effects on mitochondrial cytochrome c oxidase. Experimental and observational studies have subsequently demonstrated that the inhibition of cytochrome c oxidase and other enzymes leads to the generation superoxide radicals and cellular peroxides. Cellular

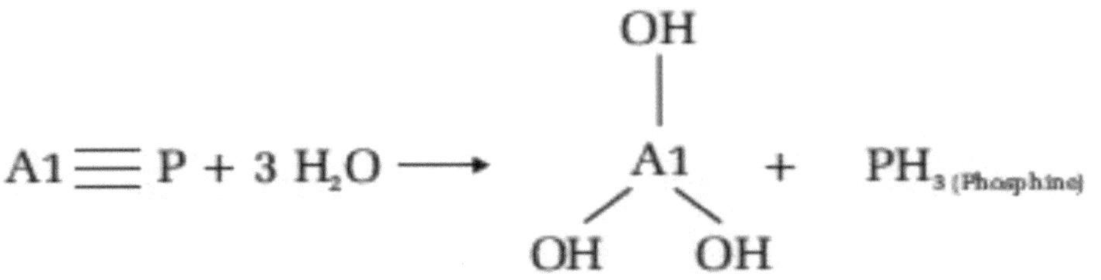

Fig. 1. Aluminum phosphide and liberation of phosphine gas. Al≡P : aluminum phosphide ; PH_3: phosphine gas

injury subsequently occurs through lipid peroxidation and other oxidant mechanisms **(Chugh et al., 1996).** Indeed, significant decreases in glutathione concentrations were shown in different tissues during AlP poisoning **(Hsu et al., 2002).** Glutathione is known to be an important factor protecting against oxidation by catalyzing the reduction of the oxygen peroxide in O_2 and H_2O.
Mutagenic effects resulting from oxidative damage to DNA have been reported in vitro. A cytogenetic study of phosphide fumigant applicators reported a significantly higher incidence of chromatid gaps and deletions in comparison to controls **(Hsu et al., 1998).**
Very little information is available relating to the toxicokinetics of PH_3 in humans. In an investigation of a series of patients with acute AlP poisoning , indicators of oxidative stress (malonydialdehyde levels, superoxide dismutase and catalase activity) appeared to peak within 48 hours of exposure, with normalization of most indicators occurring by day 5 **(Chugh et al., 1996a).** Chugh et al. reported that, serum PH_3 levels correlate positively with the severity of poisoning and levels equal to or less than 1.067 ± 0.16 mg % appear to be the limit of PH_3 toxicity **(Chugh et al., 1996b).**
A bedside test has been described for the diagnosis of AlP ingestion, using gastric aspirates and paper strips impregnated with silver nitrate. The test was found to be positive in 100% of cases of AlP ingestion **(Chugh et al., 1994).** The same test was also investigated to detect PH_3 gas in the exhaled air of patients with intoxication with AlP ingestion, and the results were positive in 50 % of cases.

3. Acute aluminum phosphide poisoning

3.1 Clinical features of AAlPP

AAlPP results in the rapid onset of gastrointestinal signs and symptoms, including epigastric pain and recurrent, profuse vomiting. Characteristic garlic smell of PH_3 in the patient's expired breath. Cardiovascular manifestations include hypotention and profound circulatory collapse. Neurological manifestations following acute poisoning include headache, anxiety and dizziness, frequently accompanied by a normal mental state **(National Institute of occupational Safety and Health [NIOSH], 2003).** Pulmonary injury and oedema have been described. Acute renal and liver injury can also develop. The prognosis from suicidal ingestion of AlP is poor.
The major lethal consequence of AAlPP, myocardial suppression with profound circulatory collapse, is reportedly secondary to toxins generated, which lead to direct effects on cardiac myocytes, fluid loss induced by several episodes of vomiting and adrenal gland damage. The AAlPP is involving young patients without history of cardiac diseases. However,

clinical, biological, electrical and histological observations suggest that myocardial involvement is responsible for the acute circulatory insufficiency **(Lall et al., 1997).**

3.2 Biological abnormalities in AAIPP

Increased CK with raised cardiac marker CK-MB fraction has been previously reported point to severe myocardial damage **(Nakakita et al., 2009).** Controversies exist about the magnesium level and prognosis of AAlPP. Some studies seem to suggest that there is hypomagnesaemia associated with AAlPP and that there is a direct relationship between abnormal electrocardiographic findings and low magnesium levels. They report reduced mortality rates with magnesium therapy in these patients **(Chugh et al., 1991).** However other studies have shown no such benefits and some have even demonstrated hypermagnesaemia in patients with AAlPP **(Singh et al., 1991).** The pathogenesis of magnesium level abnormalities was not clear.

3.3 Histological injury in AAIPP

PH_3 also has corrosive effects on tissues. Louriz et al investigated microscopic changes in vital organs of the body, liver, heart and kidneys **(Louriz et al., 2009).** These changes were found to be suggestive of cellular hypoxia. Other recent studies with more patients were performed and showed congestion, edema and leukocytie or leukocyte infiltration in the liver, kidneys, heart, stomach, lungs, brain and adrenals **(Arora et al., 1995; Sinha et al., 2005).**

Nakakita studied the histology of the heart. Histopathological finding of myocyte vacuolation and myocytolysis and degeneration are both suggestive of myocardial injury. The areas of increased waviness of myocardial fibers indicate an episode of myocardial infarction **(Nakakita et al., 2009).**

3.4 Cardiotoxicity of AIP

The toxicity of AlP is systemic and can affect all organs, but particularly cardiac and vascular tissues. Myocardial injury following AlP poisoning has been documented on electrocardiograms in several studies. AlP induced cardiotoxicity was responsible for a high level of mortality. Cardiac toxicity due to AlP and PH_3 exposure is represented by a depression in myocardial cellular metabolism, as well as myocardial necrosis due to the release of reactive oxygen intermediates.

Several studies noted electric abnormalities in 38% to 91% of cases **(Chugh et al., 1991; Karla et al., 1991).** There are conduction disorders such as right and left bundle branch block (25%), atrioventricular block (8%) and rarely, sinoatrial block **(Karla et al., 1991).** On the other hand, cardiac dysrhythmias were described as atrial fibrillation (4% to 61%), junctional rhythm (4% to 100%), ventricular and atrial extrasyxtoles (18%) and ventricular fibrillation (2%) **(Gupta et al., 1995; Louriz et al, 2009).** Finally, re-polarization disorders were also reported, such as ST segment depression (12% to 65%), ST segment elevation (4% to 65%) and T wave inversion (36%) induced by AAlPP **(Lall et al., 1997).**

Indeed, in Shadnia's study, 39 patients admitted to the ICU with AAlPP were studied. Average time elapsed between poisoning and admission at the hospital was 3.4 ± 3.5 hours. Average ingested amount was 1.4 ± 0.9 tablets. ECG abnormalities were found in 17 (43.6%) cases at the time of admission with ST-T changes in 8 cases. Ischemic change in 3 cases and dysrhythmias in 6 cases. The nature of these dysrhythmias was not described. The mortality rate was high, about 67%. In this study, ECG abnormalities were a prognostic factor **(Shadnia et al., 2010).**

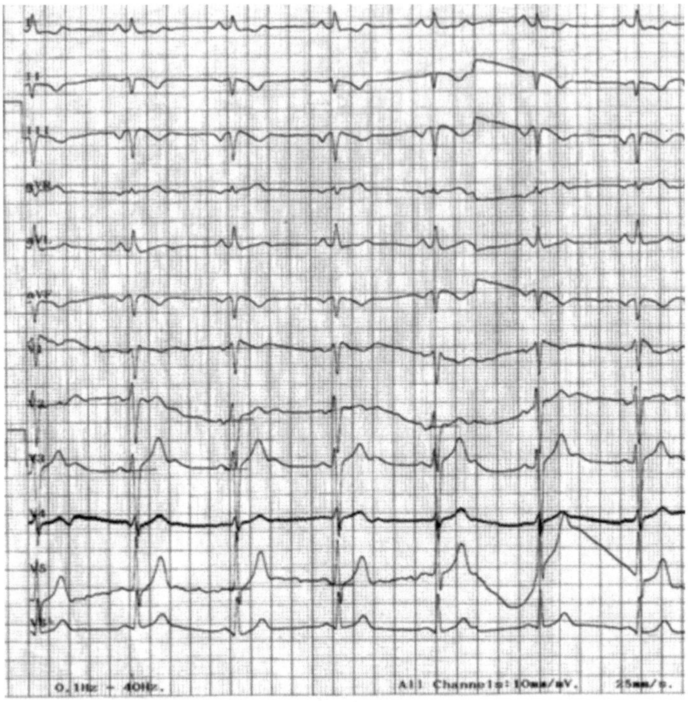

A)

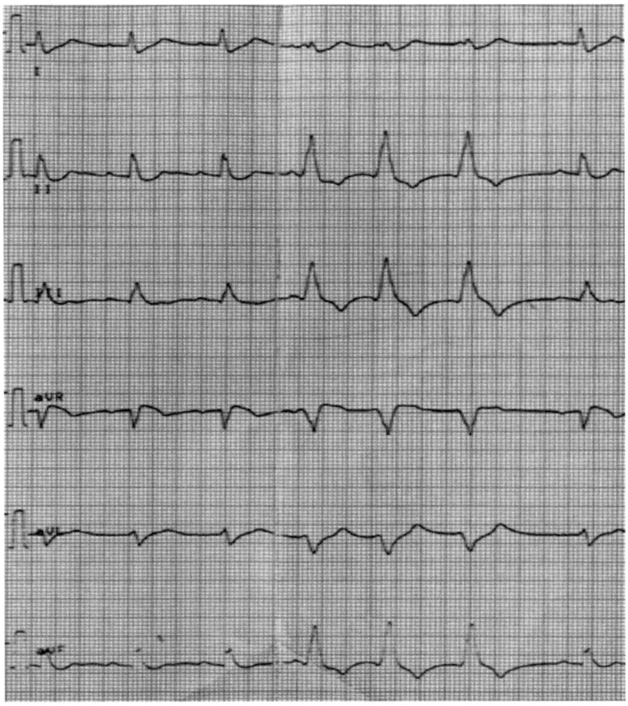

B)

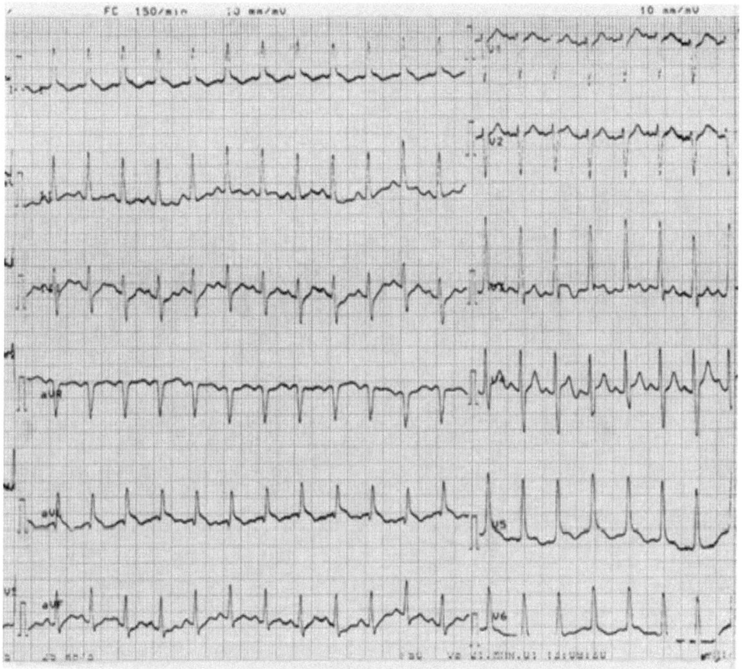

C)

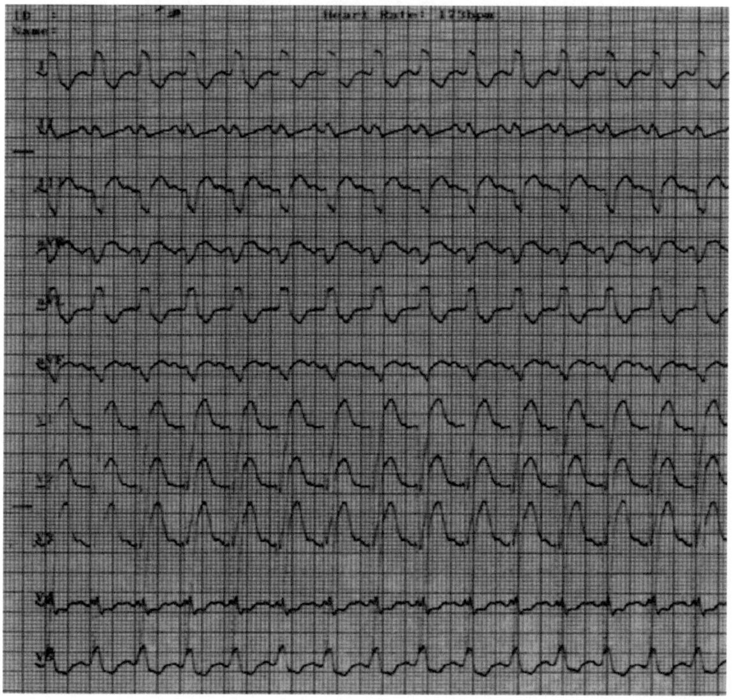

D1)

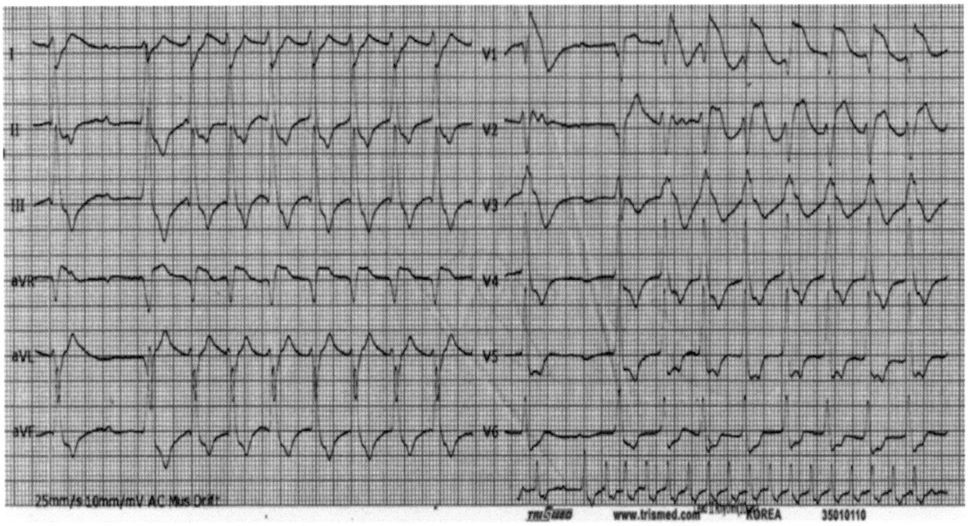

D2)

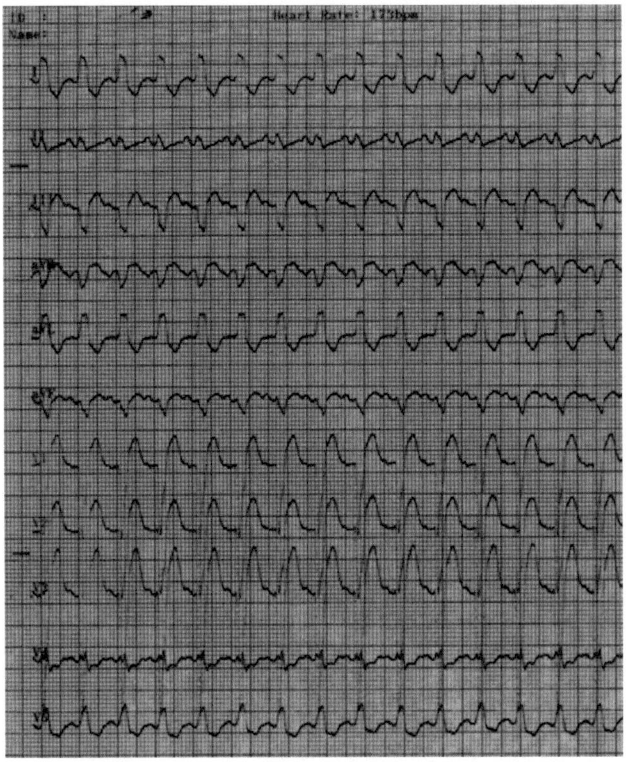

D3)

Fig. 2. Electrocardiographic changes following aluminium phosphide poisoning. 12-leads surface ECG recorded on admission showing: (A) Sinusal bradycardia (B) Ventricular extrasystoles (C) Sinusal tachycardia with ST segment depression in the leads D_1, aVL, V_5 and V_6 (D1, D2 &D3) Sinusal tachycardia with ST-T changes.

In Louriz's study, 49 patients were enrolled. The ingested dose was 1.2 ± 0.7 grams. The time between ingestion and admission to the medical ICU was 9.1 ± 10.7 hours. The ECG was abnormal in 28 cases (58.7%) at the time of admission with myocardial ischemia in 21 cases, atrial fibrillation in 6 cases, ventricular extrasystoles in 9 cases and ventricular fibrillation in one case. The mortality rate was 49%. In this study, ECG abnormalities were also a prognostic factor **(Louriz et al., 2009).**

In Mathai's study, 27 patients with AAlPP were admitted into the ICU. One and half grams of poison was consumed. There was a mean delay of 2.1 ± 1.55 hours before presenting to the hospital. Thirteen (48.1%) patients had dysrhythmia at admission of which the majority (69%) of supraventricular origin. Ventricular arythmias was found in 4 cases. The mortality rate was 59.3%. In this study, the presence of ECG abnormalities did not predict mortality **(Mathai et al., 2010).**

In these 3 studies cited above, there wasn't any association between the dose of poison consumed or the time delay in presentation to the hospital with the mortality. All the ECG abnormalities found in these studies were recorded at the admission to the hospital. However, other ECG changes could be found during the hospitalization.

Indeed, Bogle et al described a case of a lethal AAlPP caused by deliberate ingestion of AlP. ECG showed a sinus tachycardia 2 hours after ingestion of a 10 g sachet of pesticide with 56% of AlP. ECG recorded 12 hours after ingestion showed extreme widening of the QRS complexe despite amiodarone therapy. The rate of ECG abnormalities resulting of AAlPP might be under estimated **(Bogle et al., 2006).**

Some electrical abnormalities noted in our practice are reported in Figure 2.

In several studies, echocardiography showed a global hypokinesis of the left ventrivule **(Akkaoui et al., 2007; Bajaj et al., 1988)** (Figure 3).

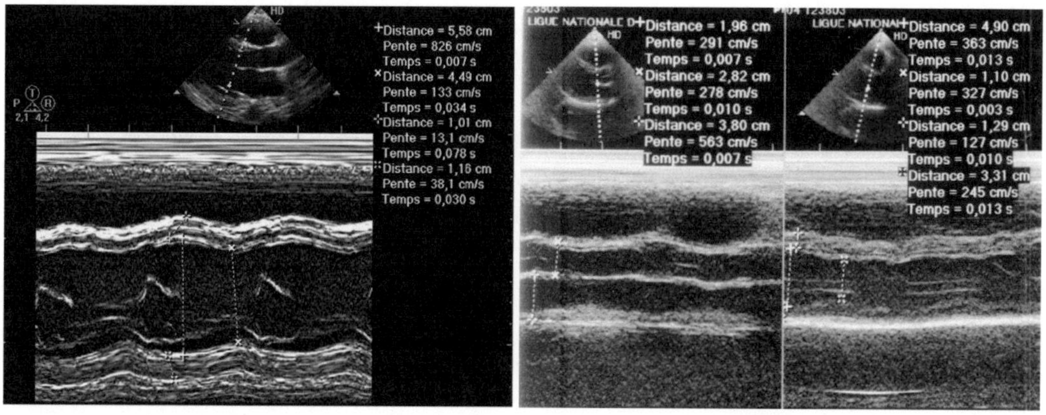

A) B)

Fig. 3. Echocardiographically parasternal long axis depicted improvement of ventricle function following aluminum phosphide poisoning . A) Echocardiogram obtained on the second day after admission depicts global hypokinesis with LVEF of 30% and dilatation of LV. B) Echocardiogram taken eight days after admission showed improvement of ventricle function.

Indeed, Bahsin et al showed a generalized hypokinesis of left ventricle wall and interventricular septum in 80% of their cases. This study revealed akinesis and pericarditis in 3% and 35% of the cases, respectively **(Bhasin et al., 1991).** Thus, Bajaj et al showed a global hypokinesis of the left ventricle in the three patients that underwent serial ventriculography **(Bajaj et al., 1988).** However, other authors have described a focal myocardial necrosis **(Singh et al., 1991; Wilson et al., 1980).** At a patient hospitalized in our intensive care unit, we observed an unusual and important dilation of right cardiac cavities explained partially by hypokinesia of the left ventricle but probably also by the direct toxicity of the AlP on the right ventricle (Figure 4).

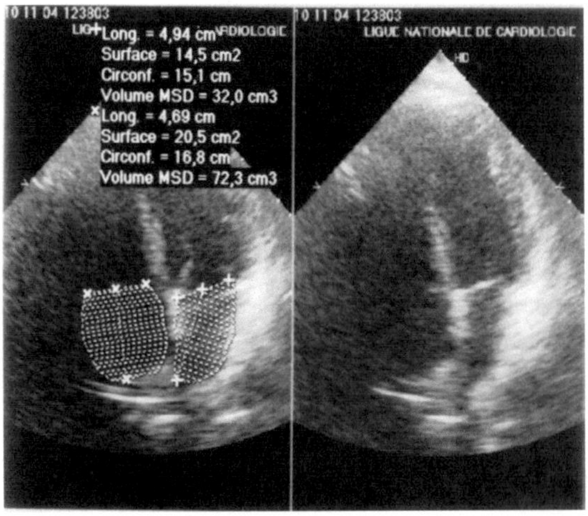

Fig. 4. Echocardiography parasternal long axis depicted improvement of ventricule function. Echocardiogram obtained at admission depicts global hypokinesis with left ventricle ejection fraction (LVEF) of 40% and important dilation of right ventricle and auricle.

4. Conclusion

The severity of the poisoning is judged by the cardiac failure and the unavailability of an antidote. Myocardial injury following AAlPP is responsible for significant mortality. Despite all intensive medical care efforts in supportive therapy, the prognosis of AAlPP is poor. Therefore the use and availability of the pesticide aluminium phosphide should be restricted as much as possible.

5. References

Abder-Rahman H. (1999). Effect of aluminum phosphide on blood glucose level. *Vet Human Toxicol,* No.41, pp.31-32

Akkaoui M, Achour S, Abidi K, Himdi B, Madani N, Zeggwagh AA & Abouqal R. (2007). Reversible myocardial injury associated with aluminum phosphide poisoning. *Clin Toxicol,* No.45, pp. 728-31

Arora B, Punia RS, Karla R, Chugh SN & Arora DR. (1995). Histopathological changes in aluminum phosphide poisoning. *J Indian Med Assoc,* No. 93, pp. 380-81.

Bajaj R, Wasir HS, Agarwal R, Malhotra A, Chopra P & Bhatia ML. (1988). Aluminum phosphide poisoning.Clinical toxicity and outcome in eleven intensively monitored patients. *Natl Med J India*, No.1, pp. 270-274

Bogle RG, Theron P, Brooks P, Dargan PI & Redhead J. (2006). Aluminium phosphide poisoning. *Emerg Med J*, No.23, pp.e3

Chugh SN, Dushayant K, Ram S & Arora B. (1991). Incidence and outcome of aluminum phosphide poisoning in a hospital study. *Indian J Med Res*, No.94, pp. 232-35.

Chugh SN, Chung K, Ram S & Malhotra KC. (1991). Electrocardiographic abnormalities in aluminum phosphide poisoning with special reference to its incidence, pathogenesis, mortality and hisptopathology. *J Indian Med Assoc* ,No.89, pp. 32-35

Chugh SN, Jaggal KL, Sharma A, Arora B & Malhotra KC. (1991). Magnesium levels in acute cardiotoxicity due to aluminum phosphide poisoning. *Indian J Med Res*, No.94, pp. 437-9.

Chugh SN, Kamar P, Sharma A, Chugh K, Mittal A & Arora B. (1994). Magnesium status and parenteral magnesium sulphate therapy in acute aluminium phosphide intoxication. *Magnes Res*, No. 7, pp. 289-94.

Chugh SN, Arora V, Sharma A & Chugh K (1996). Free radical scavengers and lipid peroxidation in acute aluminum phosphide poisoning. *Indian J Med Res* 1996a, No104, pp. 190-3.

Chugh SN, Pal R, Singh V& Seth S. (1996). Serial blood phosphine levels in acute aluminum phosphide poisoning. *J Assoc Physicians India* 1996b, No.44, pp. 184-5

Cienki JJ. (2001). *Non-anticoagulant rodenticides*. (Ford MD, Delaney KA, Ling LJ, Erickson T). *Clinical Toxicology*, 858. Philadelphia.

Gupta MS, Malik A & Shama VK. (1995). Cardiovascular manifestations in aluminum phosphide poisoning with especial reference to echocardiographic changes. *J Assoc Physicians India*, No.43, pp. 774-780

Hsu CH, Quistad GB & Casida JE. (1998). Phosphine-induced oxidative stress in Hepa 1c1c7cells. *Toxicol Sci*, No.46, pp. 204

Hsu C-H, CHiB-C, Liu J-H, Chen C-J & Chen R-Y. (2002). phosphine induced oxidative damage in rats: Role of glutathione. *Toxicology*, No.179, pp.1-8

Karla GS, Anand IS, Jit I, Bushnurmath B &Wahi PL. (1991) Aluminum phosphide poisoning haemodynamic observations. *Indian Heart J*, No.43, pp. 175-8

Lall SB,Sinha K, Mittra S & Seth SD. (1997). An experimental study on cardiotoxicity of aluminum phosphide. *Indian J Exp Biol*, No.35, pp. 1060-1064

Louriz M, Dendane T, Abidi K, Madani N, Abouqal R & Zeggwagh AA. (2009). Prognostic factors of acute aluminum phosphide poisoning. *Indian J Med Sci*, No.63, pp. 227-34

Mathai A & Bhanu MS. (2010). Acute aluminium phosphide poisoning: can we predict mortality ? *Indian J Anaesth*, No.54, pp. 302-307

Mehrpour O, Alfred S, Shadnia S, Keyler DE, Soltaninejad K & Chalaki N. (2008). Hyperglycemia in acute aluminum phosphide poisoning as a potential prognostic factor. *Hum Exp Toxicol* , No.27, pp.591-5.

Nakakita, H.a , Katsumata, Y.b & Ozawa, T.b . (2009). The effect of phosphine on respiration of rat liver mitochondria. *Indian Journal of Critical Care Medicine*, No.13, pp. 41-43

National Institute of occupational Safety and Health. NIOSH alert: preventing phosphine poisoning and explosions during fumigation. Columbus, OH: NIOSH,2003:99-

126,1-16Proudfoot AT. (2009). Aluminum and Zinc phosphide poisoning. *Cli Toxicol* , No.47, pp. 89-100

Sasser SM. (1998). Rodenticides. In: Viccellio P, BaniaT, Brent J, Hoffman RS, Kulig KW, Mofenson HC, et al, editors. Emergency toxicology. 2end ed. Philadelphia, PA: Lippincott-Ravec; P. 433.

Shadnia S, Mehrpour O & Soltaninejad K. (2010). A simplified acute physiology score in the prediction of acute aluminium phosphide poisoning outcome. *Indian J Med Sci* , No.64, pp. 532-539

Sinha US, Kapoor AK, Singh AK, Gupta A & Mehrotra R. (2005). Histopathological changes in casesof aluminum phosphide poisoning. *Indian J Pathol Microbiol*, No.48, pp. 177-180

Singh RB, Singh RG & Singh U. (1991). Hyperglicemia following aluminum phosphide poisoning. *Int J Clin Pharmacol Ther Toxicol*, No.29, pp. 82-85

Sudakin DL. (2005). Occupational exposure to aluminum phosphide and phosphine gas ? A suspected case report and review of the literature. *Human and experimental toxicology*, No.24, pp. 27-33

Wilson R, Lovejoy FH, Jaeger RJ & Landrigan PL. (1980). Acute phosphine poisoning aboard a grain freighter Epidemiologic, clinical and pathological finding. *JAMA*, No.244, pp. 148-150